HEALTH CARE REFORM

HEALTH CARE REFORM

WHAT IT IS, WHY IT'S NECESSARY, HOW IT WORKS

Jeff –
Enjoy!

JONATHAN GRUBER

WITH **HP NEWQUIST**

ILLUSTRATED BY **NATHAN SCHREIBER**

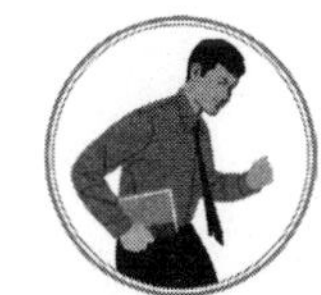

A NOVEL GRAPHIC FROM HILL AND WANG
A DIVISION OF FARRAR, STRAUS AND GIROUX
NEW YORK

HILL AND WANG
A DIVISION OF FARRAR, STRAUS AND GIROUX

THIS IS A Z FILE, INC. BOOK

DISTRIBUTED IN CANADA BY D&M PUBLISHERS, INC.
PRINTED IN THE UNITED STATES OF AMERICA
PUBLISHED SIMULTANEOUSLY IN HARDCOVER AND PAPERBACK
FIRST EDITION, 2011

LIBRARY OF CONGRESS CATALOGING-IN-PUBLICATION DATA
GRUBER, JONATHAN.
HEALTH CARE REFORM : WHAT IT IS, WHY IT'S NECESSARY, HOW IT WORKS / JONATHAN GRUBER, HARVEY NEWQUIST ; ILLUSTRATED BY NATHAN SCHREIBER.
P. CM
ISBN 978-0-8090-9462-2 (HARDBACK)
ISBN 978-0-8090-5397-1 (PAPERBACK)
1. HEALTH CARE REFORM--UNITED STATES. 2. MEDICAL POLICY--UNITED STATES. 3. MEDICAL CARE--UNITED STATES. I. NEWQUIST, HP (HARVEY P.) II. TITLE.

RA395.A3G78 2011
362.1'042DC23

2011020495

ART BY NATHAN SCHREIBER
ART ASSISTANT: BLUE DELLIQUANTI
DESIGNED BY RICHARD AMARI
EDITED BY HOWARD ZIMMERMAN

WWW.FSGBOOKS.COM

7 9 10 8 6

THIS BOOK IS DEDICATED TO MY WONDERFUL FAMILY, ANDREA, SAM, JACK, AND AVA, WHO CONVINCED ME TO TAKE ON THE PROJECT AND WHO HAVE BEEN MY BIGGEST CHEERLEADERS THROUGHOUT ITS COMPLETION.

CONTENTS

HEALTH CARE REFORM

CHAPTER 1 A CURE FOR WHAT AILS US

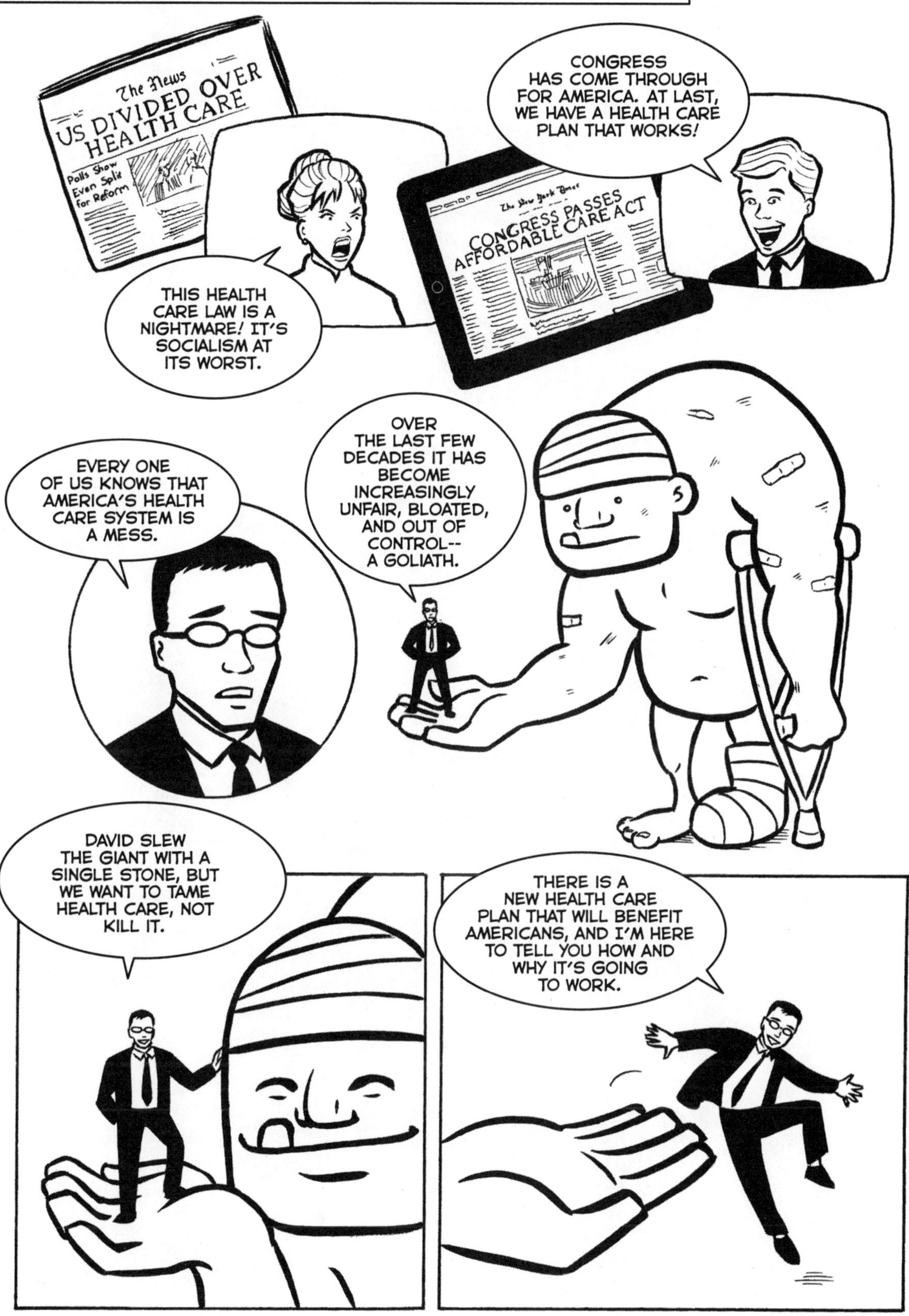
The News
US DIVIDED OVER HEALTH CARE
Polls Show Even Split for Reform
THIS HEALTH CARE LAW IS A NIGHTMARE! IT'S SOCIALISM AT ITS WORST.
The New York Times
CONGRESS PASSES AFFORDABLE CARE ACT
CONGRESS HAS COME THROUGH FOR AMERICA. AT LAST, WE HAVE A HEALTH CARE PLAN THAT WORKS!
EVERY ONE OF US KNOWS THAT AMERICA'S HEALTH CARE SYSTEM IS A MESS.
OVER THE LAST FEW DECADES IT HAS BECOME INCREASINGLY UNFAIR, BLOATED, AND OUT OF CONTROL-- A GOLIATH.
DAVID SLEW THE GIANT WITH A SINGLE STONE, BUT WE WANT TO TAME HEALTH CARE, NOT KILL IT.
THERE IS A NEW HEALTH CARE PLAN THAT WILL BENEFIT AMERICANS, AND I'M HERE TO TELL YOU HOW AND WHY IT'S GOING TO WORK.

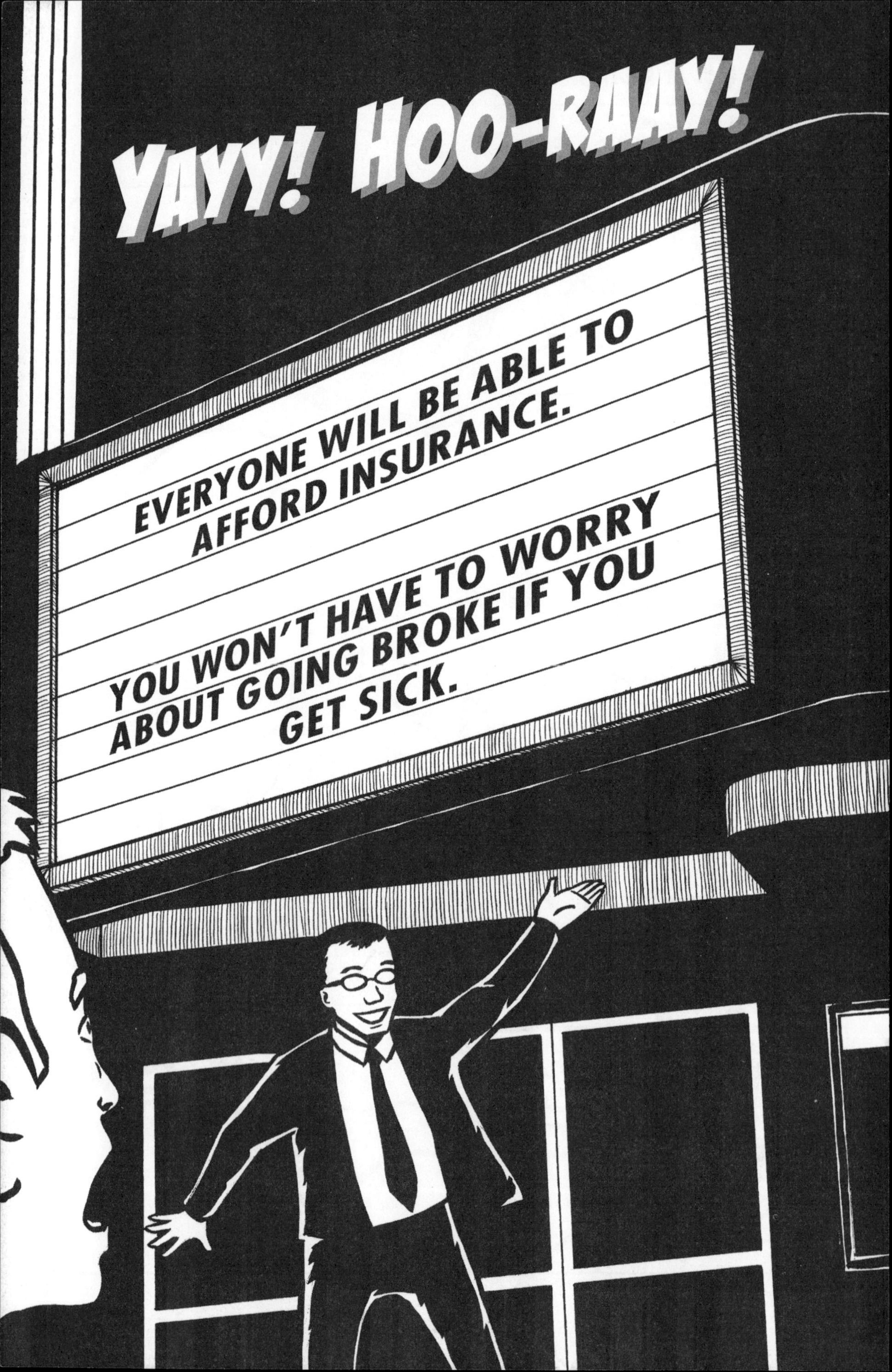

YAYY! HOO-RAAY!

EVERYONE WILL BE ABLE TO
AFFORD INSURANCE.

YOU WON'T HAVE TO WORRY
ABOUT GOING BROKE IF YOU
GET SICK.

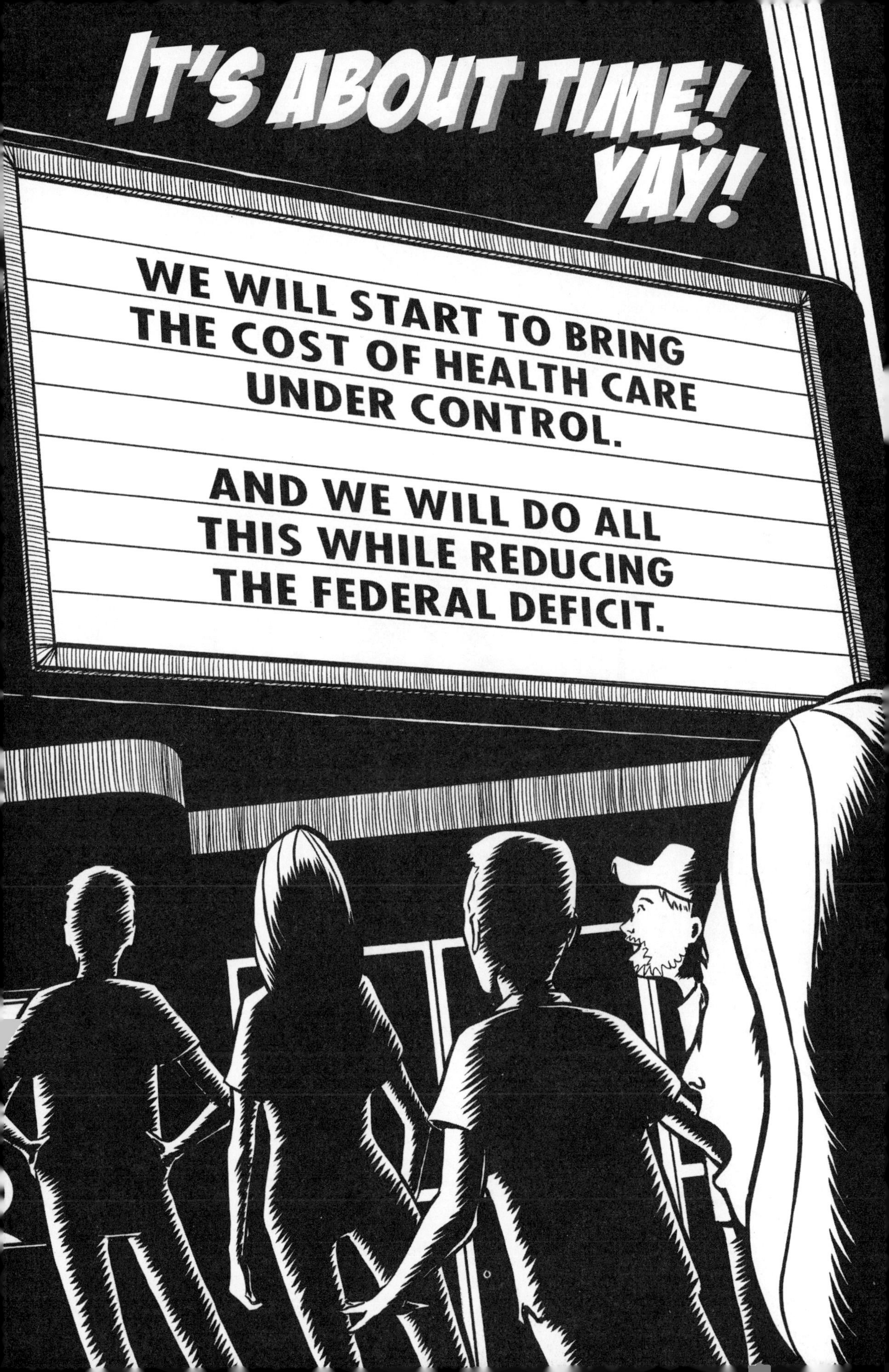

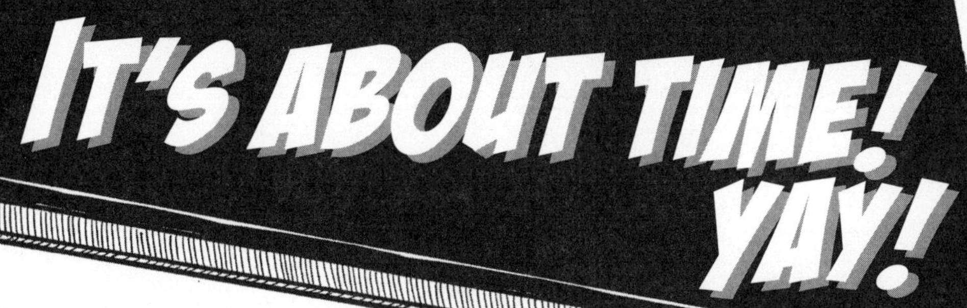
IT'S ABOUT TIME! YAY!
WE WILL START TO BRING THE COST OF HEALTH CARE UNDER CONTROL.
AND WE WILL DO ALL THIS WHILE REDUCING THE FEDERAL DEFICIT.

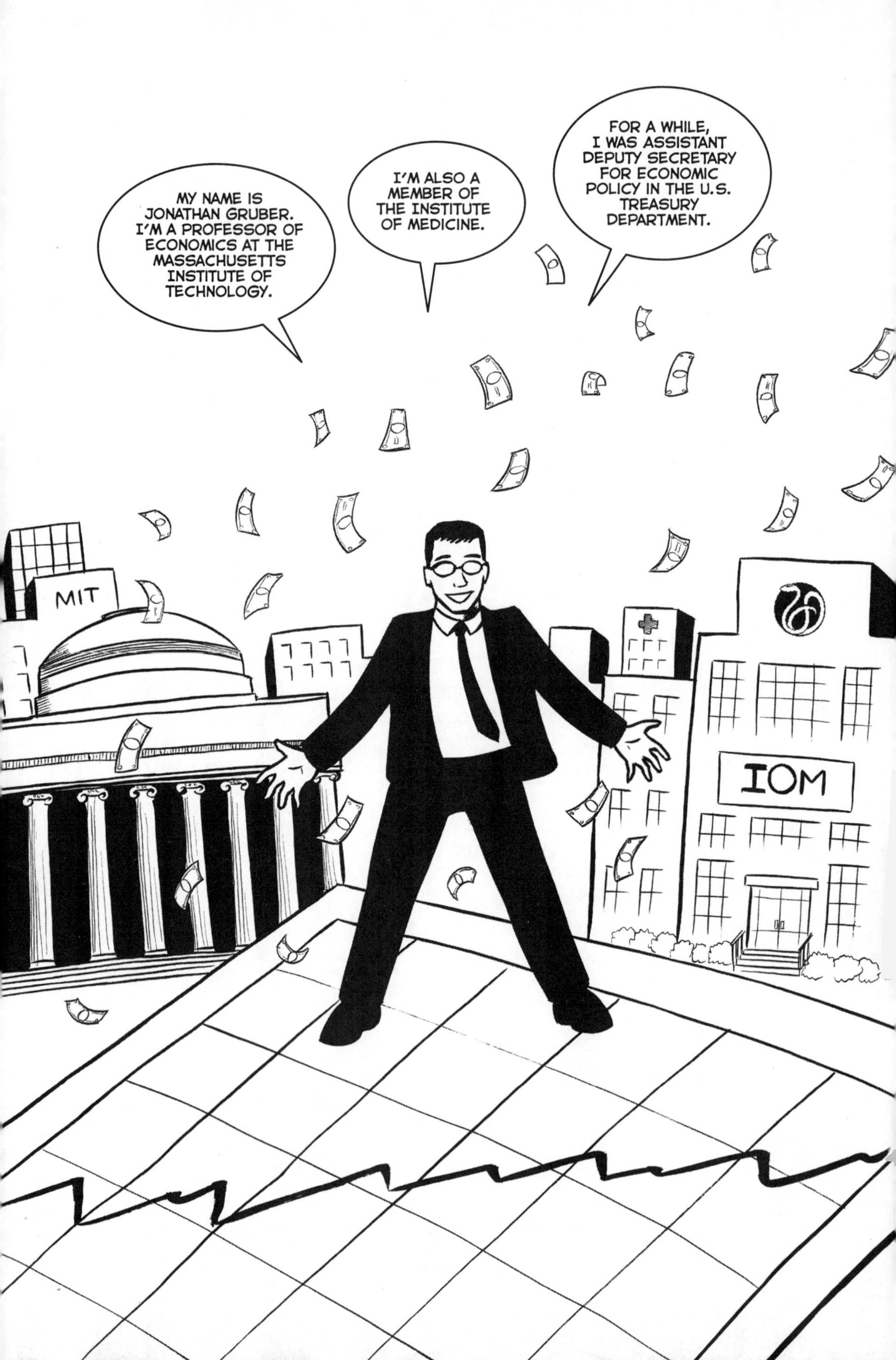
MY NAME IS JONATHAN GRUBER. I'M A PROFESSOR OF ECONOMICS AT THE MASSACHUSETTS INSTITUTE OF TECHNOLOGY.
I'M ALSO A MEMBER OF THE INSTITUTE OF MEDICINE.
FOR A WHILE, I WAS ASSISTANT DEPUTY SECRETARY FOR ECONOMIC POLICY IN THE U.S. TREASURY DEPARTMENT.
MIT
IOM

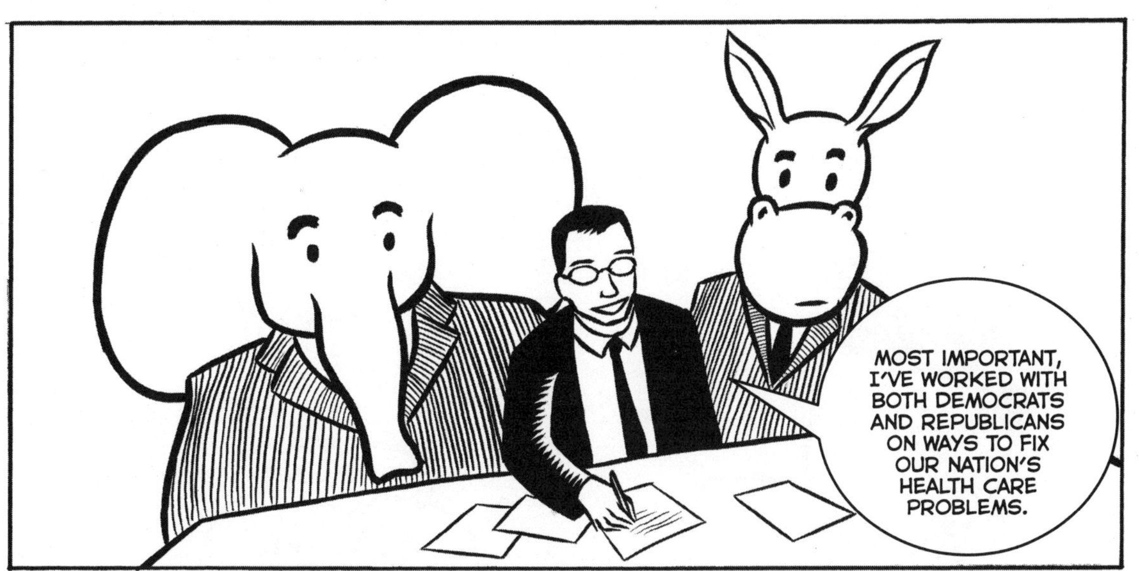
MOST IMPORTANT, I'VE WORKED WITH BOTH DEMOCRATS AND REPUBLICANS ON WAYS TO FIX OUR NATION'S HEALTH CARE PROBLEMS.

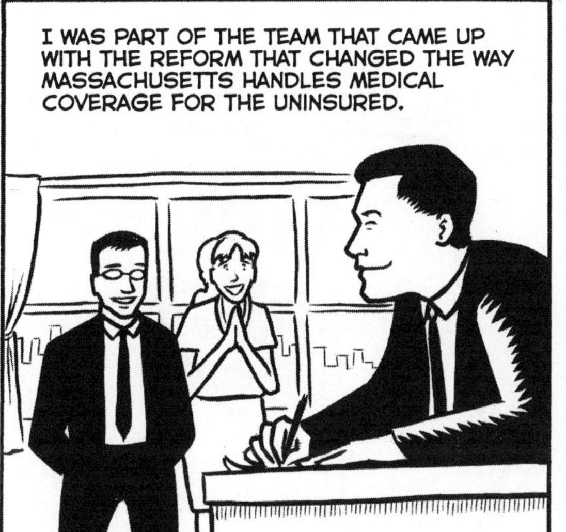
I WAS PART OF THE TEAM THAT CAME UP WITH THE REFORM THAT CHANGED THE WAY MASSACHUSETTS HANDLES MEDICAL COVERAGE FOR THE UNINSURED.

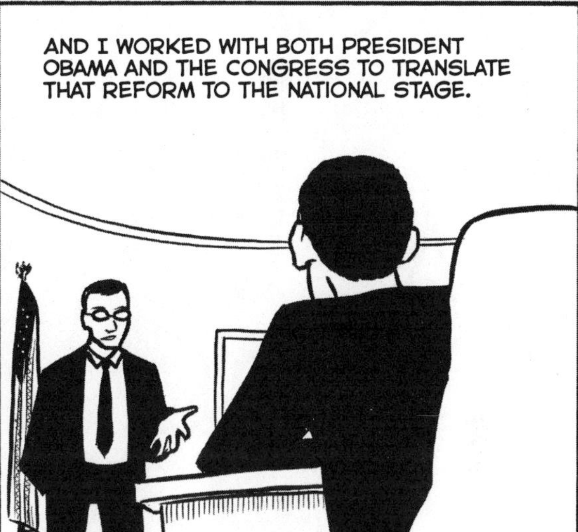
AND I WORKED WITH BOTH PRESIDENT OBAMA AND THE CONGRESS TO TRANSLATE THAT REFORM TO THE NATIONAL STAGE.

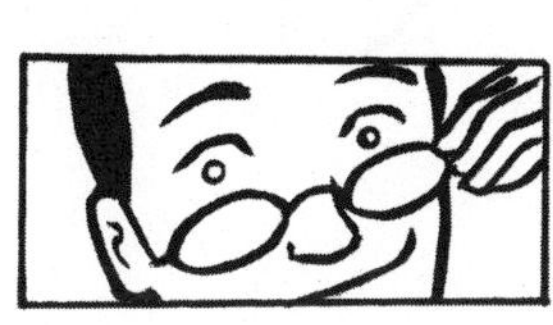
SO I'VE GOT A LITTLE EXPERIENCE IN THIS AREA.

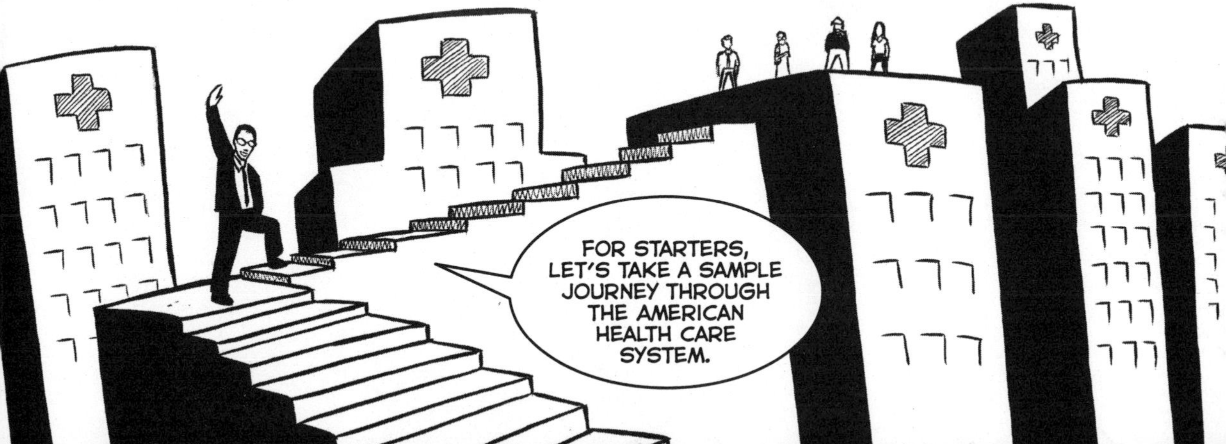
FOR STARTERS, LET'S TAKE A SAMPLE JOURNEY THROUGH THE AMERICAN HEALTH CARE SYSTEM.

LET ME INTRODUCE YOU TO FOUR TYPICAL AMERICANS.

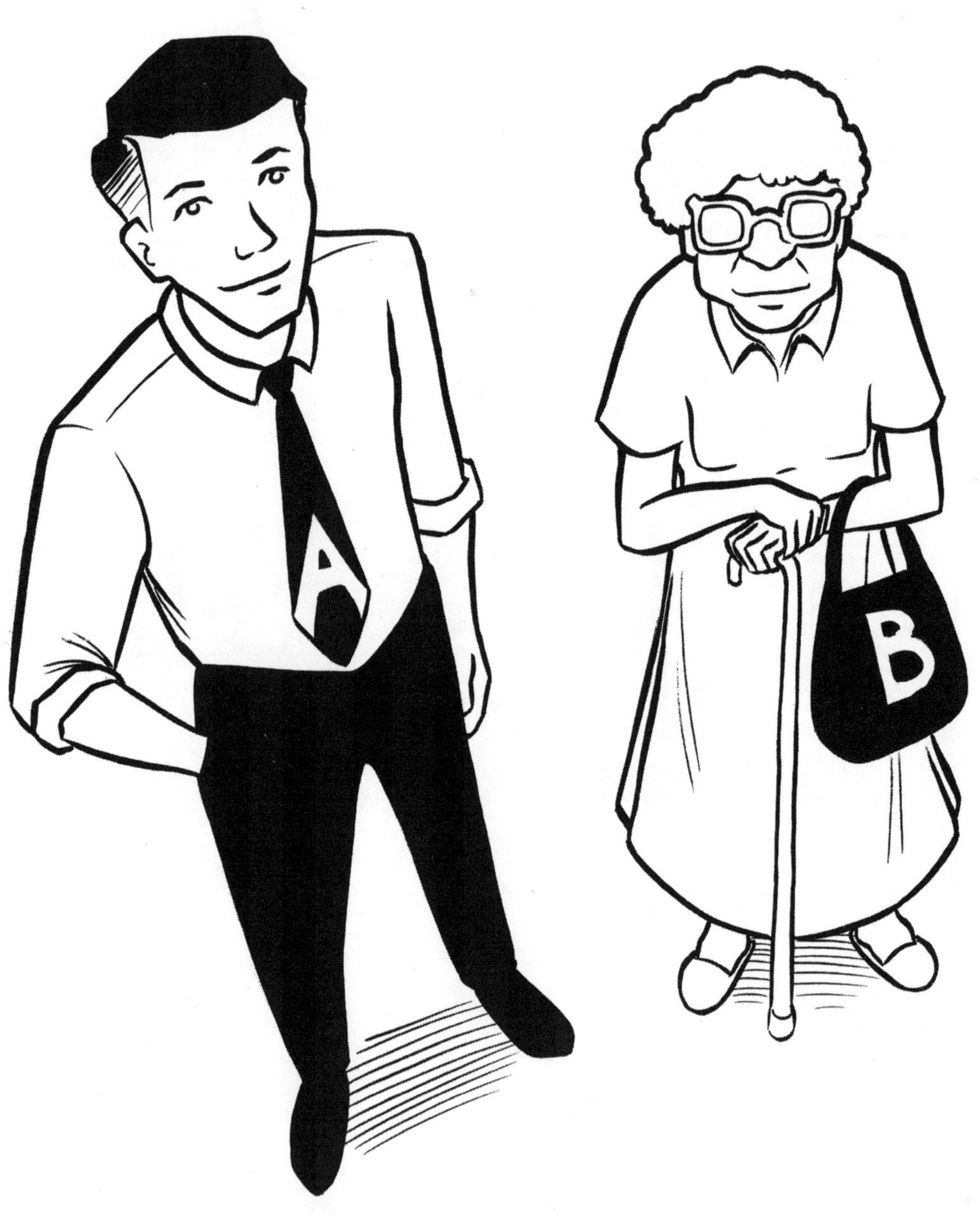

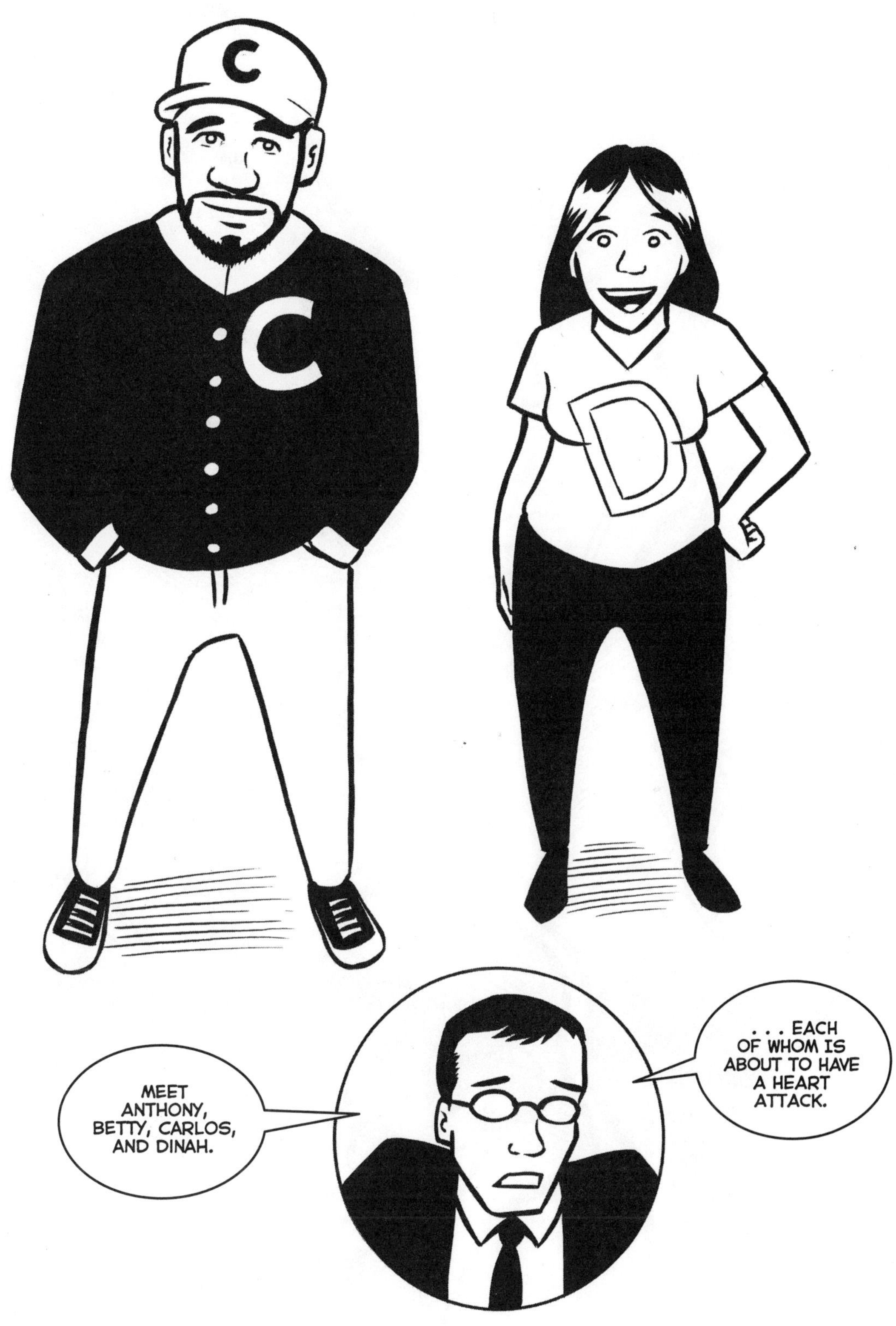
MEET ANTHONY, BETTY, CARLOS, AND DINAH.
. . . EACH OF WHOM IS ABOUT TO HAVE A HEART ATTACK.

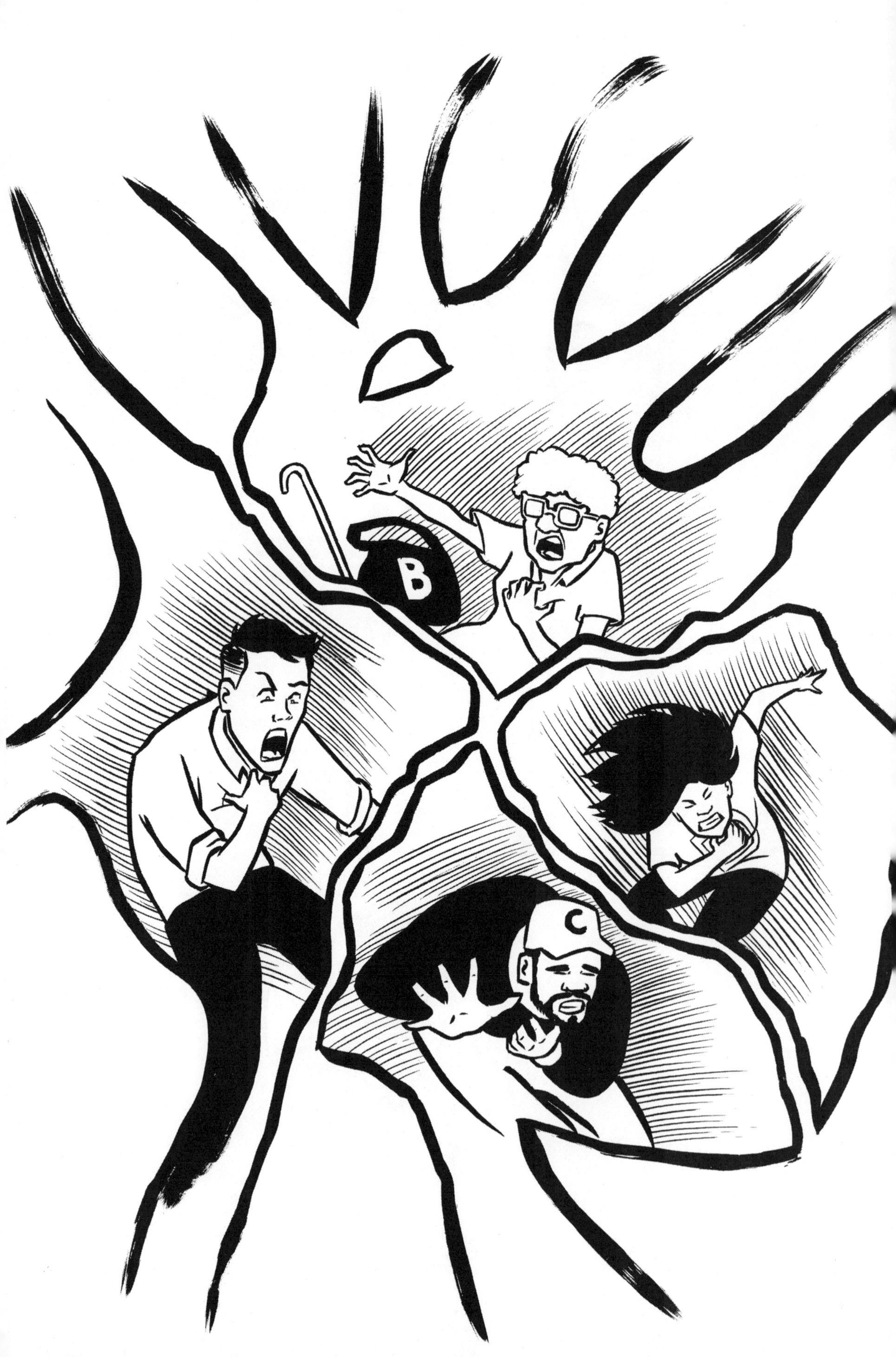

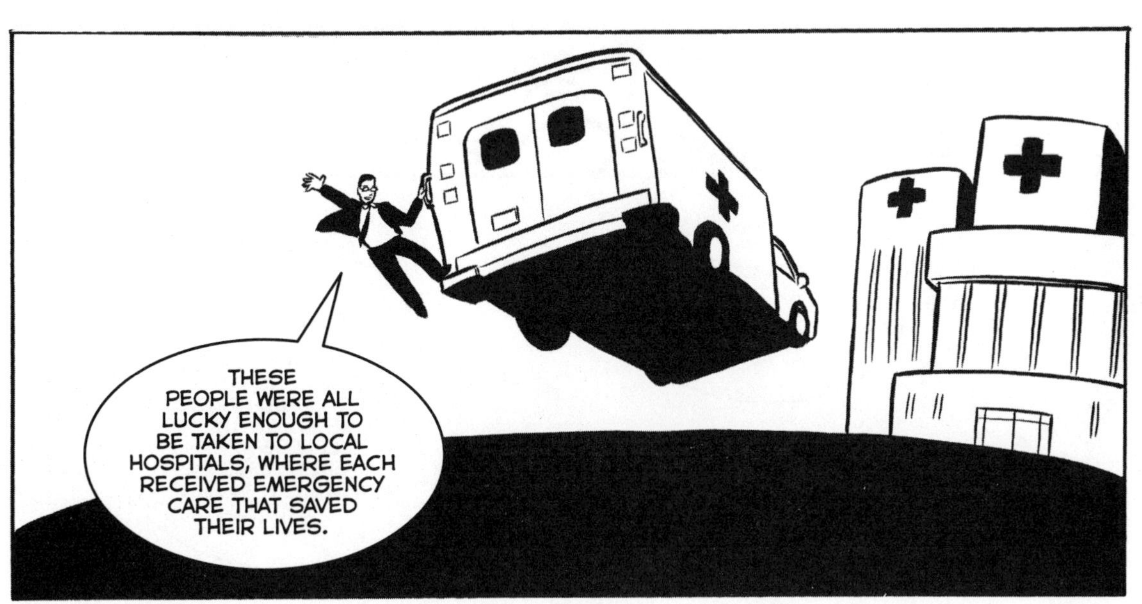
THESE PEOPLE WERE ALL LUCKY ENOUGH TO BE TAKEN TO LOCAL HOSPITALS, WHERE EACH RECEIVED EMERGENCY CARE THAT SAVED THEIR LIVES.

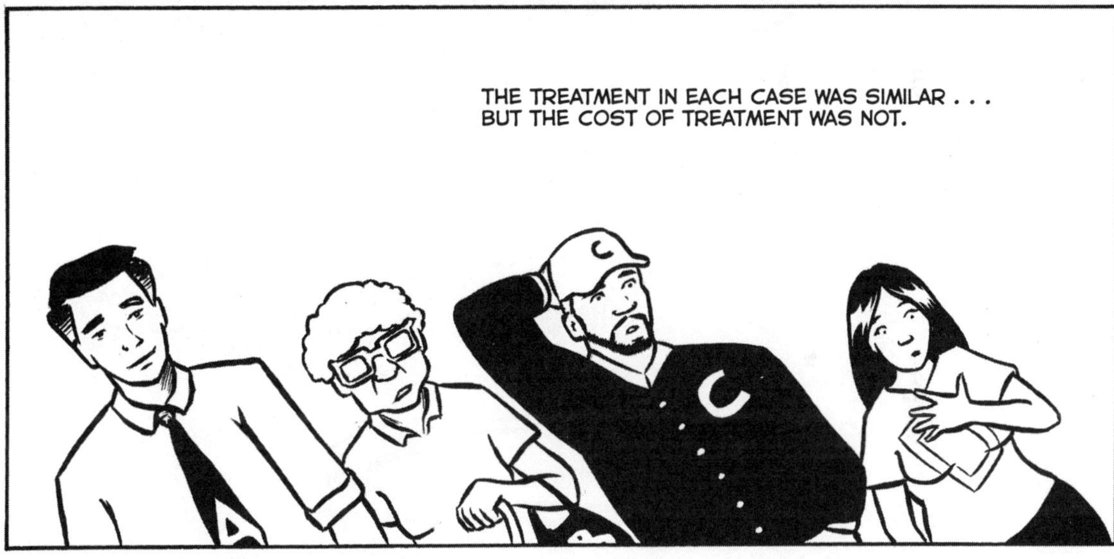
THE TREATMENT IN EACH CASE WAS SIMILAR . . .
BUT THE COST OF TREATMENT WAS NOT.

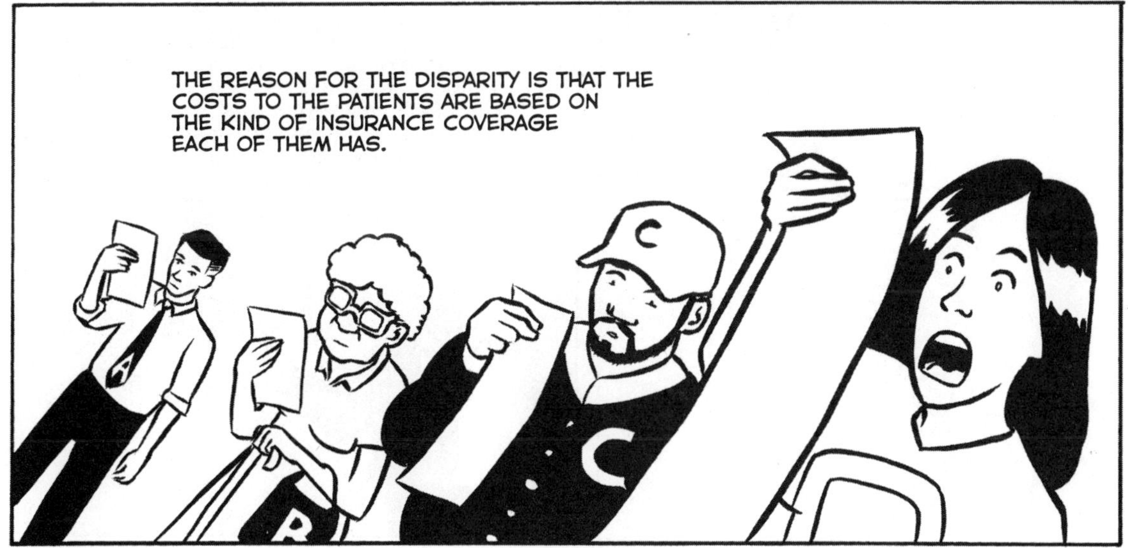
THE REASON FOR THE DISPARITY IS THAT THE COSTS TO THE PATIENTS ARE BASED ON THE KIND OF INSURANCE COVERAGE EACH OF THEM HAS.

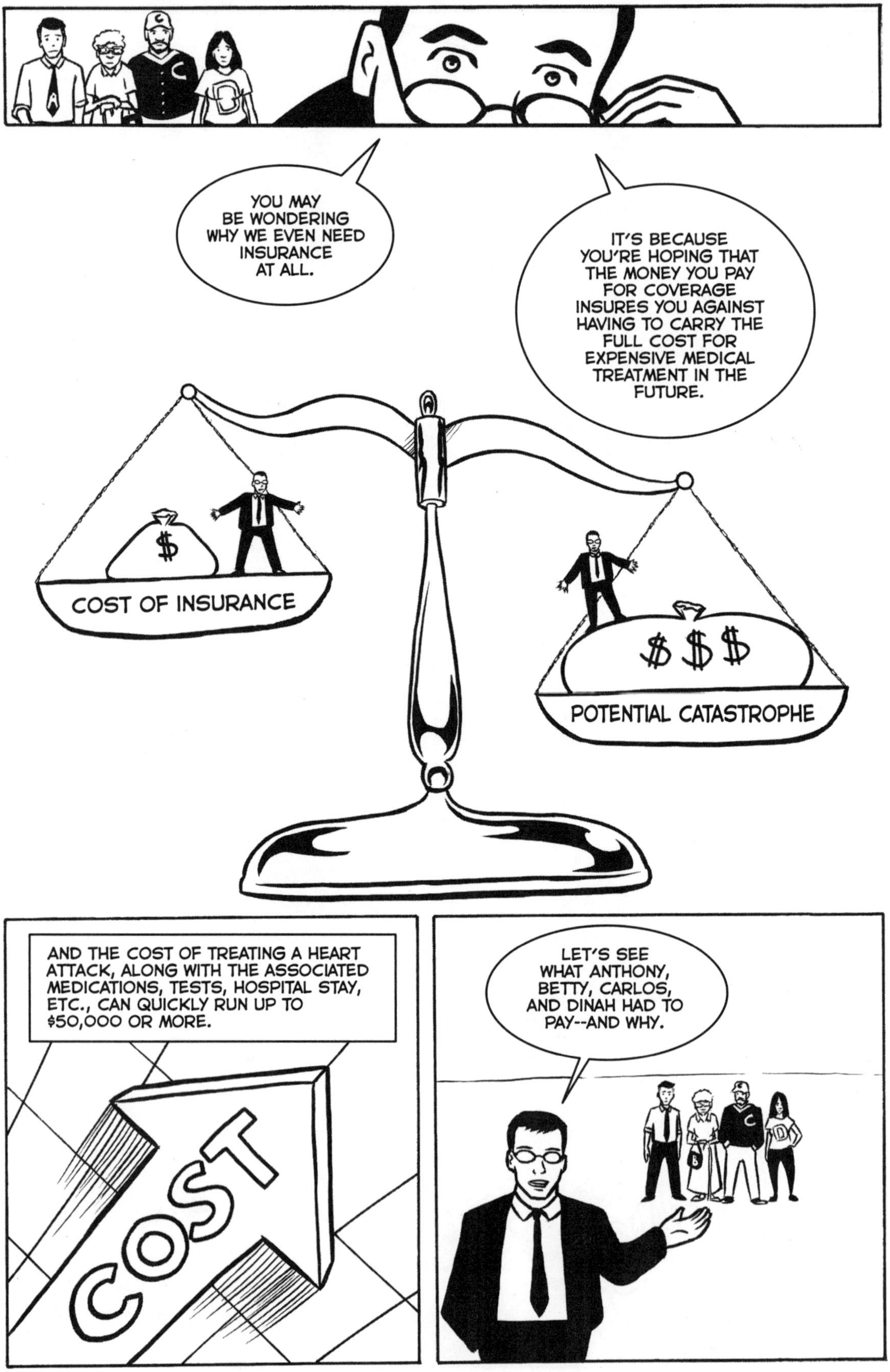

YOU MAY BE WONDERING WHY WE EVEN NEED INSURANCE AT ALL.

IT'S BECAUSE YOU'RE HOPING THAT THE MONEY YOU PAY FOR COVERAGE INSURES YOU AGAINST HAVING TO CARRY THE FULL COST FOR EXPENSIVE MEDICAL TREATMENT IN THE FUTURE.

$

COST OF INSURANCE

$$$

POTENTIAL CATASTROPHE

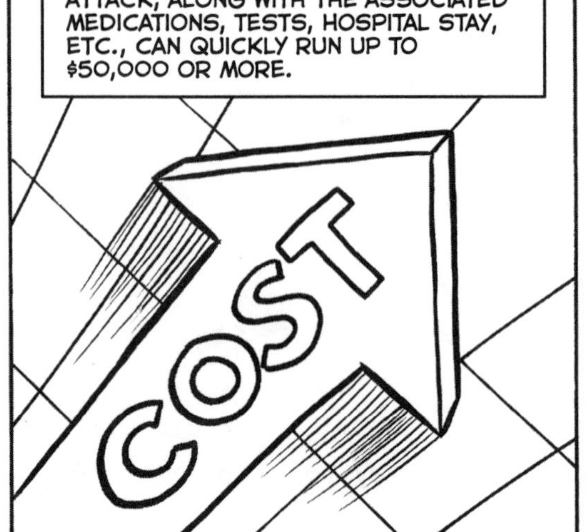

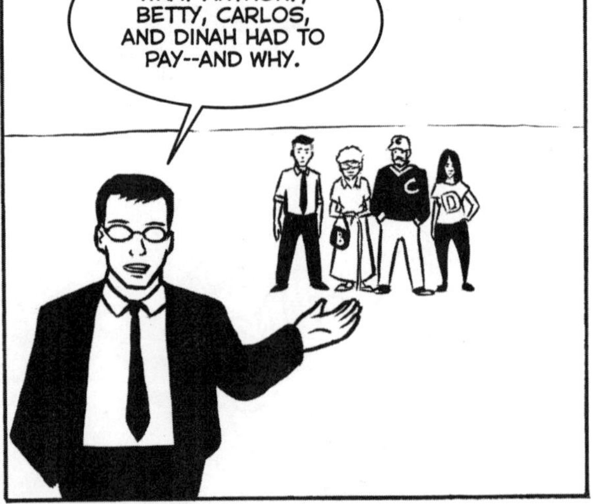
LET'S SEE WHAT ANTHONY, BETTY, CARLOS, AND DINAH HAD TO PAY--AND WHY.

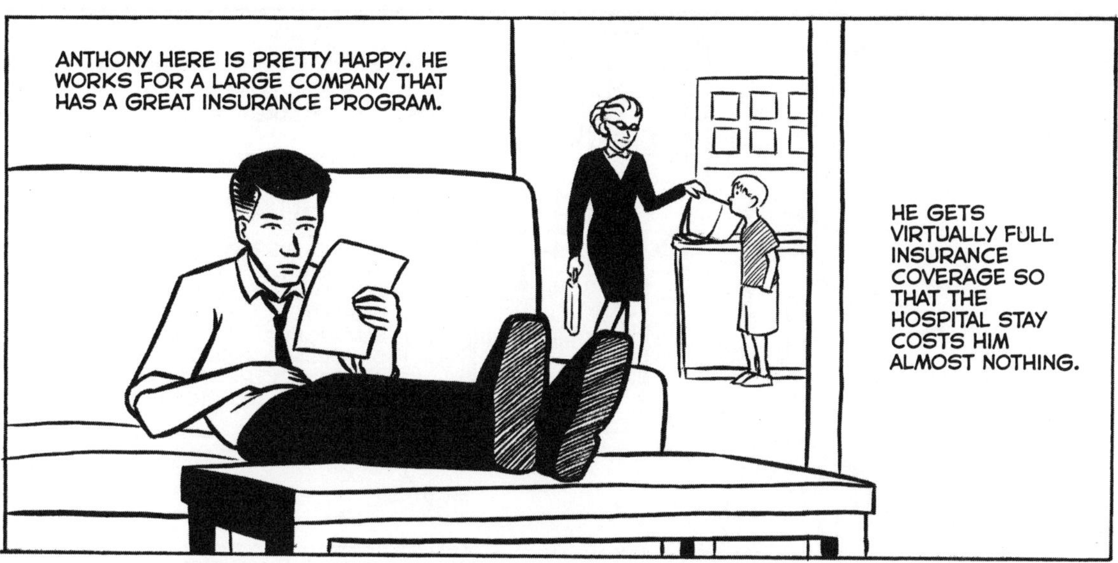
ANTHONY HERE IS PRETTY HAPPY. HE WORKS FOR A LARGE COMPANY THAT HAS A GREAT INSURANCE PROGRAM.
HE GETS VIRTUALLY FULL INSURANCE COVERAGE SO THAT THE HOSPITAL STAY COSTS HIM ALMOST NOTHING.

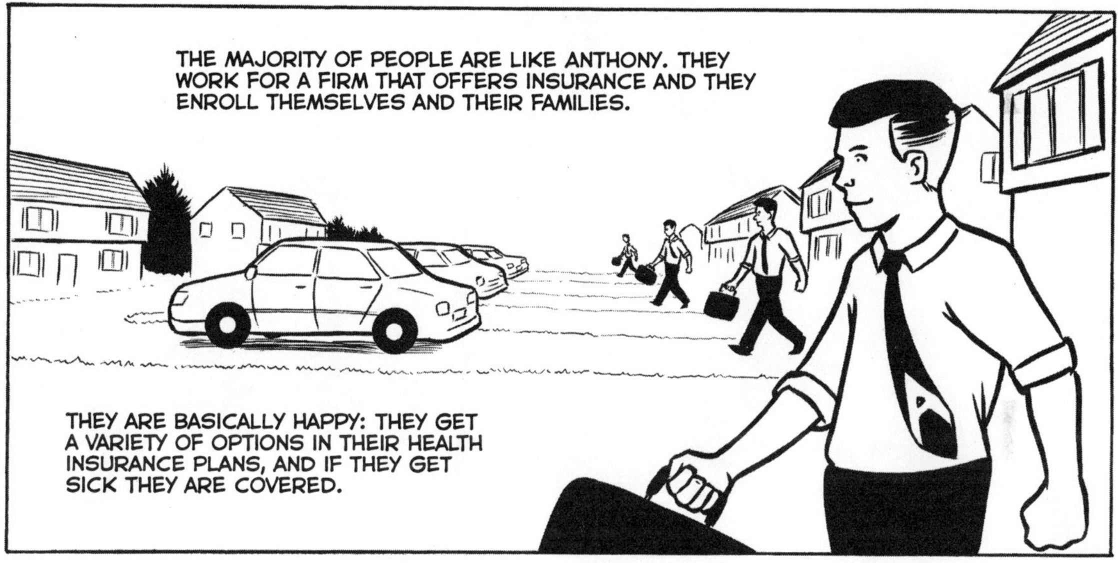
THE MAJORITY OF PEOPLE ARE LIKE ANTHONY. THEY WORK FOR A FIRM THAT OFFERS INSURANCE AND THEY ENROLL THEMSELVES AND THEIR FAMILIES.
THEY ARE BASICALLY HAPPY: THEY GET A VARIETY OF OPTIONS IN THEIR HEALTH INSURANCE PLANS, AND IF THEY GET SICK THEY ARE COVERED.
A

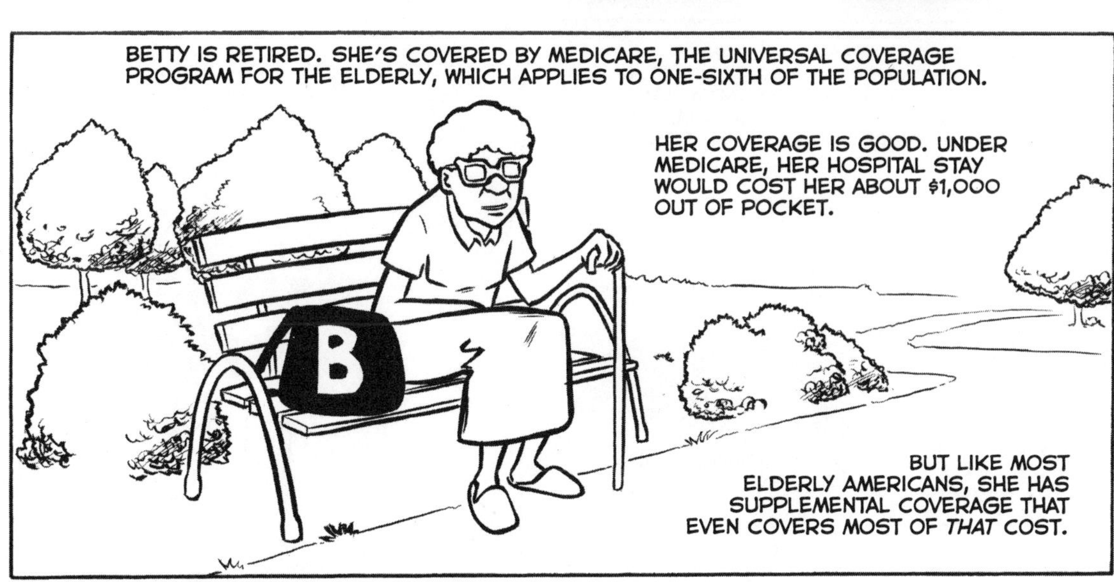
BETTY IS RETIRED. SHE'S COVERED BY MEDICARE, THE UNIVERSAL COVERAGE PROGRAM FOR THE ELDERLY, WHICH APPLIES TO ONE-SIXTH OF THE POPULATION.
HER COVERAGE IS GOOD. UNDER MEDICARE, HER HOSPITAL STAY WOULD COST HER ABOUT $1,000 OUT OF POCKET.
B
BUT LIKE MOST ELDERLY AMERICANS, SHE HAS SUPPLEMENTAL COVERAGE THAT EVEN COVERS MOST OF *THAT* COST.

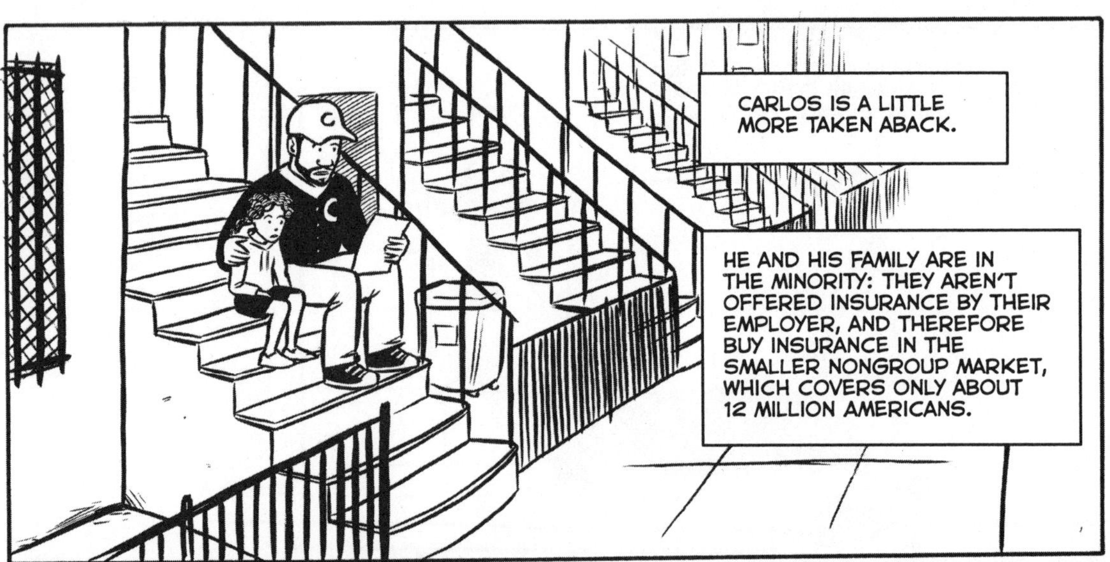
CARLOS IS A LITTLE MORE TAKEN ABACK.
HE AND HIS FAMILY ARE IN THE MINORITY: THEY AREN'T OFFERED INSURANCE BY THEIR EMPLOYER, AND THEREFORE BUY INSURANCE IN THE SMALLER NONGROUP MARKET, WHICH COVERS ONLY ABOUT 12 MILLION AMERICANS.

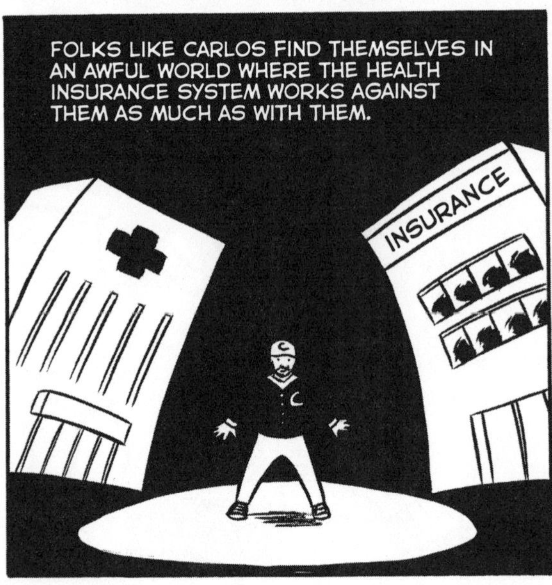
FOLKS LIKE CARLOS FIND THEMSELVES IN AN AWFUL WORLD WHERE THE HEALTH INSURANCE SYSTEM WORKS AGAINST THEM AS MUCH AS WITH THEM.
INSURANCE

THE PREMIUMS ARE MUCH HIGHER THAN FOR THOSE WITH EMPLOYER INSURANCE OR MEDICARE, AND THE COVERAGE IS MUCH WORSE. A TYPICAL PERSON LIKE CARLOS WILL PAY $2,500 OR MORE FOR A HOSPITAL STAY.

PREMIUMS

COVERAGE

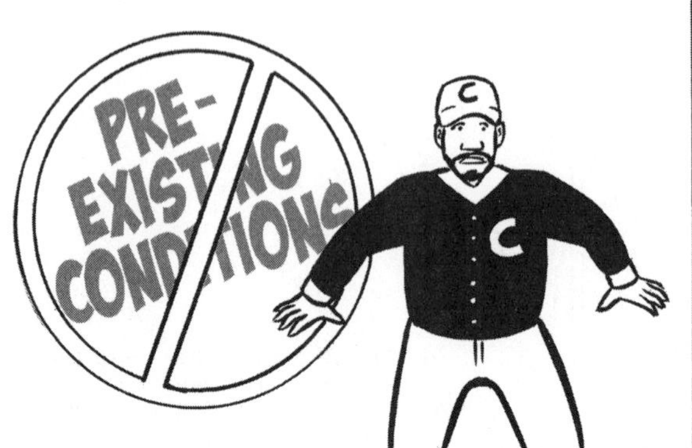
MOREOVER, HIS HEALTH INSURANCE COVERAGE DOESN'T COVER PREEXISTING CONDITIONS. SO IF CARLOS HAD A HEART CONDITION BEFORE THIS HEART ATTACK, HE WILL BE LIABLE FOR THE FULL COST OF TREATMENT.
PRE-EXISTING CONDITIONS

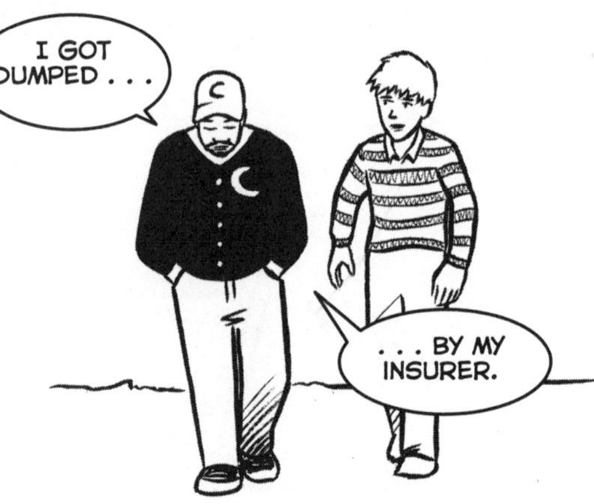
AND EVEN IF THIS IS ONLY HIS FIRST HEART ATTACK, AFTER THIS IS OVER THE INSURER CAN RAISE HIS RATES THROUGH THE ROOF OR DROP HIM FROM COVERAGE ALTOGETHER.
I GOT DUMPED . . .
. . . BY MY INSURER.

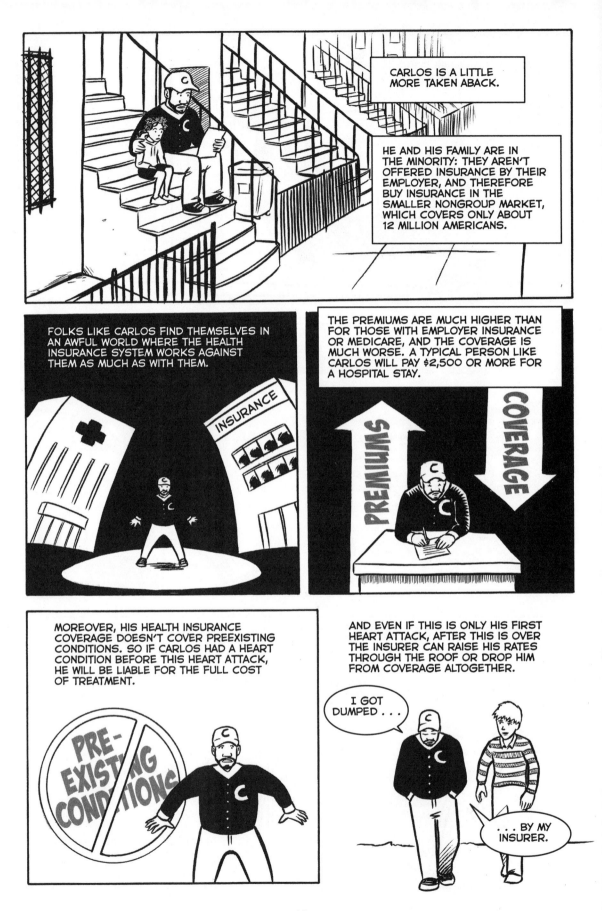

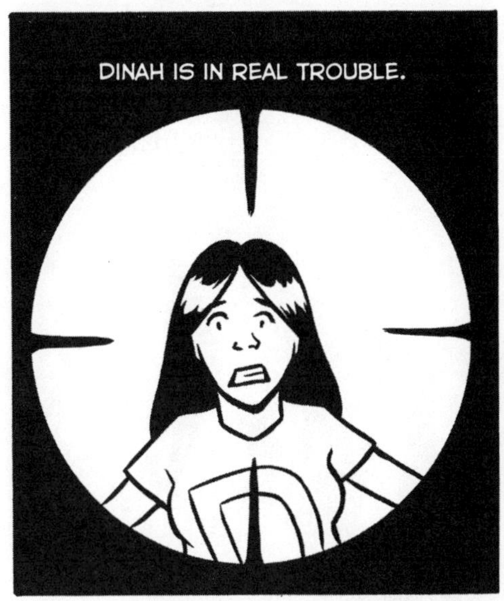
DINAH IS IN REAL TROUBLE.

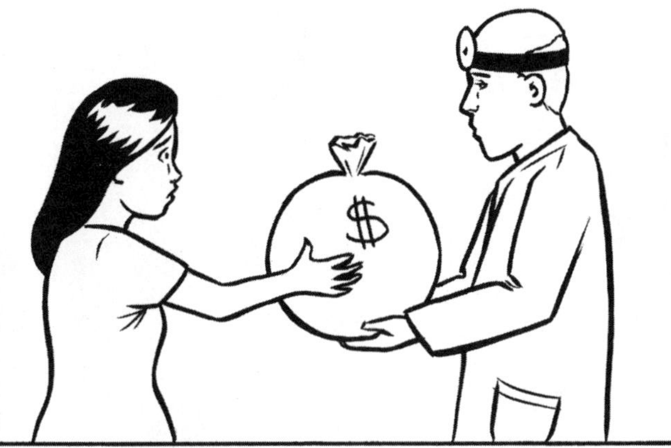
SHE DOESN'T HAVE HEALTH CARE COVERAGE, AND THE COST OF HER TREATMENT IS UP TO HER TO PAY--IN TOTAL.
$

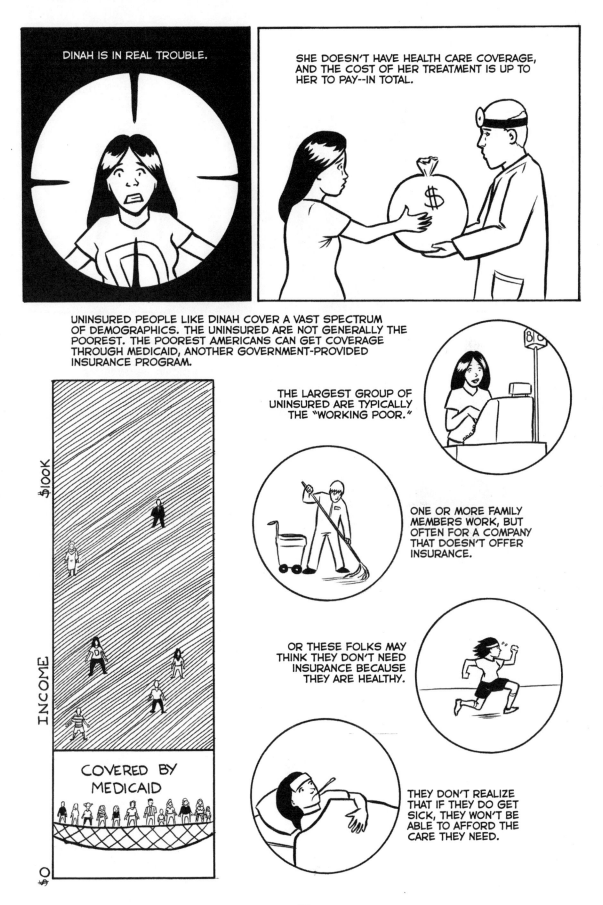

UNINSURED PEOPLE LIKE DINAH COVER A VAST SPECTRUM OF DEMOGRAPHICS. THE UNINSURED ARE NOT GENERALLY THE POOREST. THE POOREST AMERICANS CAN GET COVERAGE THROUGH MEDICAID, ANOTHER GOVERNMENT-PROVIDED INSURANCE PROGRAM.

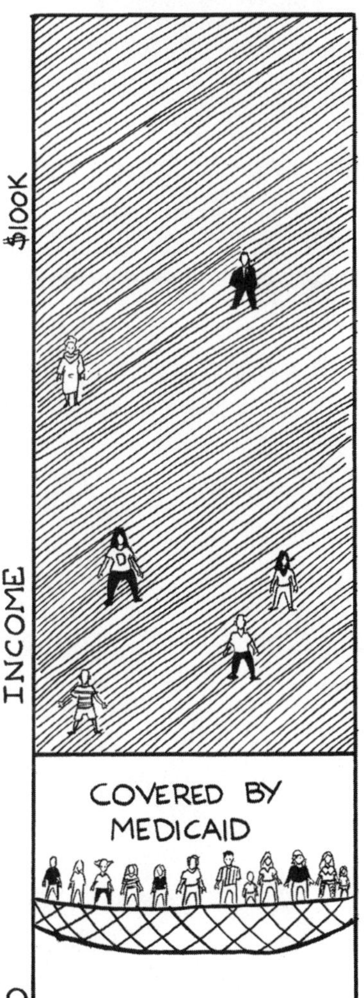
$100K
INCOME
COVERED BY MEDICAID
$0

THE LARGEST GROUP OF UNINSURED ARE TYPICALLY THE "WORKING POOR."

ONE OR MORE FAMILY MEMBERS WORK, BUT OFTEN FOR A COMPANY THAT DOESN'T OFFER INSURANCE.

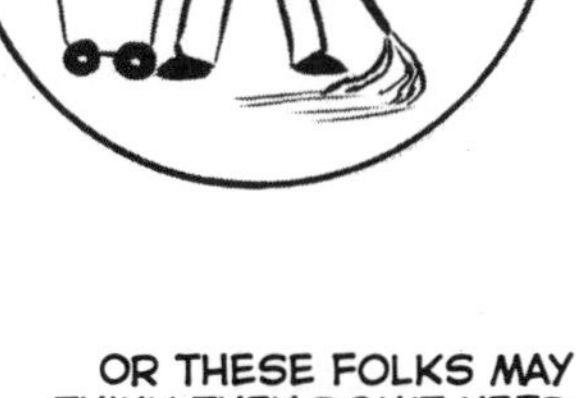

OR THESE FOLKS MAY THINK THEY DON'T NEED INSURANCE BECAUSE THEY ARE HEALTHY.

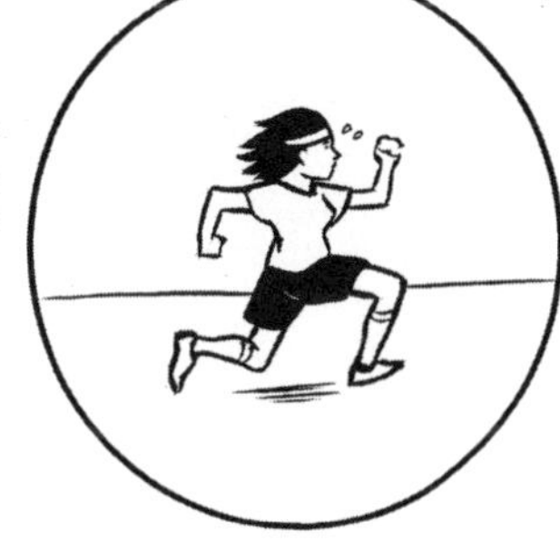

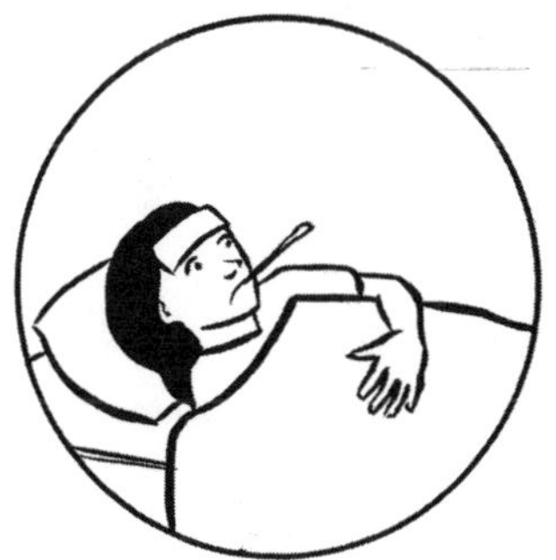

THEY DON'T REALIZE THAT IF THEY DO GET SICK, THEY WON'T BE ABLE TO AFFORD THE CARE THEY NEED.

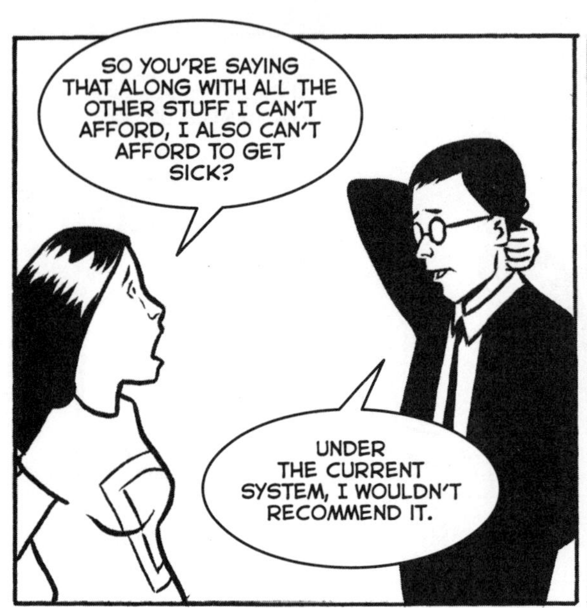
SO YOU'RE SAYING THAT ALONG WITH ALL THE OTHER STUFF I CAN'T AFFORD, I ALSO CAN'T AFFORD TO GET SICK?
UNDER THE CURRENT SYSTEM, I WOULDN'T RECOMMEND IT.

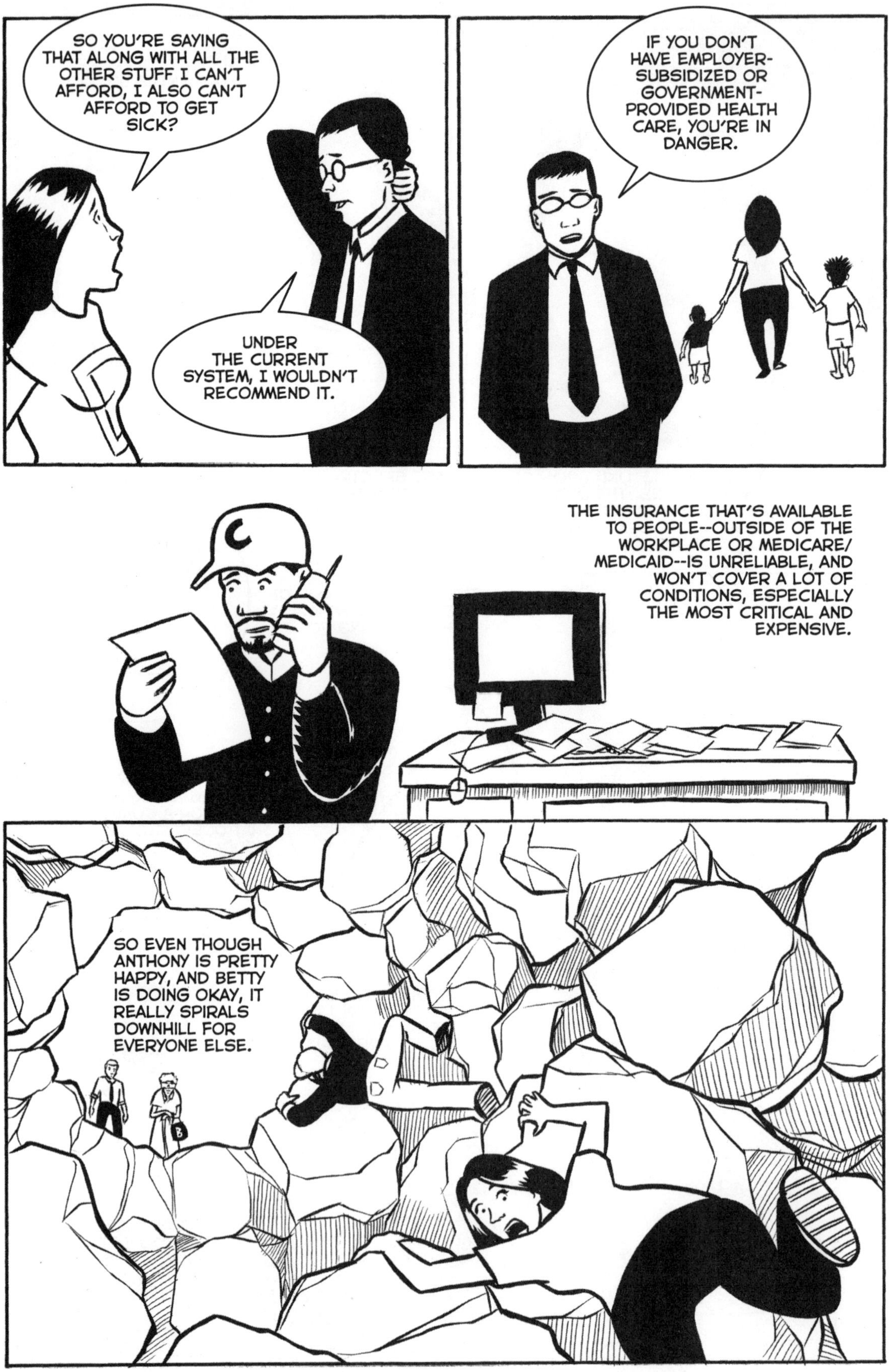

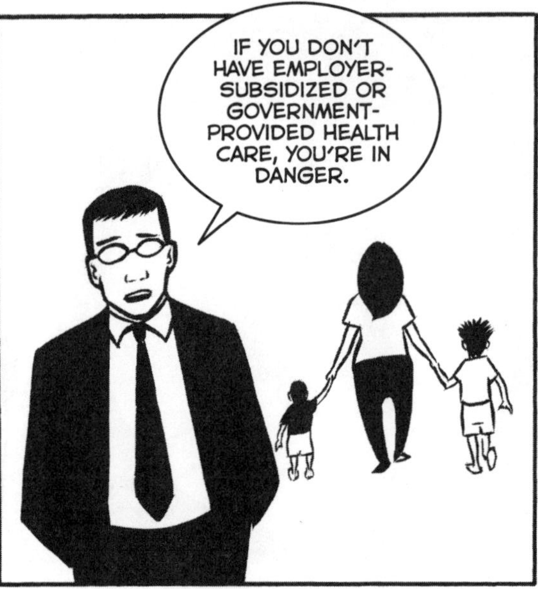
IF YOU DON'T HAVE EMPLOYER-SUBSIDIZED OR GOVERNMENT-PROVIDED HEALTH CARE, YOU'RE IN DANGER.

THE INSURANCE THAT'S AVAILABLE TO PEOPLE--OUTSIDE OF THE WORKPLACE OR MEDICARE/ MEDICAID--IS UNRELIABLE, AND WON'T COVER A LOT OF CONDITIONS, ESPECIALLY THE MOST CRITICAL AND EXPENSIVE.

SO EVEN THOUGH ANTHONY IS PRETTY HAPPY, AND BETTY IS DOING OKAY, IT REALLY SPIRALS DOWNHILL FOR EVERYONE ELSE.

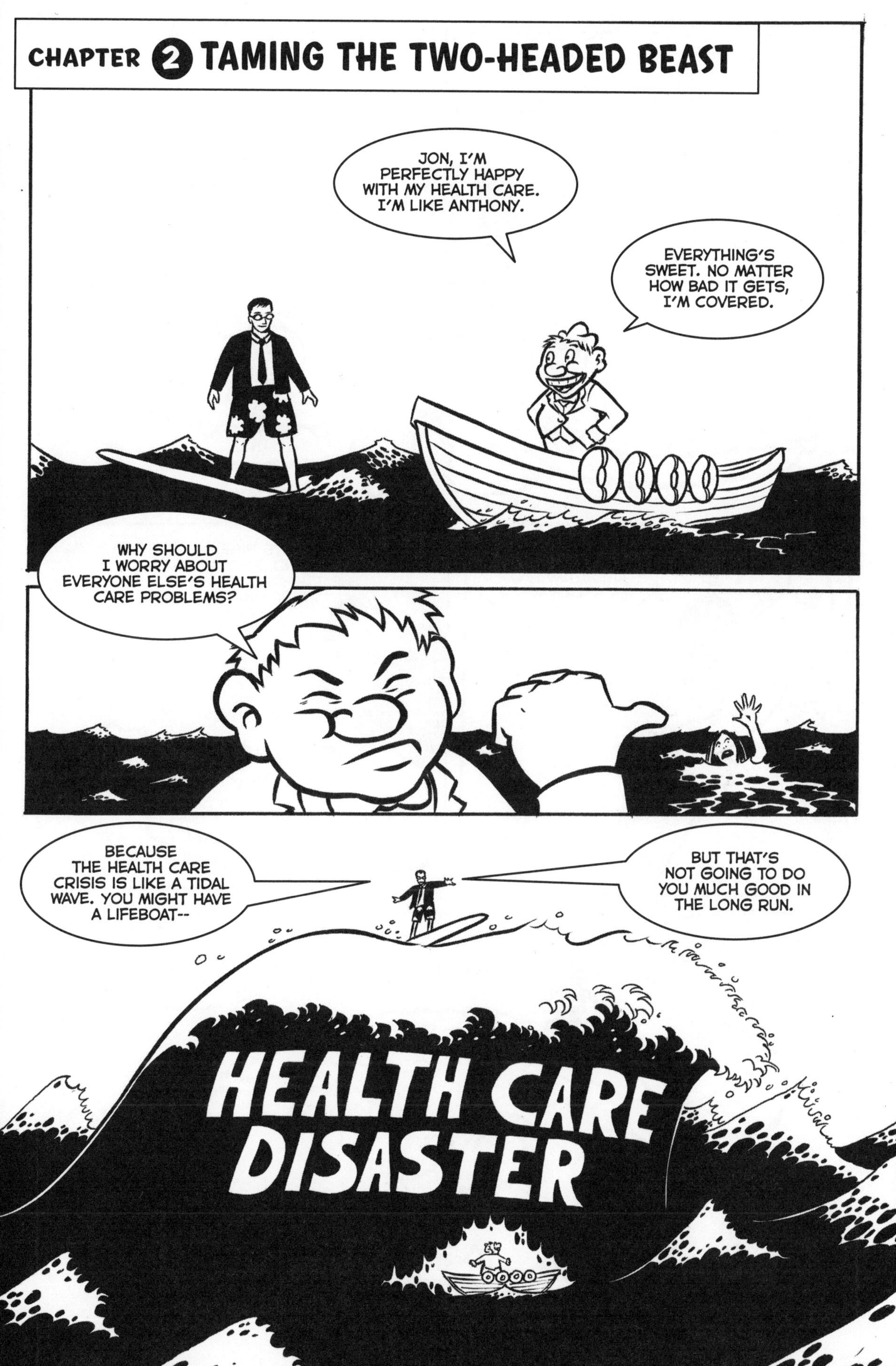
CHAPTER 2 TAMING THE TWO-HEADED BEAST
JON, I'M PERFECTLY HAPPY WITH MY HEALTH CARE. I'M LIKE ANTHONY.
EVERYTHING'S SWEET. NO MATTER HOW BAD IT GETS, I'M COVERED.
WHY SHOULD I WORRY ABOUT EVERYONE ELSE'S HEALTH CARE PROBLEMS?
BECAUSE THE HEALTH CARE CRISIS IS LIKE A TIDAL WAVE. YOU MIGHT HAVE A LIFEBOAT--
BUT THAT'S NOT GOING TO DO YOU MUCH GOOD IN THE LONG RUN.
HEALTH CARE DISASTER

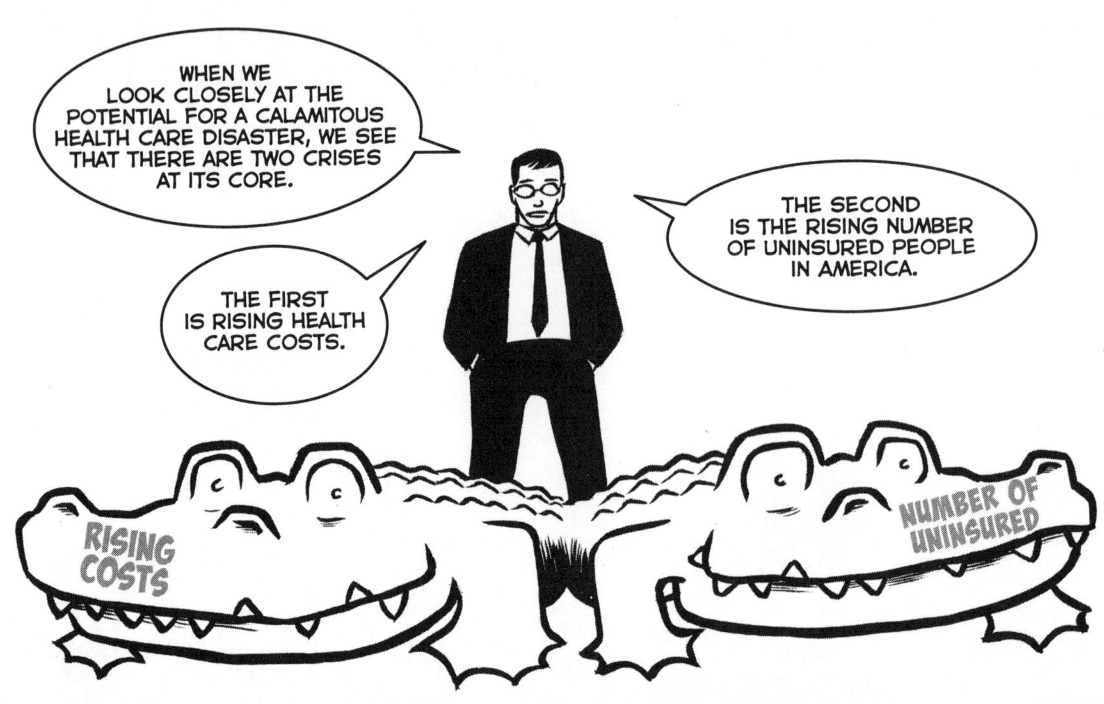
WHEN WE LOOK CLOSELY AT THE POTENTIAL FOR A CALAMITOUS HEALTH CARE DISASTER, WE SEE THAT THERE ARE TWO CRISES AT ITS CORE.
THE FIRST IS RISING HEALTH CARE COSTS.
THE SECOND IS THE RISING NUMBER OF UNINSURED PEOPLE IN AMERICA.
RISING COSTS
NUMBER OF UNINSURED

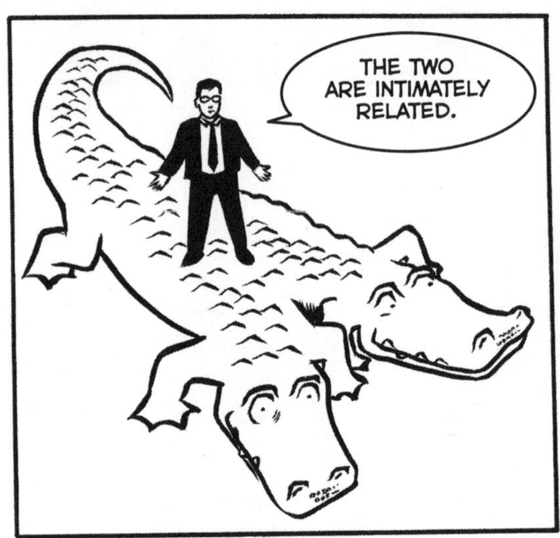
THE TWO ARE INTIMATELY RELATED.

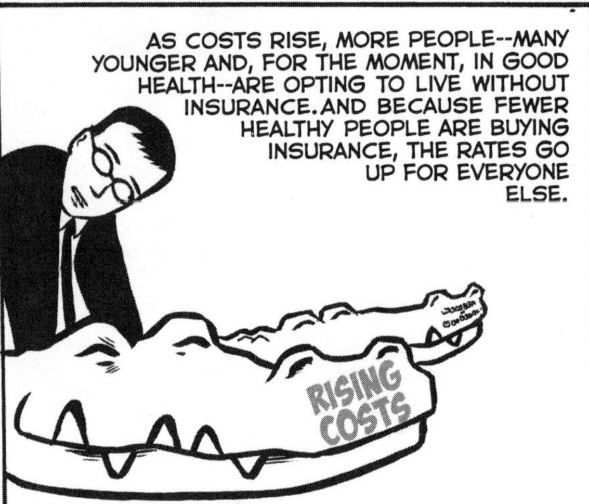
AS COSTS RISE, MORE PEOPLE--MANY YOUNGER AND, FOR THE MOMENT, IN GOOD HEALTH--ARE OPTING TO LIVE WITHOUT INSURANCE. AND BECAUSE FEWER HEALTHY PEOPLE ARE BUYING INSURANCE, THE RATES GO UP FOR EVERYONE ELSE.
RISING COSTS

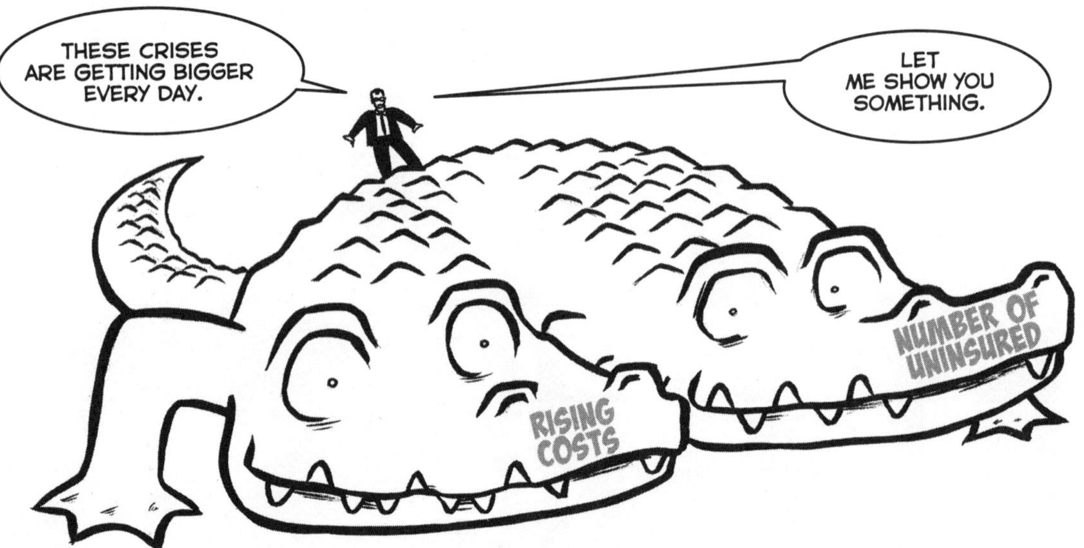
THESE CRISES ARE GETTING BIGGER EVERY DAY.
LET ME SHOW YOU SOMETHING.
RISING COSTS
NUMBER OF UNINSURED

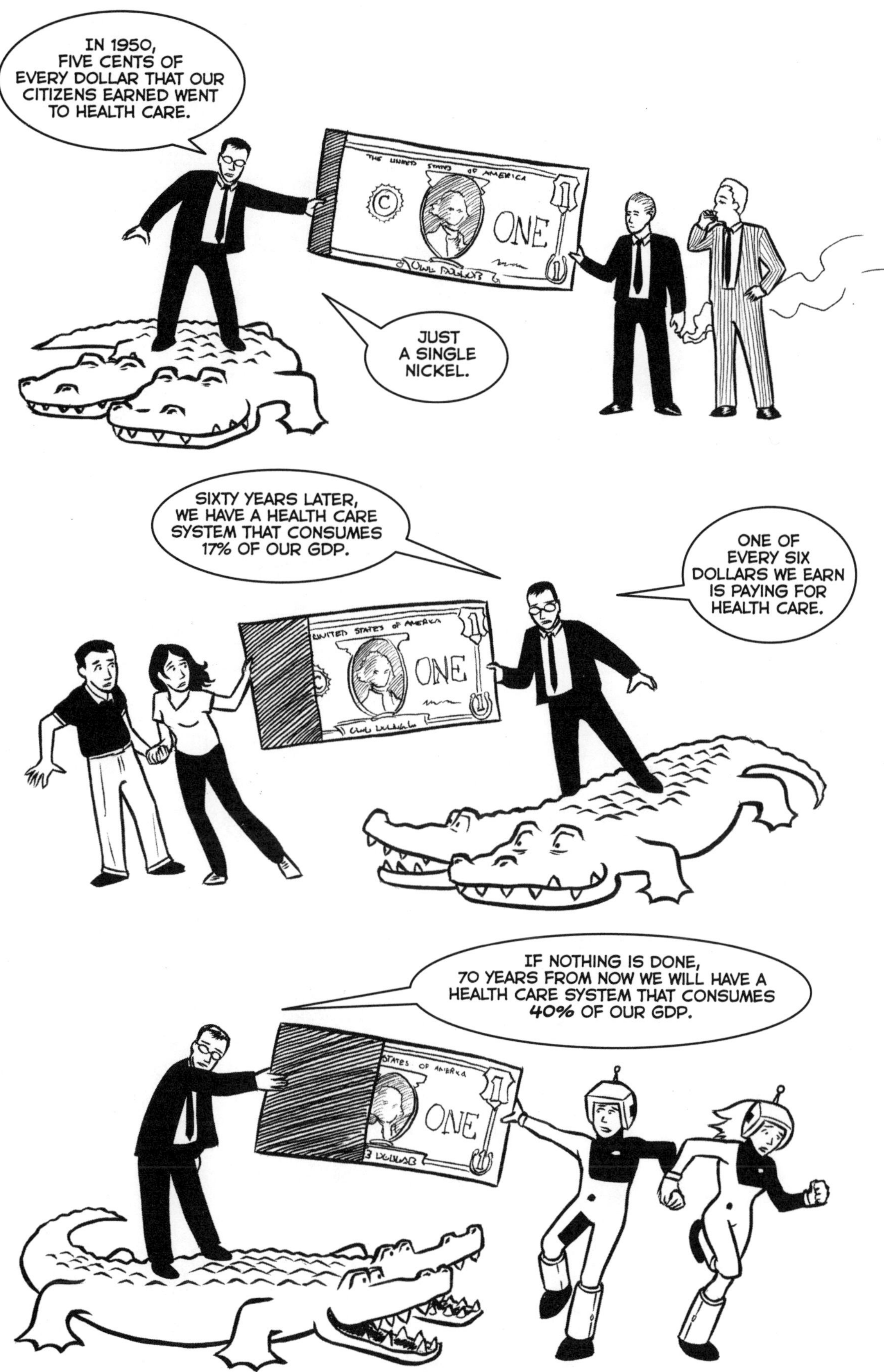
IN 1950, FIVE CENTS OF EVERY DOLLAR THAT OUR CITIZENS EARNED WENT TO HEALTH CARE.
JUST A SINGLE NICKEL.
SIXTY YEARS LATER, WE HAVE A HEALTH CARE SYSTEM THAT CONSUMES 17% OF OUR GDP.
ONE OF EVERY SIX DOLLARS WE EARN IS PAYING FOR HEALTH CARE.
IF NOTHING IS DONE, 70 YEARS FROM NOW WE WILL HAVE A HEALTH CARE SYSTEM THAT CONSUMES **40%** OF OUR GDP.

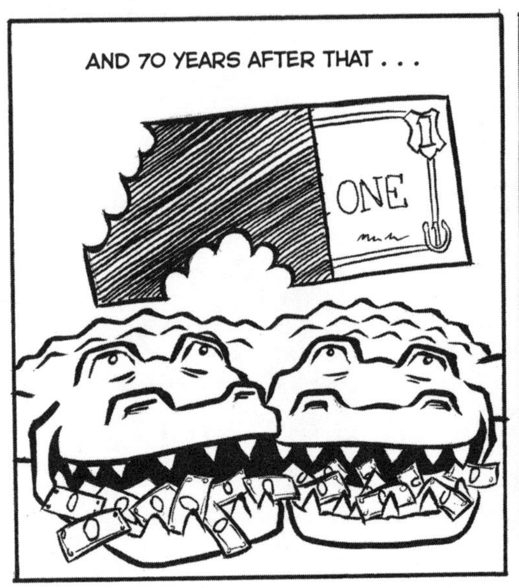
AND 70 YEARS AFTER THAT . . .
ONE

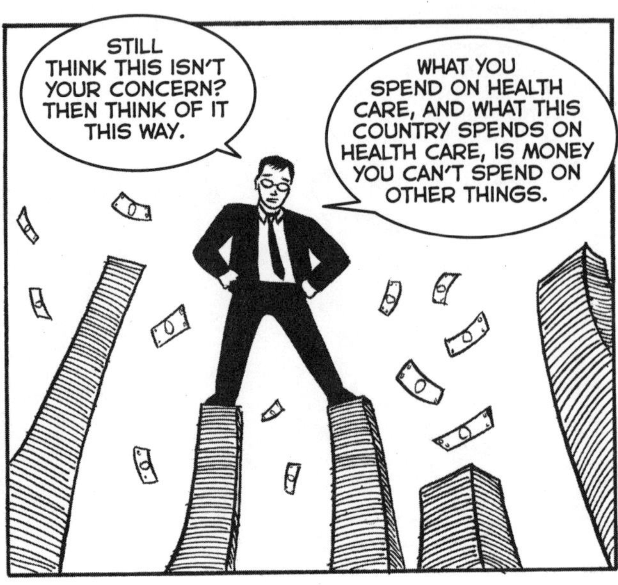
STILL THINK THIS ISN'T YOUR CONCERN? THEN THINK OF IT THIS WAY.
WHAT YOU SPEND ON HEALTH CARE, AND WHAT THIS COUNTRY SPENDS ON HEALTH CARE, IS MONEY YOU CAN'T SPEND ON OTHER THINGS.

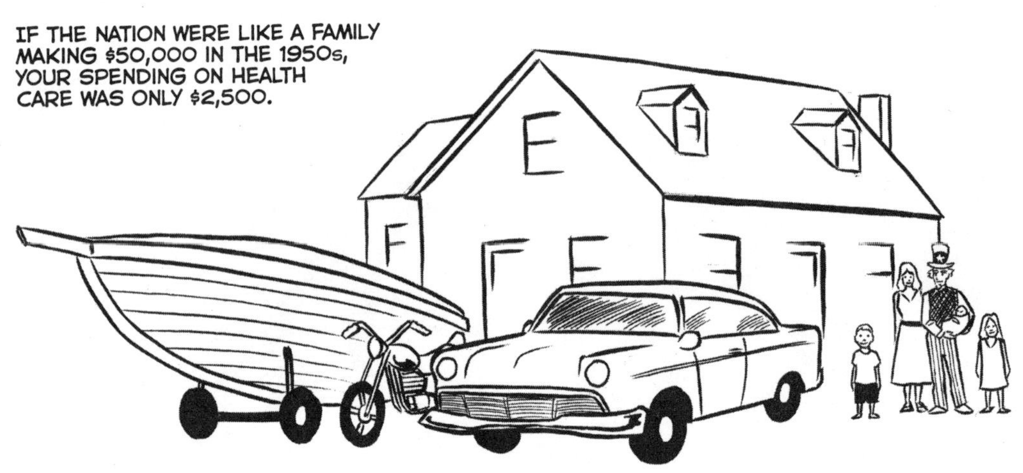
IF THE NATION WERE LIKE A FAMILY MAKING $50,000 IN THE 1950s, YOUR SPENDING ON HEALTH CARE WAS ONLY $2,500.

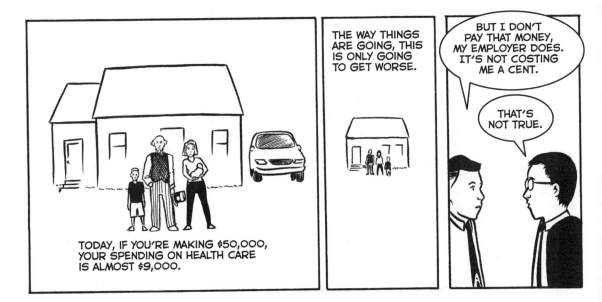

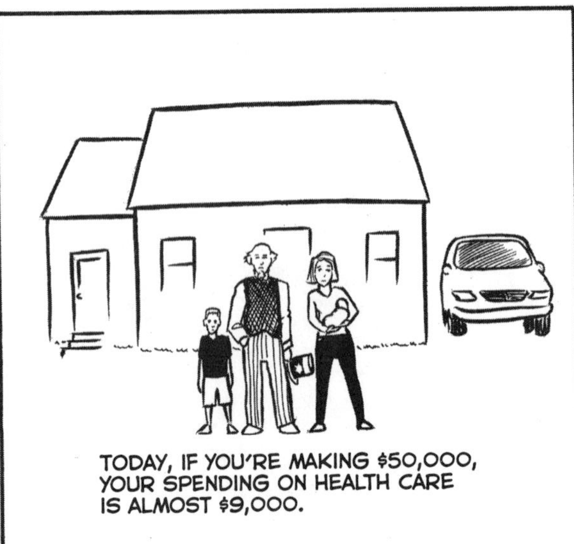
TODAY, IF YOU'RE MAKING $50,000, YOUR SPENDING ON HEALTH CARE IS ALMOST $9,000.

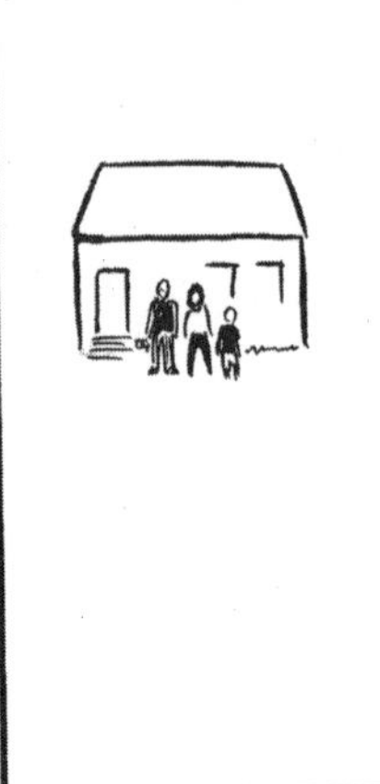
THE WAY THINGS ARE GOING, THIS IS ONLY GOING TO GET WORSE.

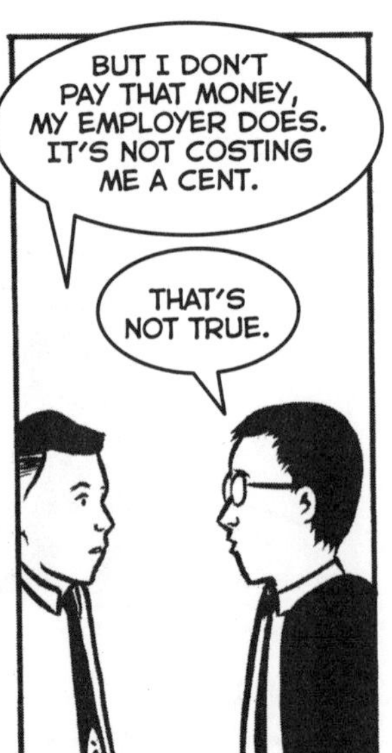
BUT I DON'T PAY THAT MONEY, MY EMPLOYER DOES. IT'S NOT COSTING ME A CENT.
THAT'S NOT TRUE.

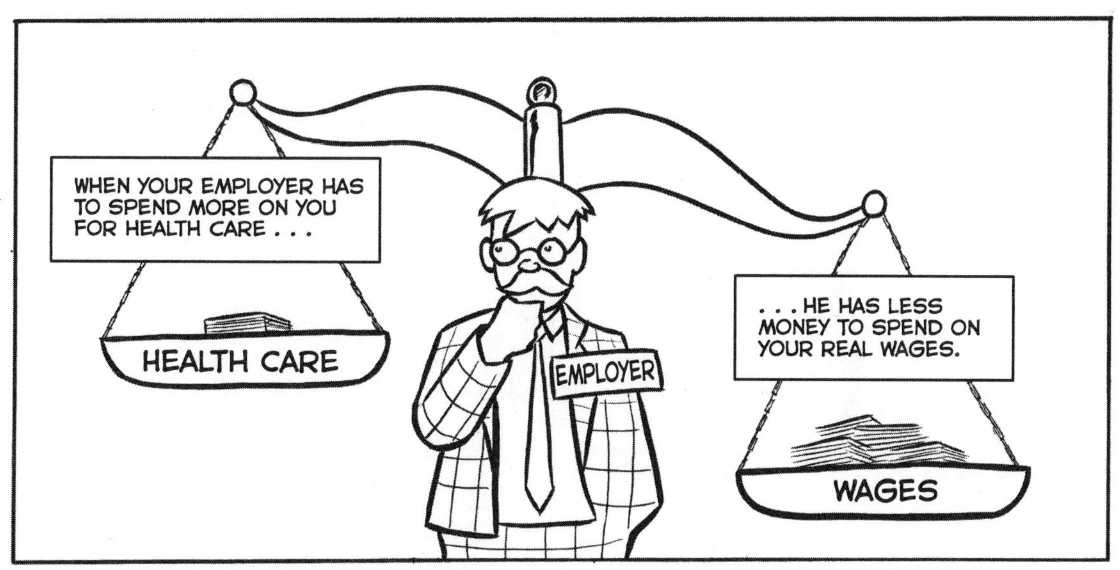
WHEN YOUR EMPLOYER HAS TO SPEND MORE ON YOU FOR HEALTH CARE . . .
HEALTH CARE
EMPLOYER
. . . HE HAS LESS MONEY TO SPEND ON YOUR REAL WAGES.
WAGES

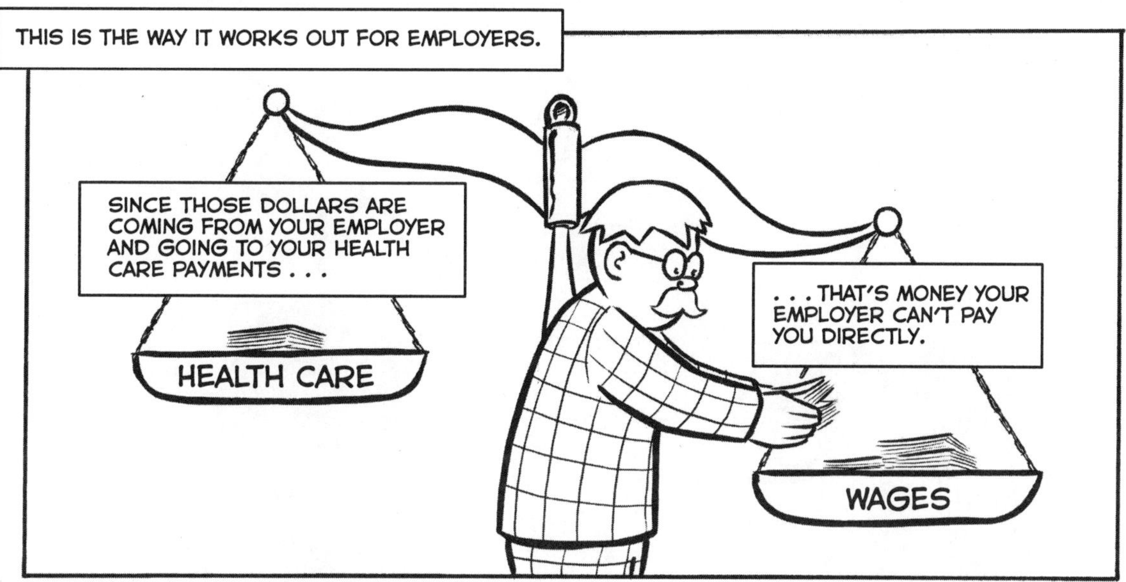
THIS IS THE WAY IT WORKS OUT FOR EMPLOYERS.
SINCE THOSE DOLLARS ARE COMING FROM YOUR EMPLOYER AND GOING TO YOUR HEALTH CARE PAYMENTS . . .
HEALTH CARE
. . . THAT'S MONEY YOUR EMPLOYER CAN'T PAY YOU DIRECTLY.
WAGES

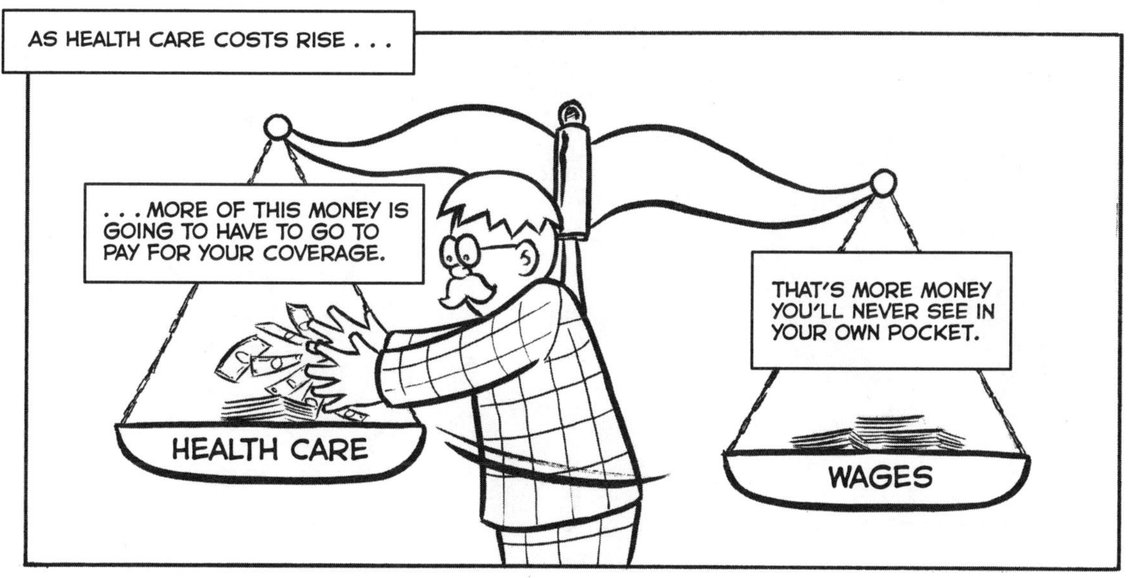
AS HEALTH CARE COSTS RISE . . .
. . . MORE OF THIS MONEY IS GOING TO HAVE TO GO TO PAY FOR YOUR COVERAGE.
HEALTH CARE
THAT'S MORE MONEY YOU'LL NEVER SEE IN YOUR OWN POCKET.
WAGES

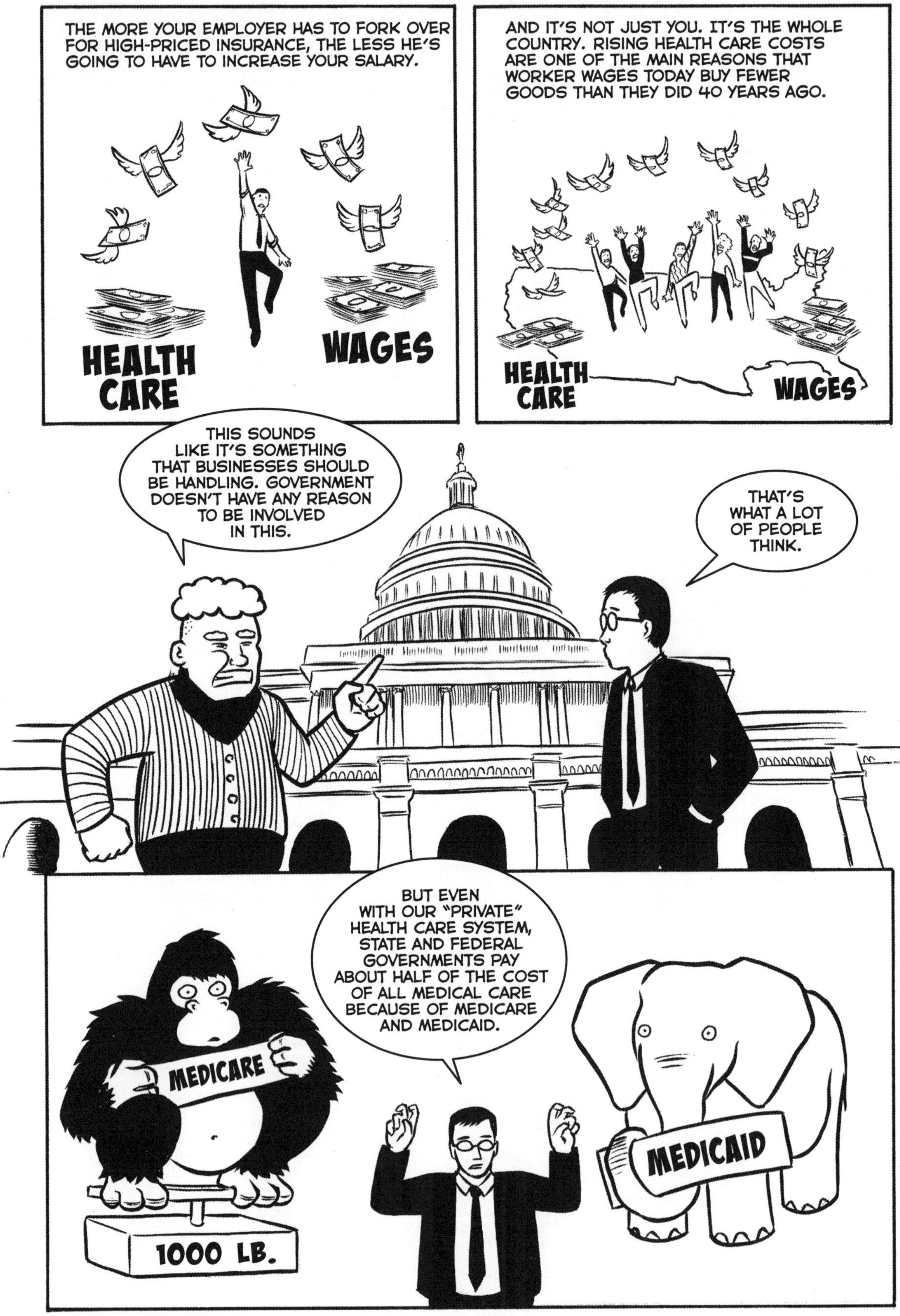

THE MORE YOUR EMPLOYER HAS TO FORK OVER FOR HIGH-PRICED INSURANCE, THE LESS HE'S GOING TO HAVE TO INCREASE YOUR SALARY.

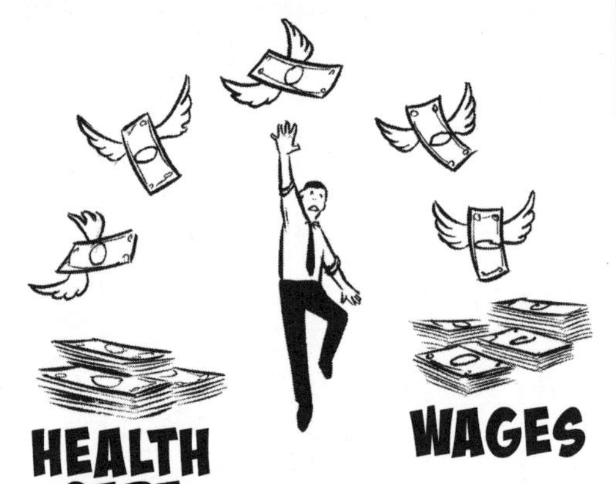

AND IT'S NOT JUST YOU. IT'S THE WHOLE COUNTRY. RISING HEALTH CARE COSTS ARE ONE OF THE MAIN REASONS THAT WORKER WAGES TODAY BUY FEWER GOODS THAN THEY DID 40 YEARS AGO.

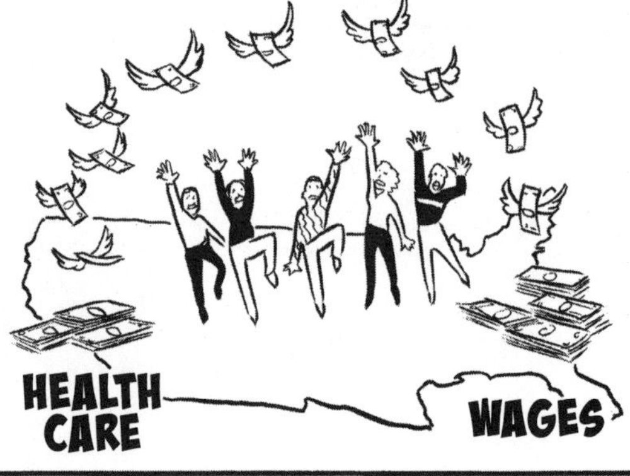

THIS SOUNDS LIKE IT'S SOMETHING THAT BUSINESSES SHOULD BE HANDLING. GOVERNMENT DOESN'T HAVE ANY REASON TO BE INVOLVED IN THIS.

THAT'S WHAT A LOT OF PEOPLE THINK.

BUT EVEN WITH OUR "PRIVATE" HEALTH CARE SYSTEM, STATE AND FEDERAL GOVERNMENTS PAY ABOUT HALF OF THE COST OF ALL MEDICAL CARE BECAUSE OF MEDICARE AND MEDICAID.

MEDICARE

1000 LB.

MEDICAID

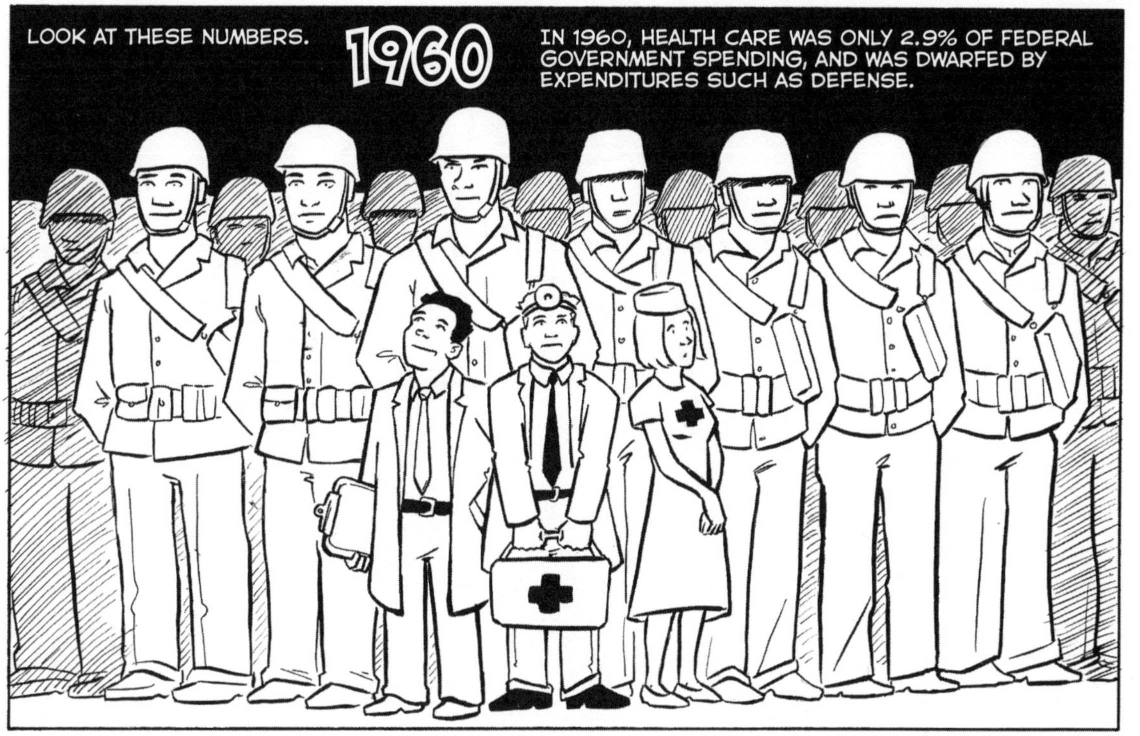

LOOK AT THESE NUMBERS.

1960

IN 1960, HEALTH CARE WAS ONLY 2.9% OF FEDERAL GOVERNMENT SPENDING, AND WAS DWARFED BY EXPENDITURES SUCH AS DEFENSE.

THE FEDERAL GOVERNMENT'S LARGEST SINGLE EXPENDITURE NOW IS ON HEALTH CARE, AND IT IS THE FASTEST GROWING AS WELL.

2007

IF NOTHING IS DONE TO CHANGE THIS, THEN OVER THE FORESEEABLE FUTURE THE FEDERAL GOVERNMENT WILL OWE NEARLY $100 TRILLION MORE IN MEDICARE PAYOUTS THAN IT EXPECTS TO COLLECT IN MEDICARE TAXES.

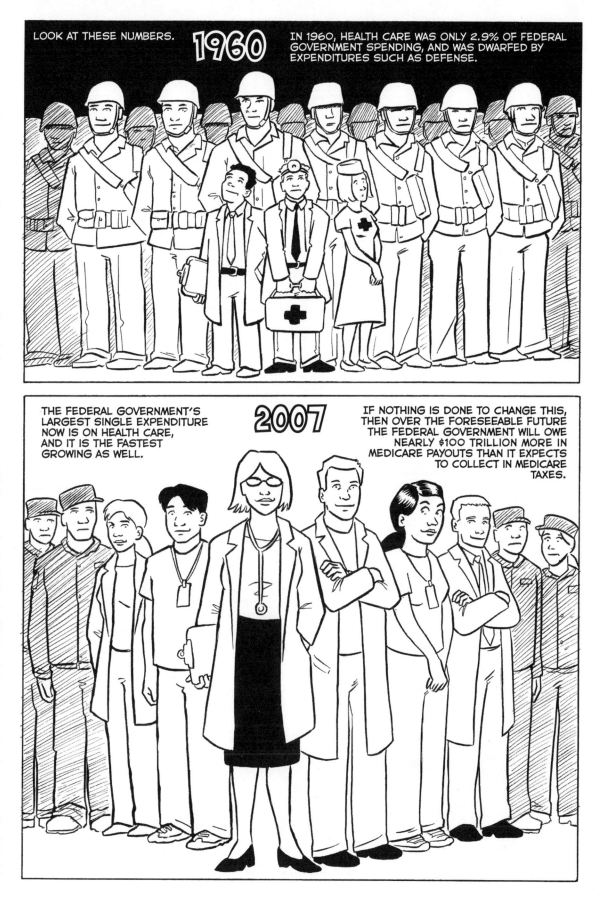

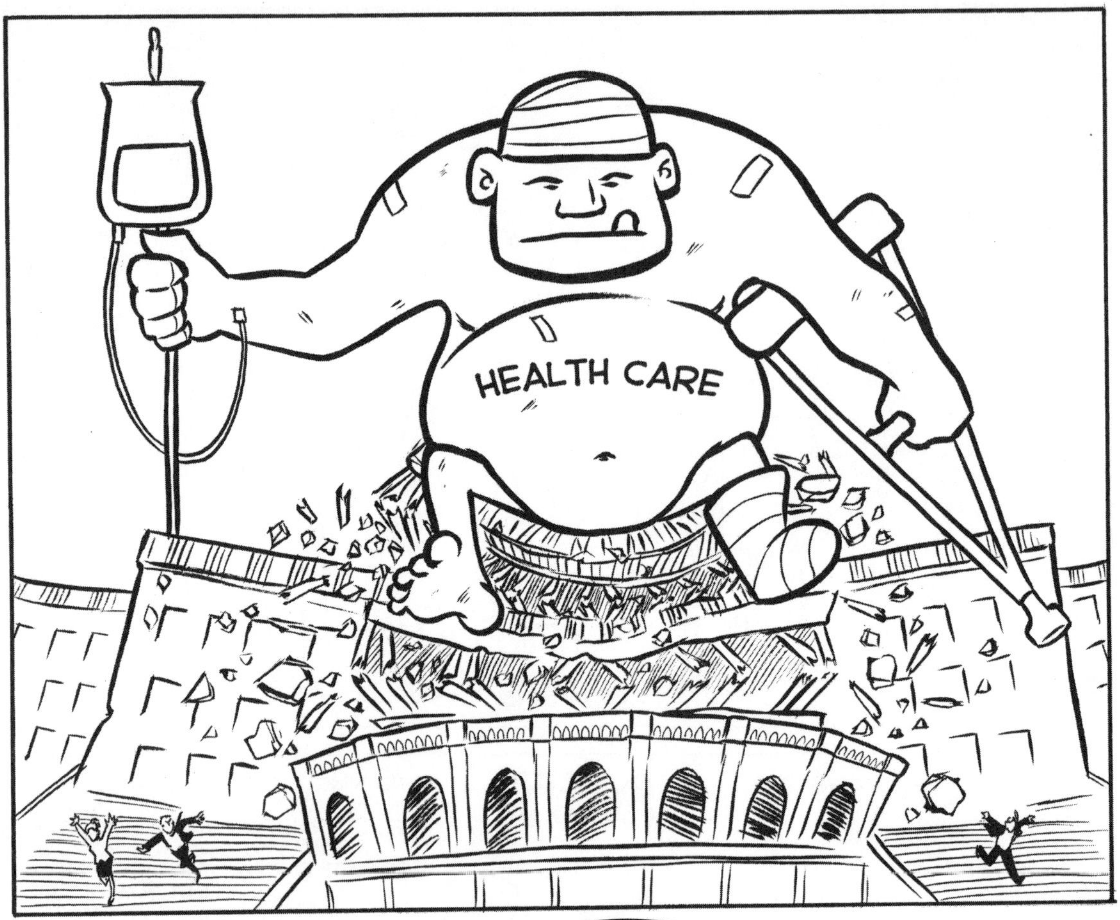

HEALTH CARE

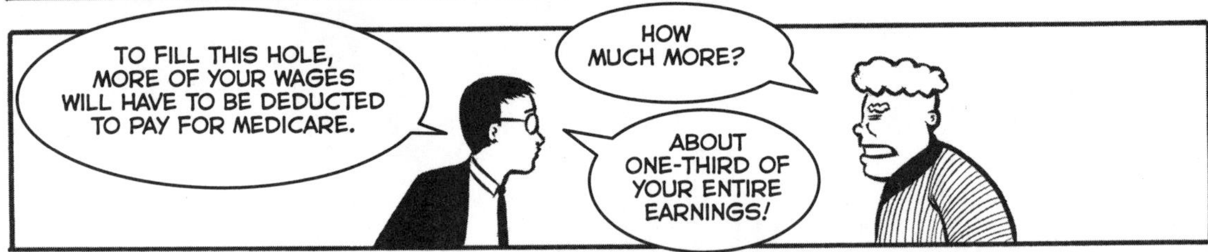
TO FILL THIS HOLE, MORE OF YOUR WAGES WILL HAVE TO BE DEDUCTED TO PAY FOR MEDICARE.
HOW MUCH MORE?
ABOUT ONE-THIRD OF YOUR ENTIRE EARNINGS!

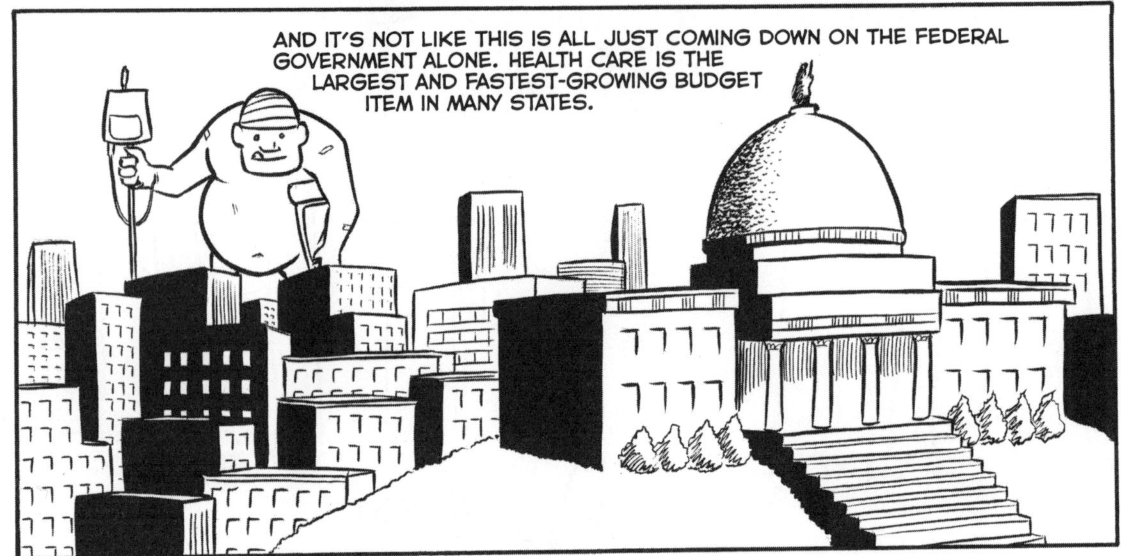
AND IT'S NOT LIKE THIS IS ALL JUST COMING DOWN ON THE FEDERAL GOVERNMENT ALONE. HEALTH CARE IS THE LARGEST AND FASTEST-GROWING BUDGET ITEM IN MANY STATES.

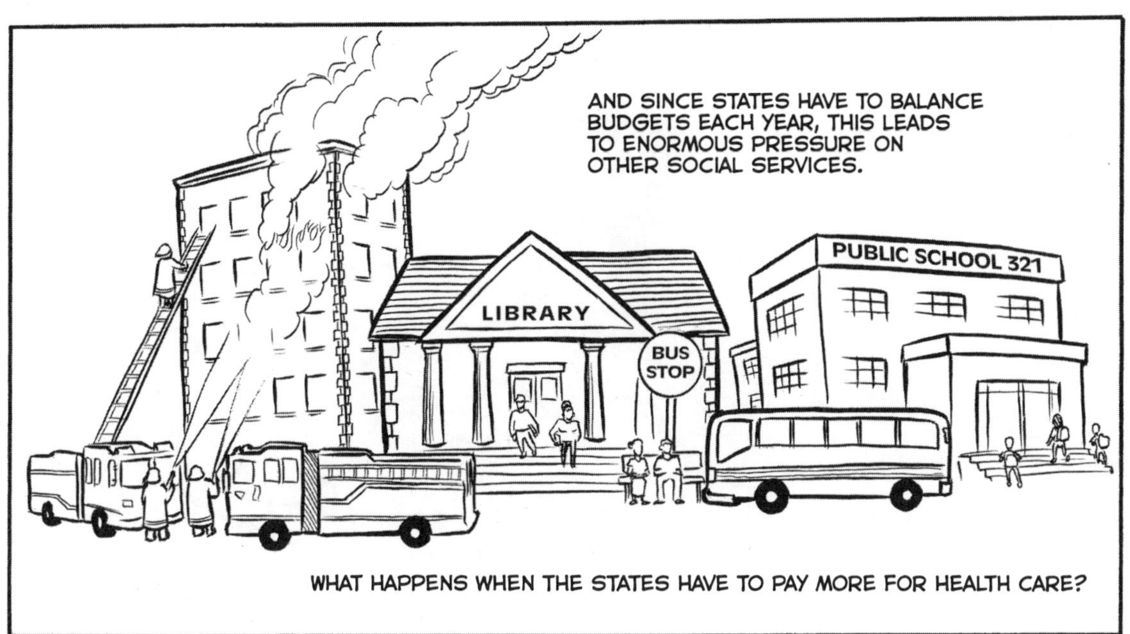
AND SINCE STATES HAVE TO BALANCE BUDGETS EACH YEAR, THIS LEADS TO ENORMOUS PRESSURE ON OTHER SOCIAL SERVICES.
PUBLIC SCHOOL 321
LIBRARY
BUS STOP
WHAT HAPPENS WHEN THE STATES HAVE TO PAY MORE FOR HEALTH CARE?

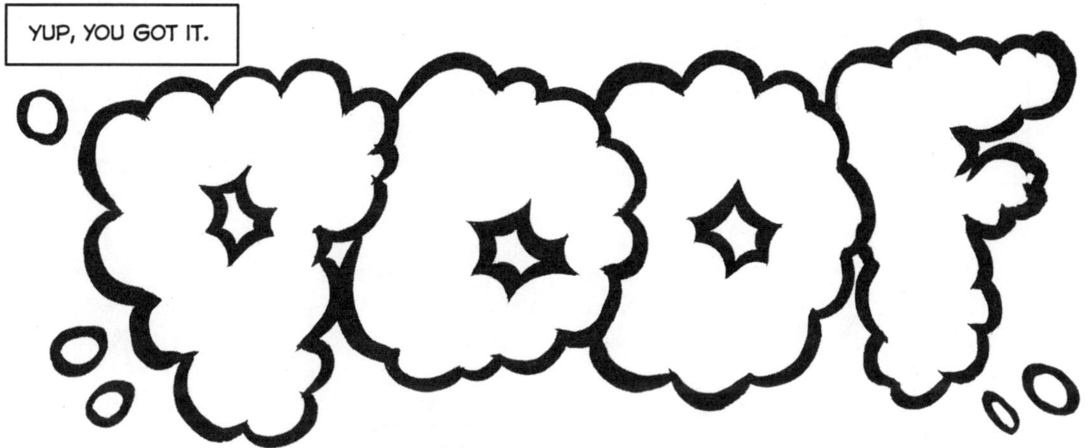
YUP, YOU GOT IT.
POOF

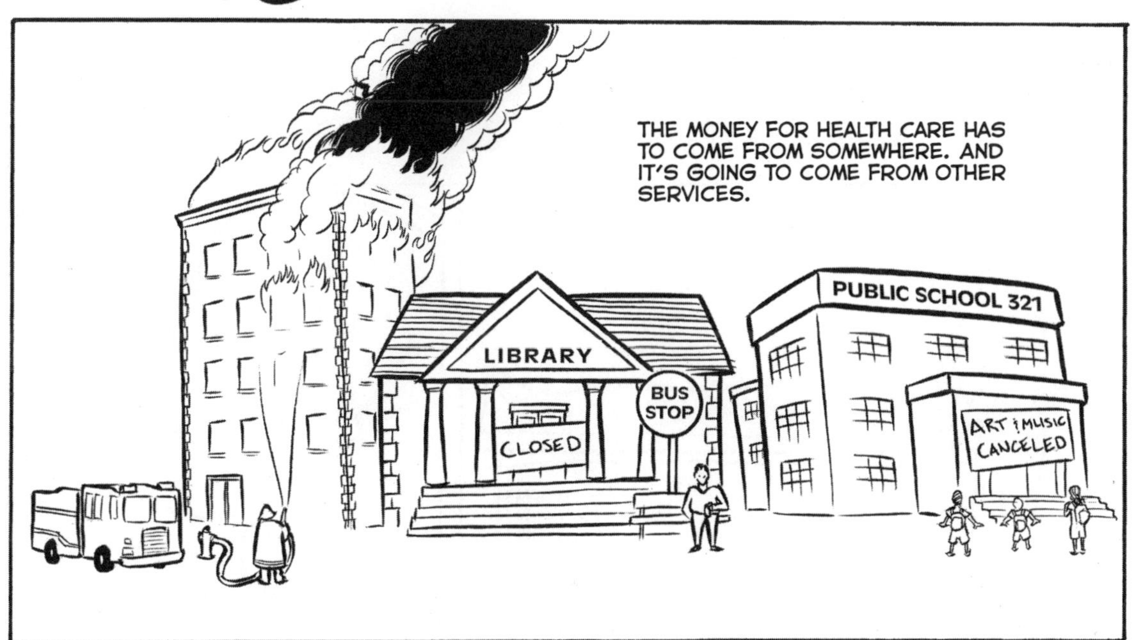
THE MONEY FOR HEALTH CARE HAS TO COME FROM SOMEWHERE. AND IT'S GOING TO COME FROM OTHER SERVICES.
PUBLIC SCHOOL 321
LIBRARY
BUS STOP
CLOSED
ART & MUSIC CANCELED

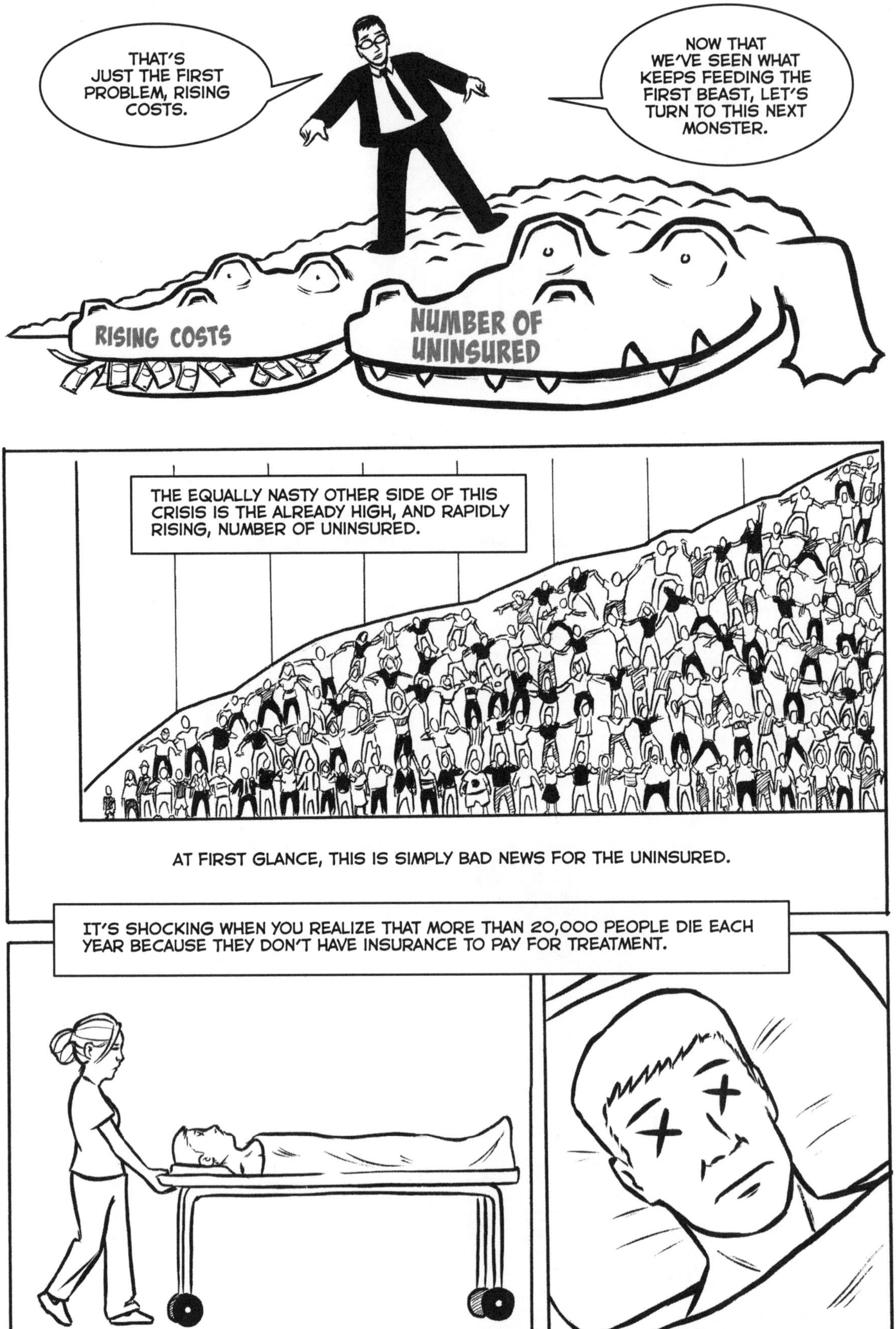

THAT'S JUST THE FIRST PROBLEM, RISING COSTS.

NOW THAT WE'VE SEEN WHAT KEEPS FEEDING THE FIRST BEAST, LET'S TURN TO THIS NEXT MONSTER.

RISING COSTS

NUMBER OF UNINSURED

THE EQUALLY NASTY OTHER SIDE OF THIS CRISIS IS THE ALREADY HIGH, AND RAPIDLY RISING, NUMBER OF UNINSURED.

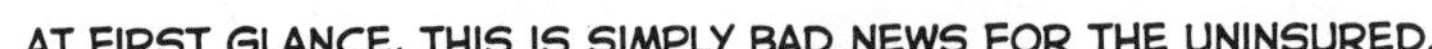
AT FIRST GLANCE, THIS IS SIMPLY BAD NEWS FOR THE UNINSURED.

IT'S SHOCKING WHEN YOU REALIZE THAT MORE THAN 20,000 PEOPLE DIE EACH YEAR BECAUSE THEY DON'T HAVE INSURANCE TO PAY FOR TREATMENT.

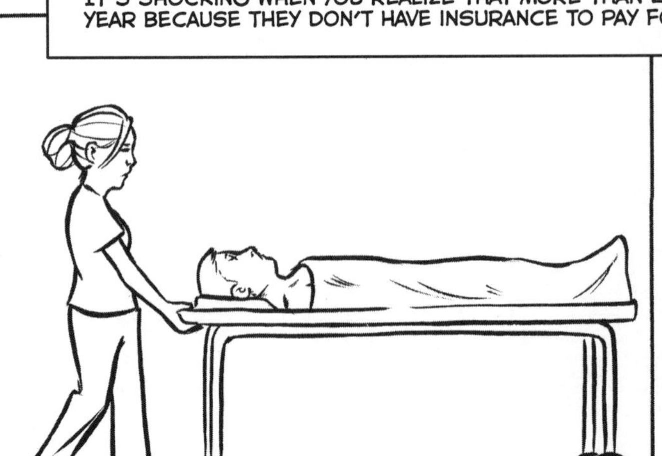

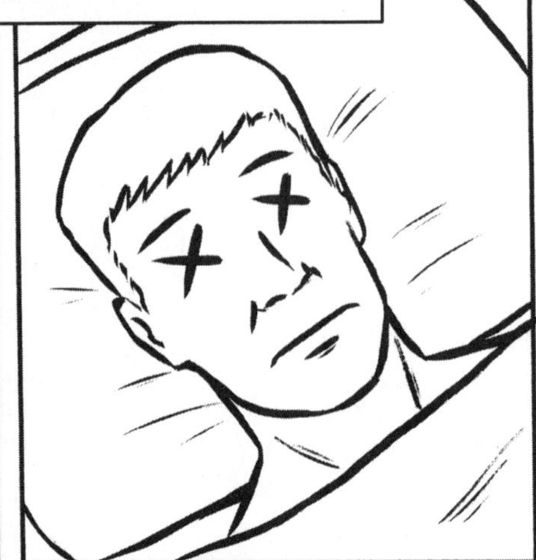

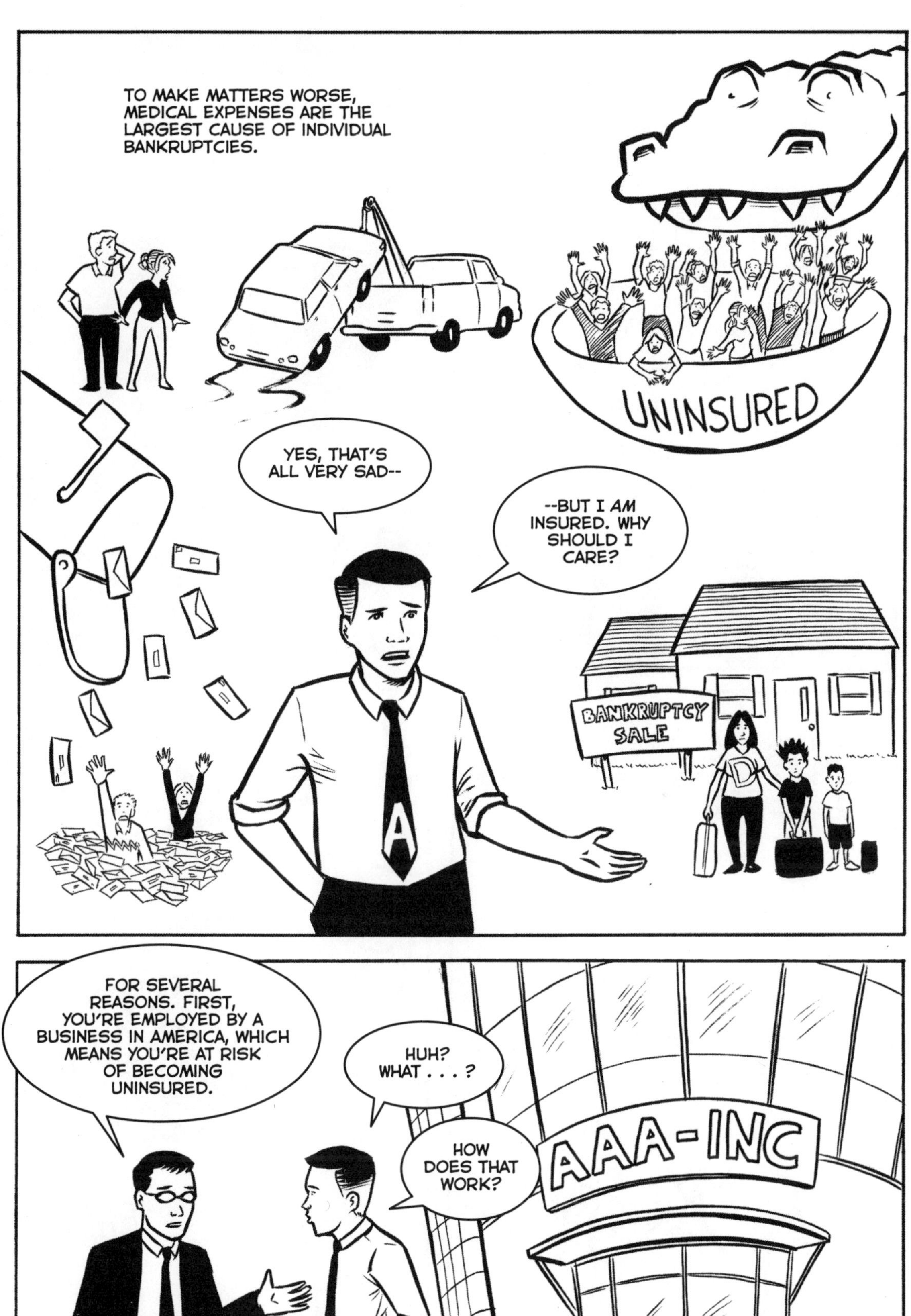
TO MAKE MATTERS WORSE, MEDICAL EXPENSES ARE THE LARGEST CAUSE OF INDIVIDUAL BANKRUPTCIES.
UNINSURED
YES, THAT'S ALL VERY SAD--
--BUT I *AM* INSURED. WHY SHOULD I CARE?
BANKRUPTCY SALE
FOR SEVERAL REASONS. FIRST, YOU'RE EMPLOYED BY A BUSINESS IN AMERICA, WHICH MEANS YOU'RE AT RISK OF BECOMING UNINSURED.
HUH? WHAT . . . ?
HOW DOES THAT WORK?
AAA-INC

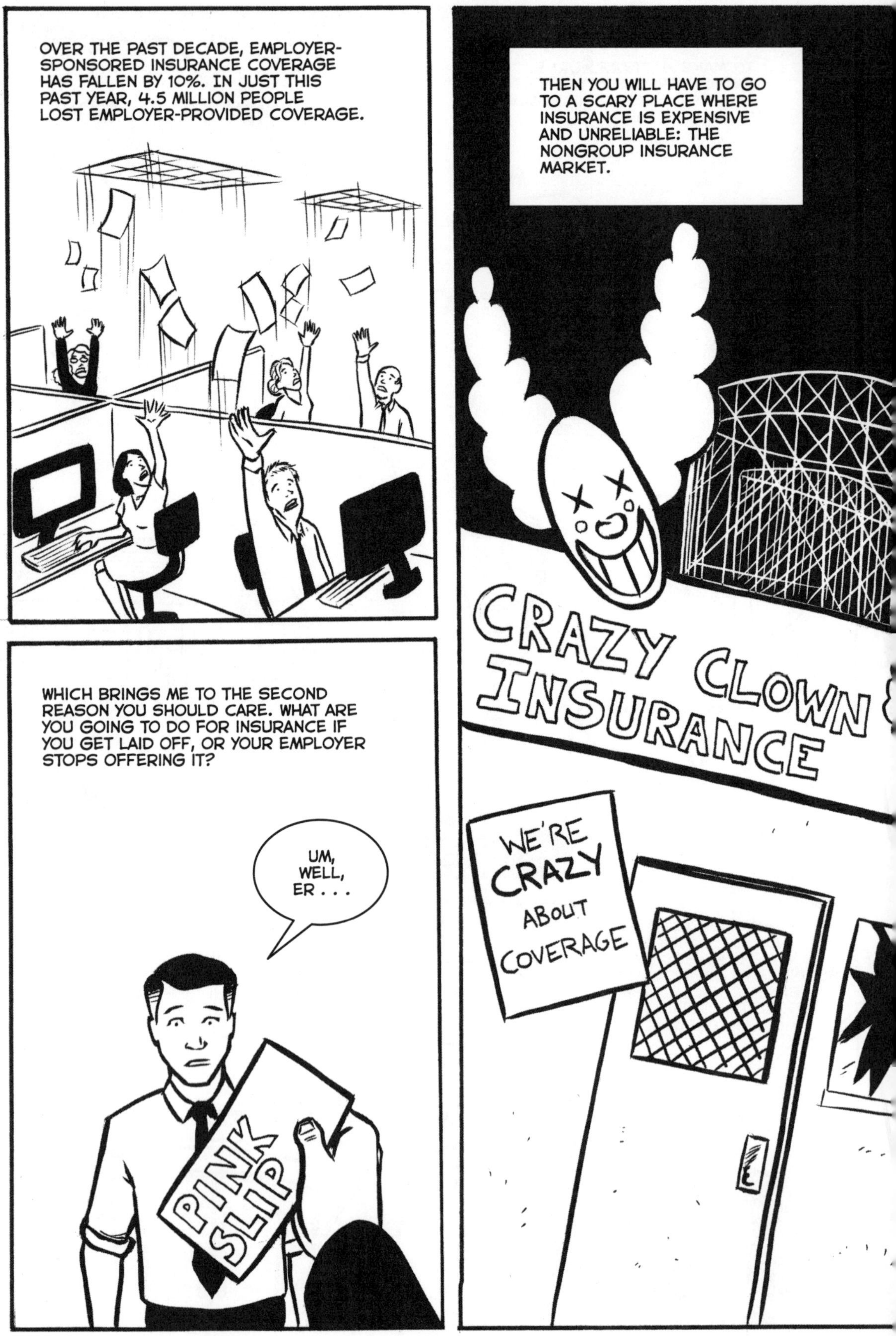

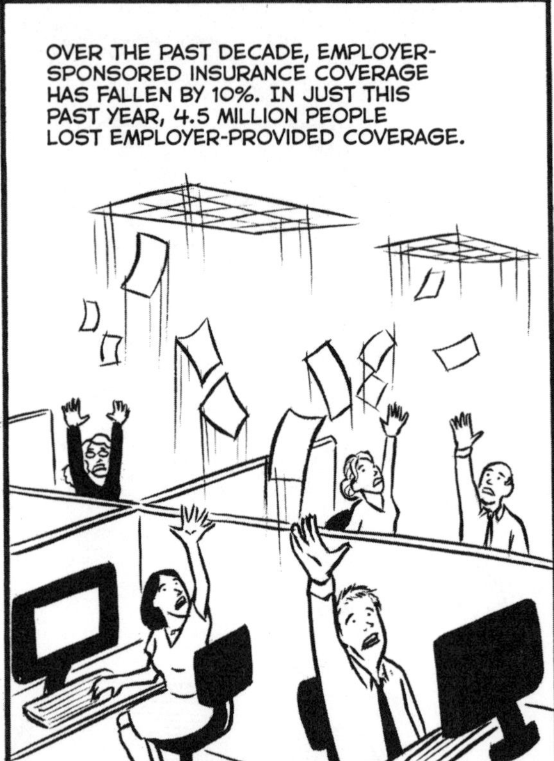

OVER THE PAST DECADE, EMPLOYER-SPONSORED INSURANCE COVERAGE HAS FALLEN BY 10%. IN JUST THIS PAST YEAR, 4.5 MILLION PEOPLE LOST EMPLOYER-PROVIDED COVERAGE.

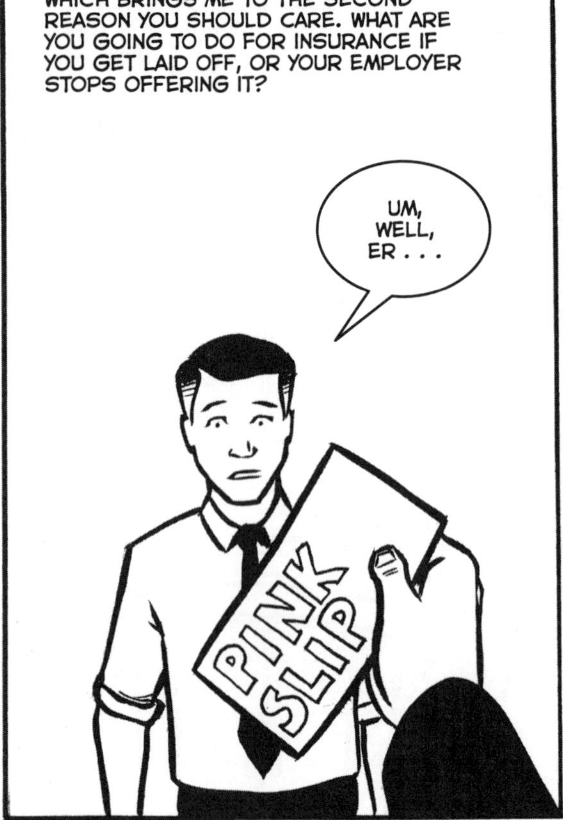

WHICH BRINGS ME TO THE SECOND REASON YOU SHOULD CARE. WHAT ARE YOU GOING TO DO FOR INSURANCE IF YOU GET LAID OFF, OR YOUR EMPLOYER STOPS OFFERING IT?
UM, WELL, ER . . .
PINK SLIP

THEN YOU WILL HAVE TO GO TO A SCARY PLACE WHERE INSURANCE IS EXPENSIVE AND UNRELIABLE: THE NONGROUP INSURANCE MARKET.

CRAZY CLOWN INSURANCE

WE'RE CRAZY ABOUT COVERAGE

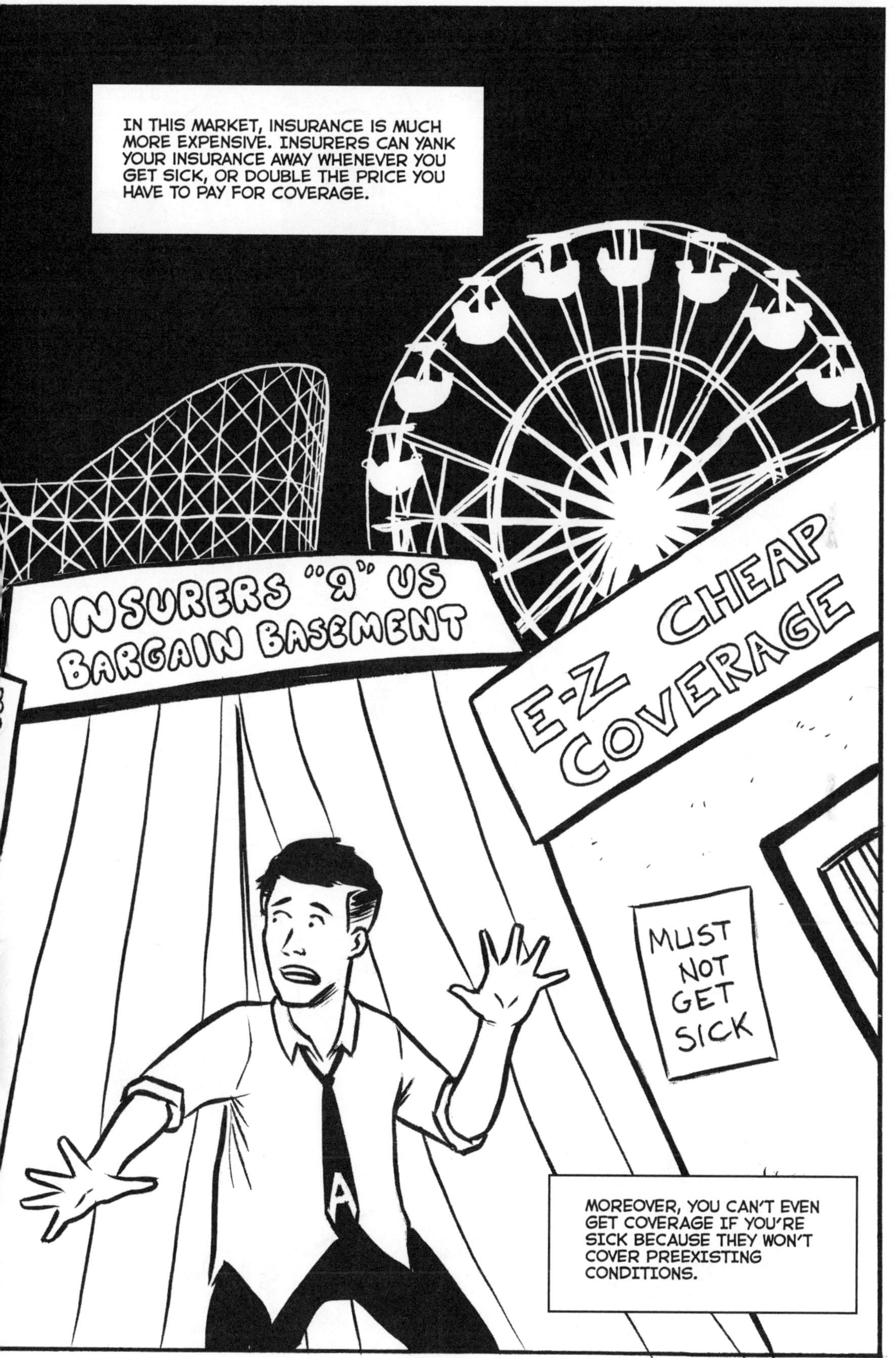
IN THIS MARKET, INSURANCE IS MUCH MORE EXPENSIVE. INSURERS CAN YANK YOUR INSURANCE AWAY WHENEVER YOU GET SICK, OR DOUBLE THE PRICE YOU HAVE TO PAY FOR COVERAGE.
INSURERS "Я" US
BARGAIN BASEMENT
E-Z CHEAP COVERAGE
MUST NOT GET SICK
A
MOREOVER, YOU CAN'T EVEN GET COVERAGE IF YOU'RE SICK BECAUSE THEY WON'T COVER PREEXISTING CONDITIONS.

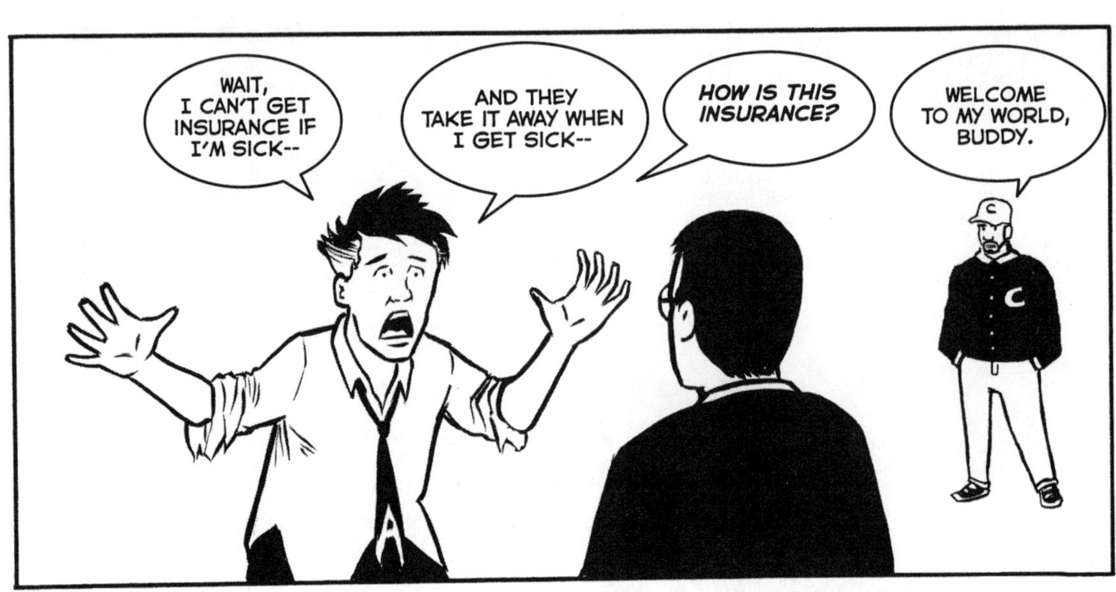
WAIT, I CAN'T GET INSURANCE IF I'M SICK--
AND THEY TAKE IT AWAY WHEN I GET SICK--
HOW IS THIS INSURANCE?
WELCOME TO MY WORLD, BUDDY.

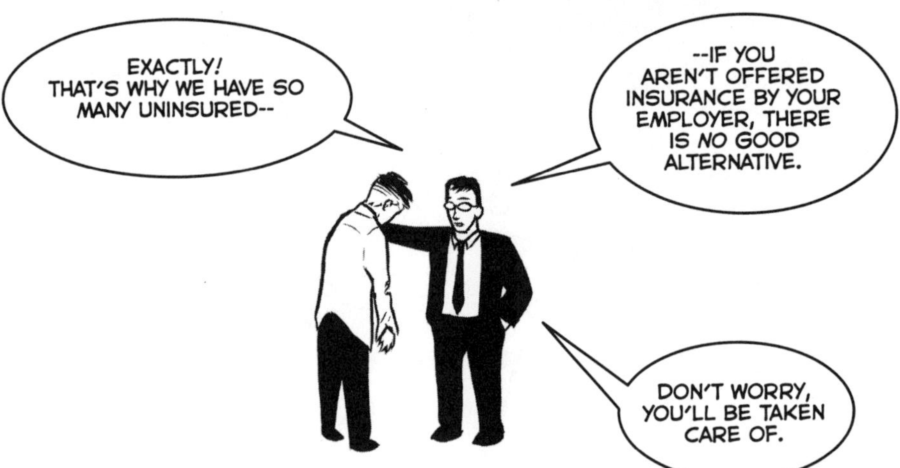
EXACTLY! THAT'S WHY WE HAVE SO MANY UNINSURED--
--IF YOU AREN'T OFFERED INSURANCE BY YOUR EMPLOYER, THERE IS *NO* GOOD ALTERNATIVE.
DON'T WORRY, YOU'LL BE TAKEN CARE OF.

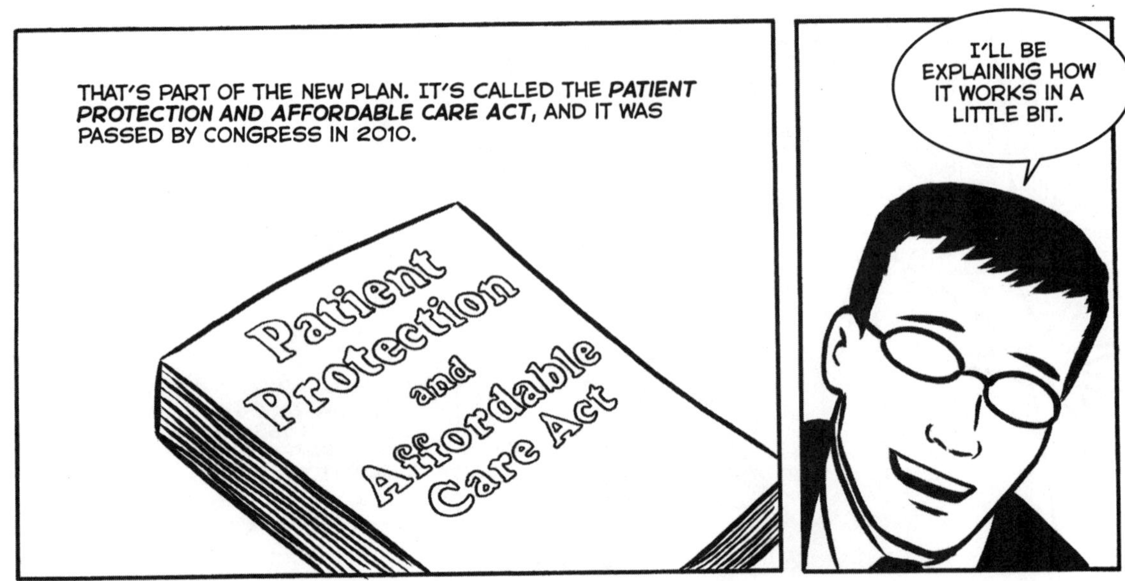
THAT'S PART OF THE NEW PLAN. IT'S CALLED THE ***PATIENT PROTECTION AND AFFORDABLE CARE ACT***, AND IT WAS PASSED BY CONGRESS IN 2010.
Patient Protection and Affordable Care Act
I'LL BE EXPLAINING HOW IT WORKS IN A LITTLE BIT.

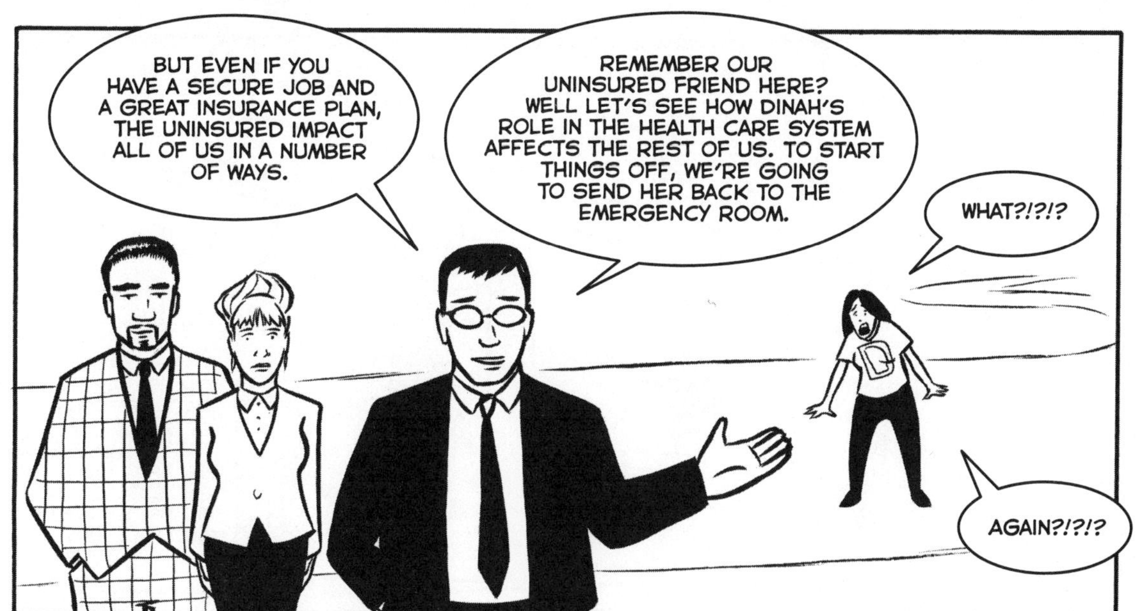
BUT EVEN IF YOU HAVE A SECURE JOB AND A GREAT INSURANCE PLAN, THE UNINSURED IMPACT ALL OF US IN A NUMBER OF WAYS.
REMEMBER OUR UNINSURED FRIEND HERE? WELL LET'S SEE HOW DINAH'S ROLE IN THE HEALTH CARE SYSTEM AFFECTS THE REST OF US. TO START THINGS OFF, WE'RE GOING TO SEND HER BACK TO THE EMERGENCY ROOM.
WHAT?!?!?
AGAIN?!?!?

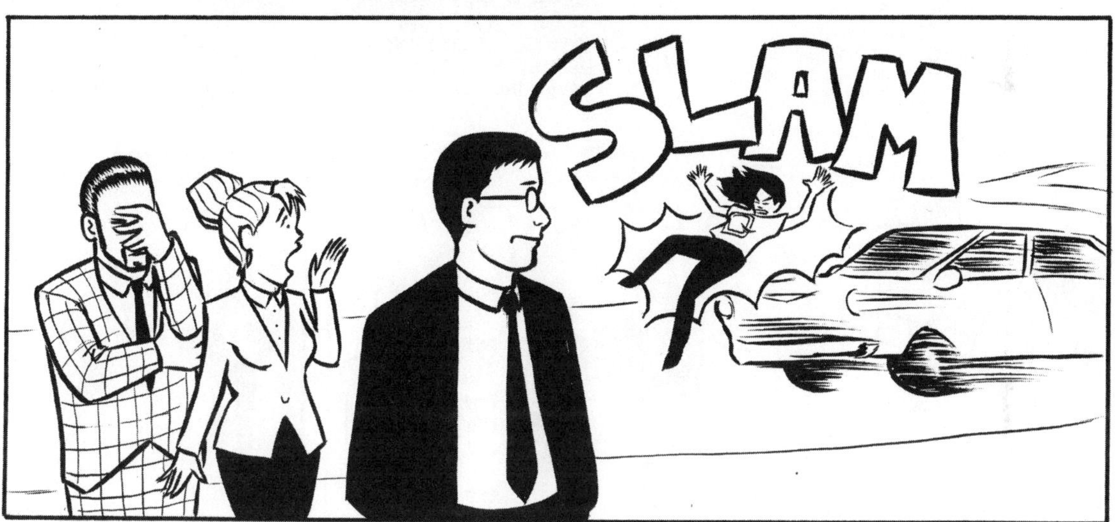
SLAM

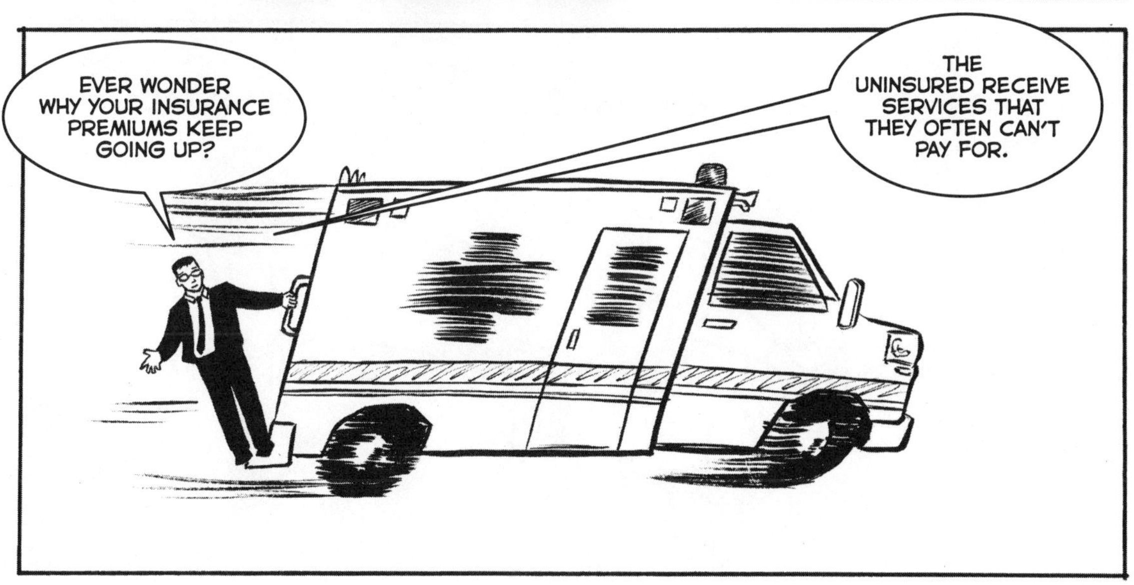
EVER WONDER WHY YOUR INSURANCE PREMIUMS KEEP GOING UP?
THE UNINSURED RECEIVE SERVICES THAT THEY OFTEN CAN'T PAY FOR.

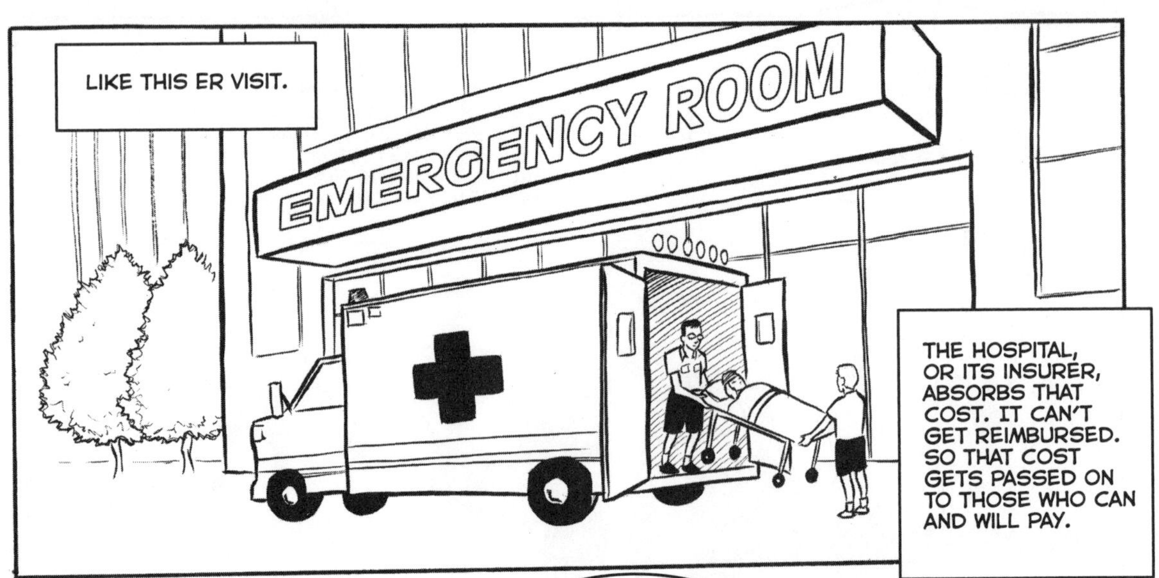
LIKE THIS ER VISIT.
EMERGENCY ROOM
THE HOSPITAL, OR ITS INSURER, ABSORBS THAT COST. IT CAN'T GET REIMBURSED. SO THAT COST GETS PASSED ON TO THOSE WHO CAN AND WILL PAY.

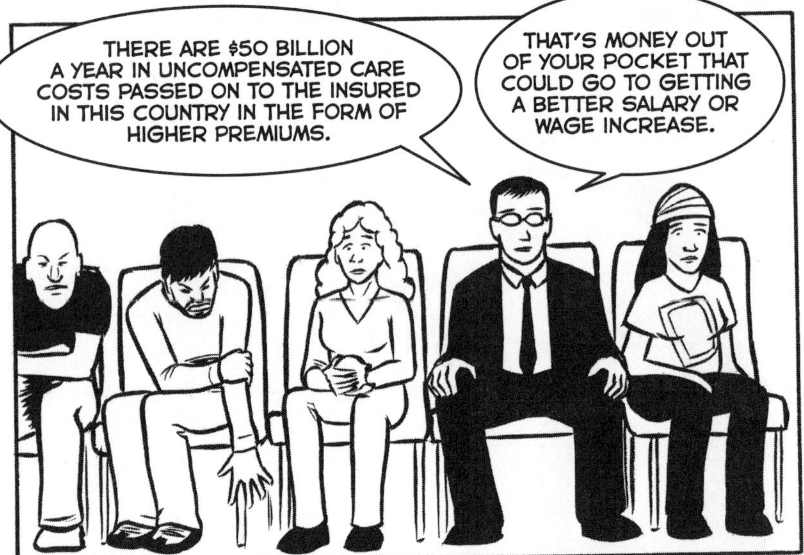
THERE ARE $50 BILLION A YEAR IN UNCOMPENSATED CARE COSTS PASSED ON TO THE INSURED IN THIS COUNTRY IN THE FORM OF HIGHER PREMIUMS.
THAT'S MONEY OUT OF YOUR POCKET THAT COULD GO TO GETTING A BETTER SALARY OR WAGE INCREASE.

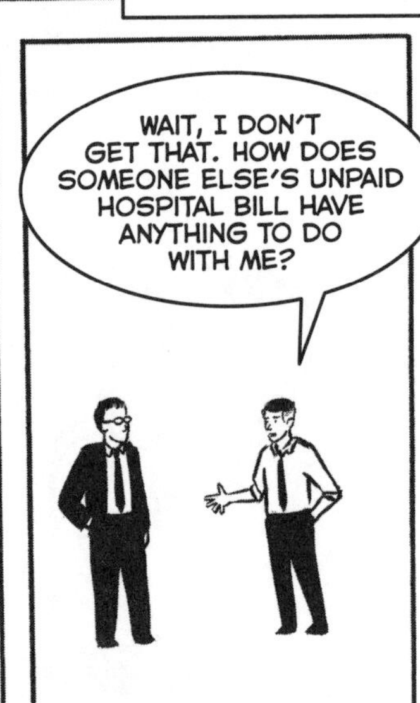
WAIT, I DON'T GET THAT. HOW DOES SOMEONE ELSE'S UNPAID HOSPITAL BILL HAVE ANYTHING TO DO WITH ME?

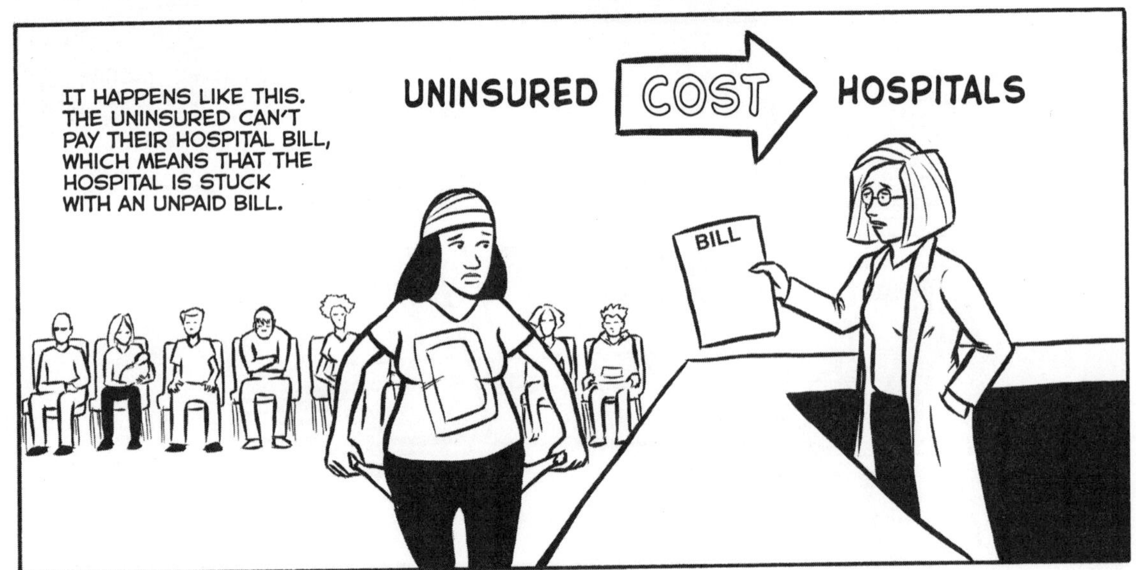
IT HAPPENS LIKE THIS. THE UNINSURED CAN'T PAY THEIR HOSPITAL BILL, WHICH MEANS THAT THE HOSPITAL IS STUCK WITH AN UNPAID BILL.
UNINSURED
COST
HOSPITALS
BILL

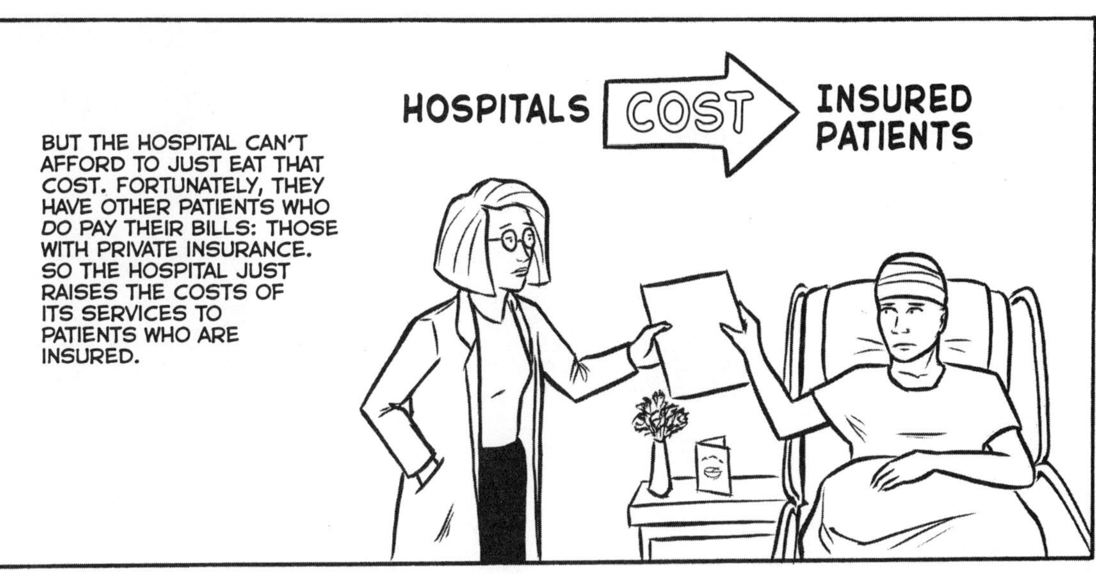
BUT THE HOSPITAL CAN'T AFFORD TO JUST EAT THAT COST. FORTUNATELY, THEY HAVE OTHER PATIENTS WHO *DO* PAY THEIR BILLS: THOSE WITH PRIVATE INSURANCE. SO THE HOSPITAL JUST RAISES THE COSTS OF ITS SERVICES TO PATIENTS WHO ARE INSURED.
HOSPITALS
COST
INSURED PATIENTS

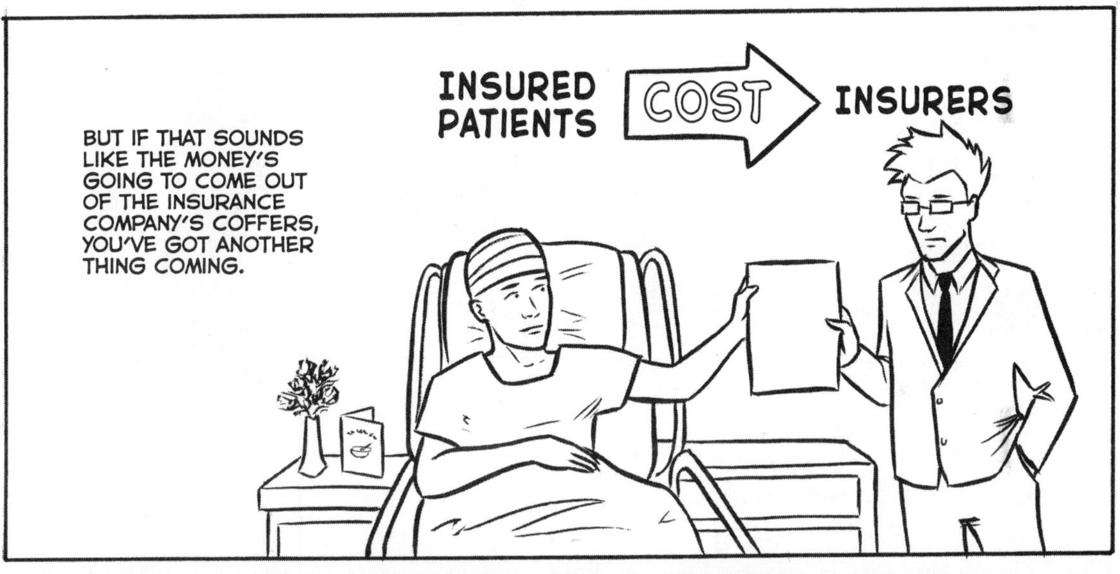
BUT IF THAT SOUNDS LIKE THE MONEY'S GOING TO COME OUT OF THE INSURANCE COMPANY'S COFFERS, YOU'VE GOT ANOTHER THING COMING.
INSURED PATIENTS
COST
INSURERS

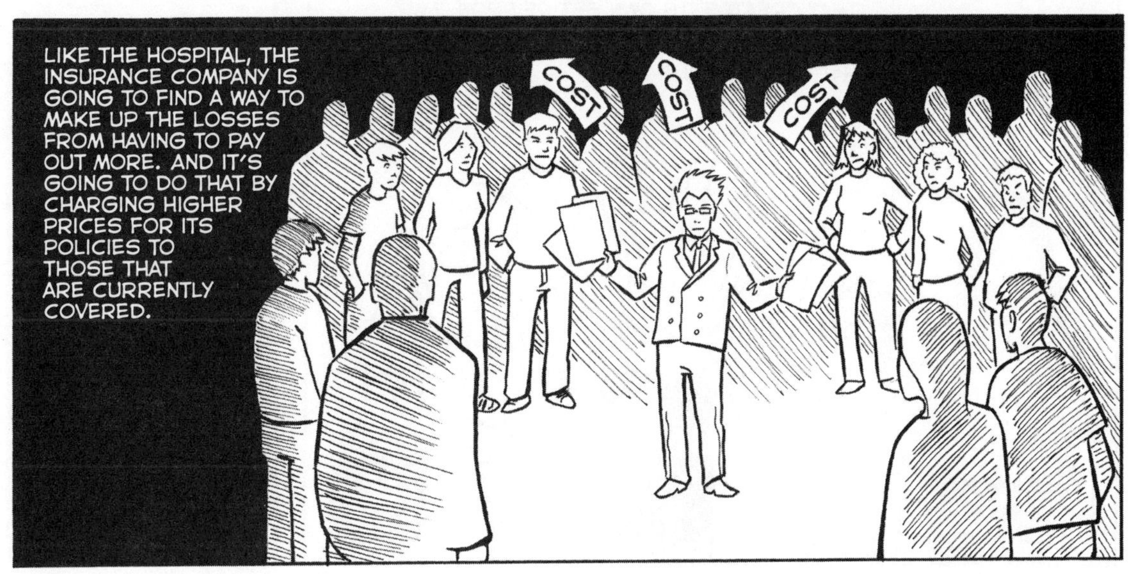
LIKE THE HOSPITAL, THE INSURANCE COMPANY IS GOING TO FIND A WAY TO MAKE UP THE LOSSES FROM HAVING TO PAY OUT MORE. AND IT'S GOING TO DO THAT BY CHARGING HIGHER PRICES FOR ITS POLICIES TO THOSE THAT ARE CURRENTLY COVERED.
COST
COST
COST

IN ADDITION, A LOT OF THE UNINSURED COME INTO THE HEALTH CARE SYSTEM ONLY WHEN THEY NEED TREATMENT, AS OPPOSED TO GETTING PREVENTIVE CARE.

THAT USUALLY MEANS THEY GO TO THE ER--EVEN FOR MINOR AILMENTS LIKE COLDS OR BUMPS AND BRUISES--WHERE COSTS ARE VERY HIGH.

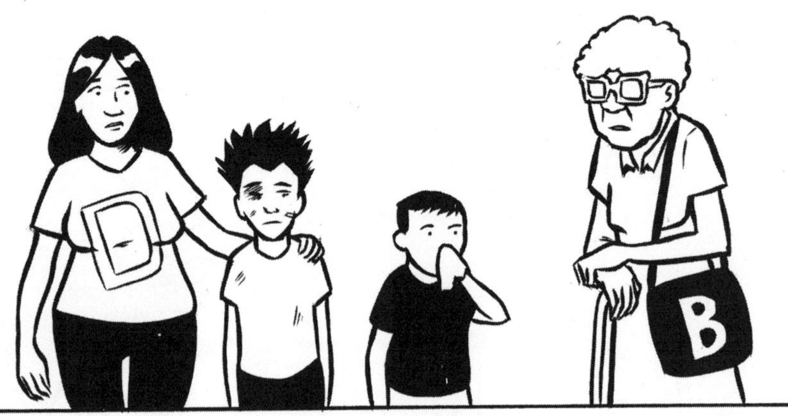

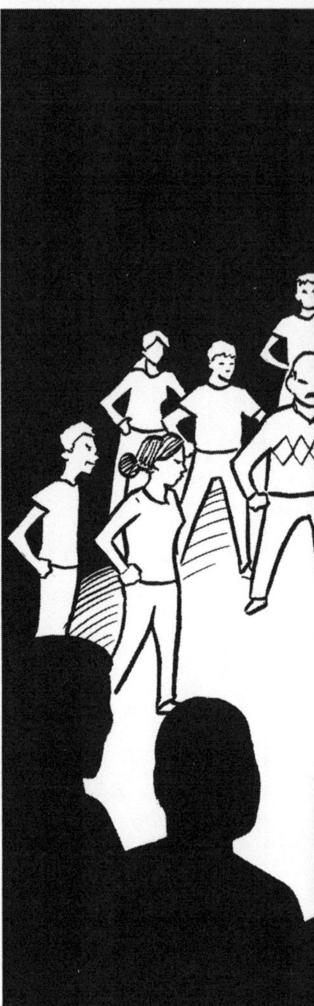

SINCE THE UNINSURED DON'T ALWAYS HAVE THE RESOURCES TO GET PREVENTIVE TREATMENT, THINGS LIKE VACCINATIONS AND FLU SHOTS, THEY COULD ALSO MAKE US SICK.

THAT CREATES ITS OWN SET OF PROBLEMS IN TERMS OF LOST WORK DAYS, TIME SPENT BEING ILL, AND EVERYTHING ELSE THAT WE HATE ABOUT BEING SICK.

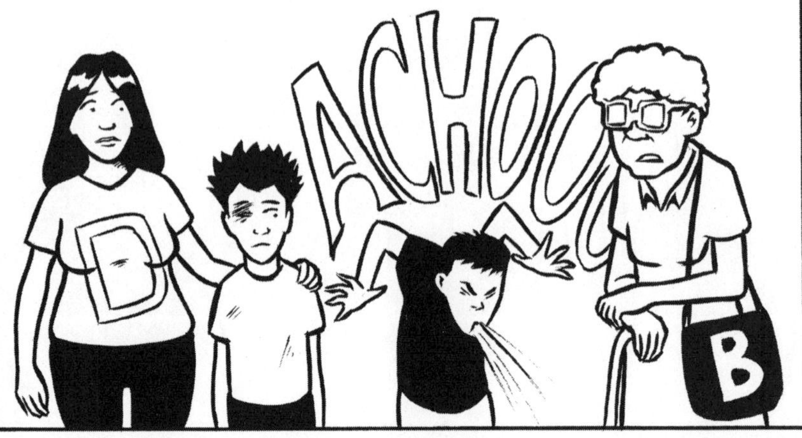

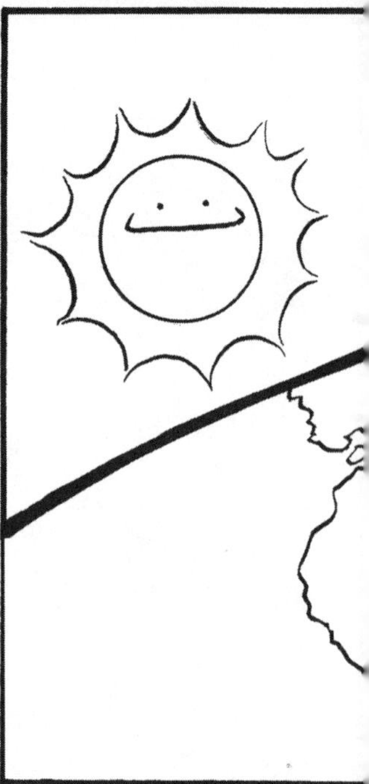

CHAPTER 3 THROUGH THE PAST, DARKLY

WELL, MR. GRUBER, AREN'T YOU JUST A CONSTANT RAY OF SUNSHINE? NO WONDER THEY CALL ECONOMICS THE "DISMAL SCIENCE!"

WHAT ARE WE SUPPOSED TO DO ABOUT THESE HUGE PROBLEMS?

GREAT QUESTION.

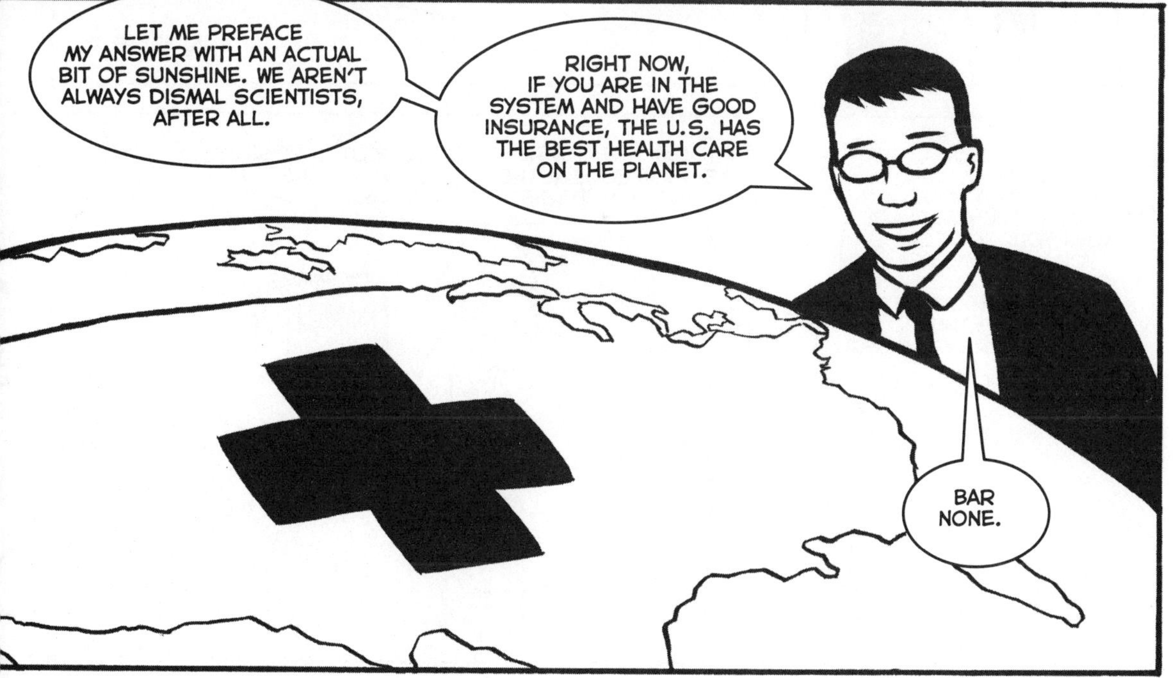
LET ME PREFACE MY ANSWER WITH AN ACTUAL BIT OF SUNSHINE. WE AREN'T ALWAYS DISMAL SCIENTISTS, AFTER ALL.
RIGHT NOW, IF YOU ARE IN THE SYSTEM AND HAVE GOOD INSURANCE, THE U.S. HAS THE BEST HEALTH CARE ON THE PLANET.
BAR NONE.

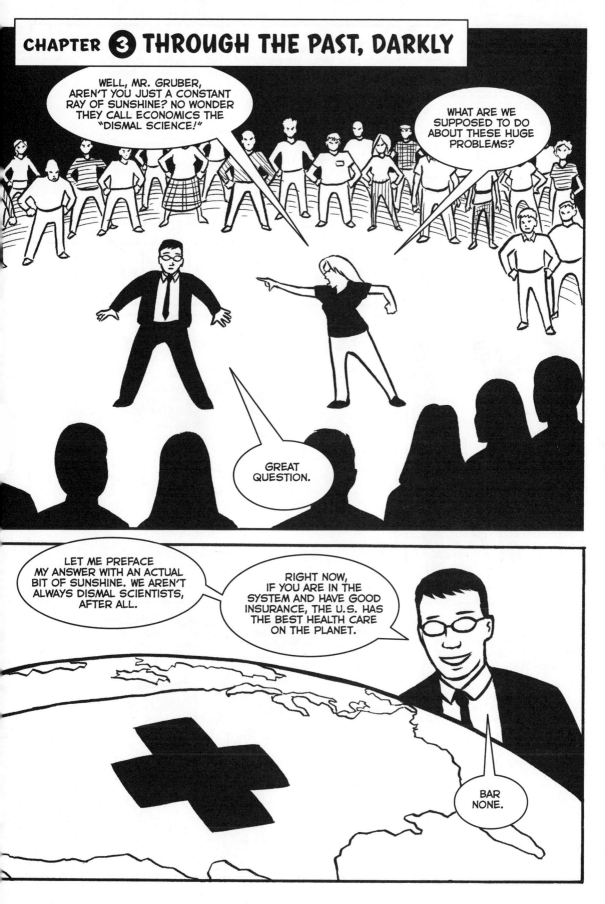

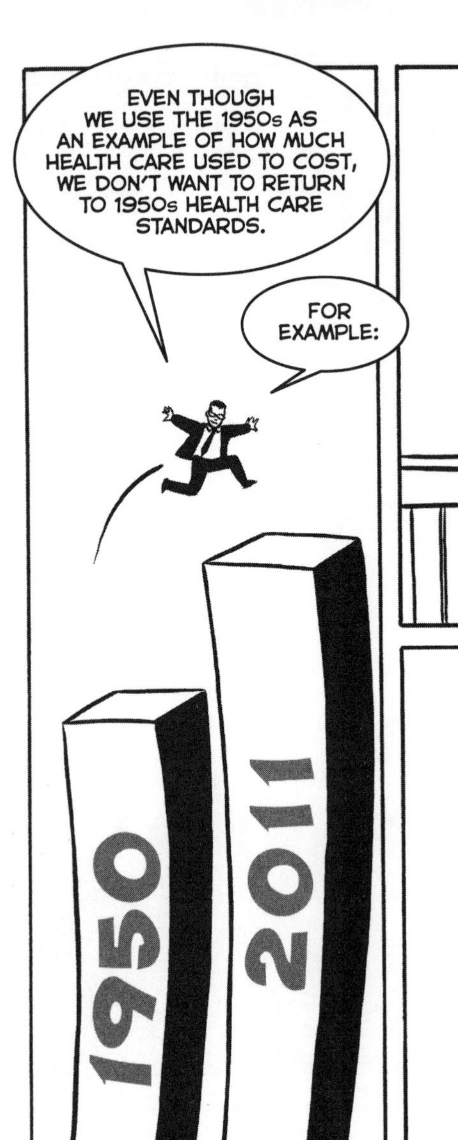
EVEN THOUGH WE USE THE 1950s AS AN EXAMPLE OF HOW MUCH HEALTH CARE USED TO COST, WE DON'T WANT TO RETURN TO 1950s HEALTH CARE STANDARDS.
FOR EXAMPLE:
1950
2011

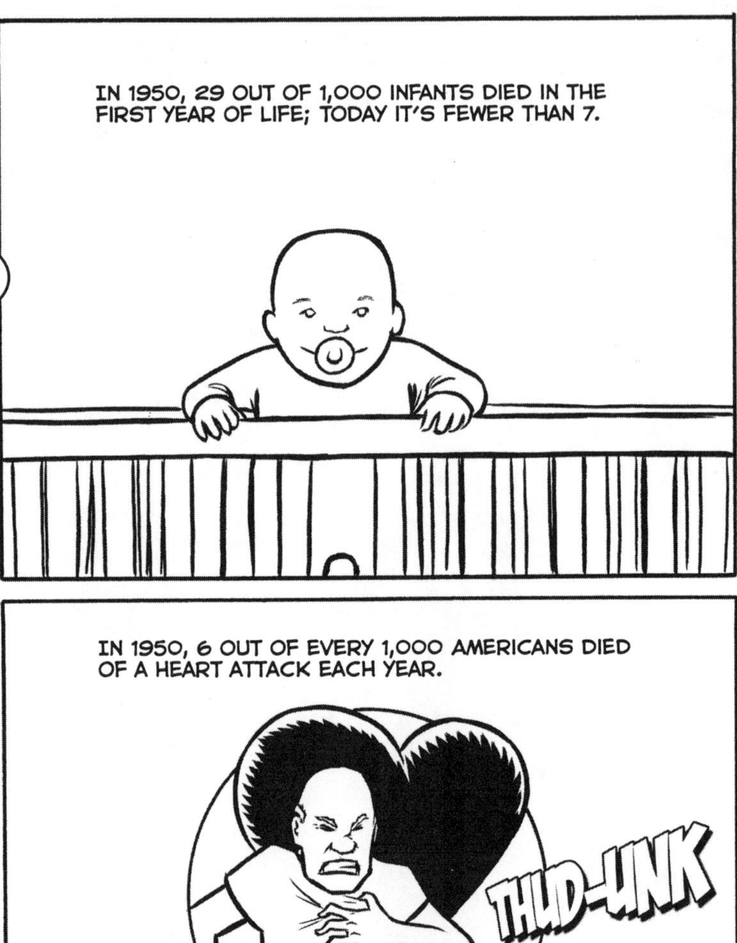
IN 1950, 29 OUT OF 1,000 INFANTS DIED IN THE FIRST YEAR OF LIFE; TODAY IT'S FEWER THAN 7.
IN 1950, 6 OUT OF EVERY 1,000 AMERICANS DIED OF A HEART ATTACK EACH YEAR.
THUD-UNK
TODAY IT IS FEWER THAN HALF THAT NUMBER.

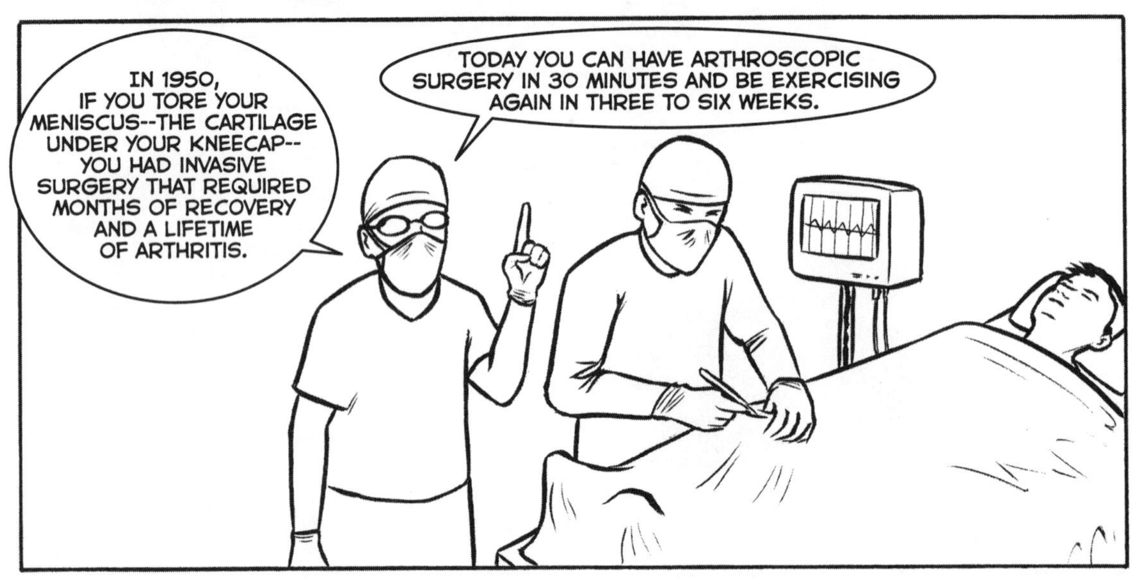
IN 1950, IF YOU TORE YOUR MENISCUS--THE CARTILAGE UNDER YOUR KNEECAP--YOU HAD INVASIVE SURGERY THAT REQUIRED MONTHS OF RECOVERY AND A LIFETIME OF ARTHRITIS.
TODAY YOU CAN HAVE ARTHROSCOPIC SURGERY IN 30 MINUTES AND BE EXERCISING AGAIN IN THREE TO SIX WEEKS.

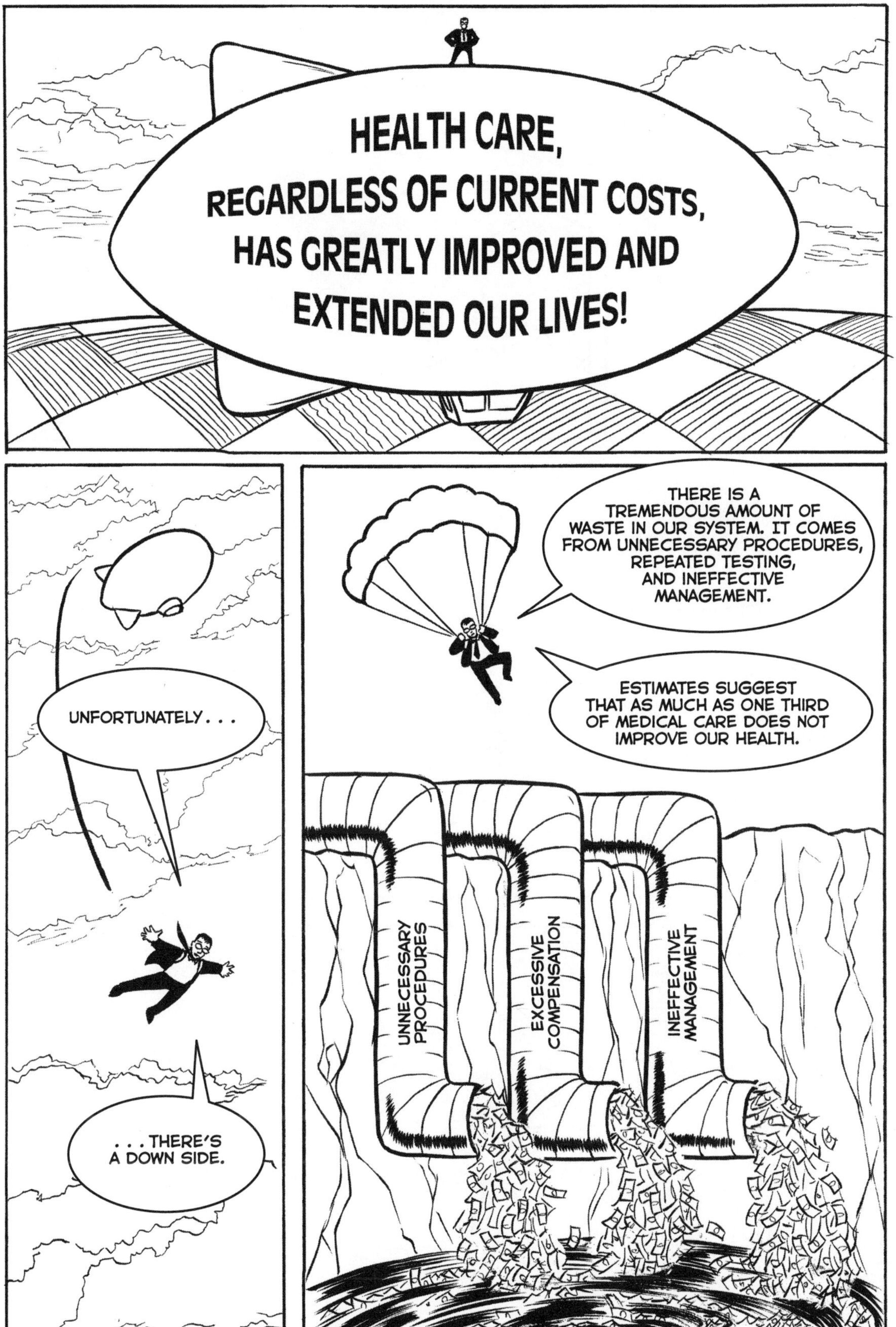

HEALTH CARE,
REGARDLESS OF CURRENT COSTS,
HAS GREATLY IMPROVED AND
EXTENDED OUR LIVES!

UNFORTUNATELY . . .

. . . THERE'S
A DOWN SIDE.

THERE IS A TREMENDOUS AMOUNT OF WASTE IN OUR SYSTEM. IT COMES FROM UNNECESSARY PROCEDURES, REPEATED TESTING, AND INEFFECTIVE MANAGEMENT.

ESTIMATES SUGGEST THAT AS MUCH AS ONE THIRD OF MEDICAL CARE DOES NOT IMPROVE OUR HEALTH.

UNNECESSARY PROCEDURES
EXCESSIVE COMPENSATION
INEFFECTIVE MANAGEMENT

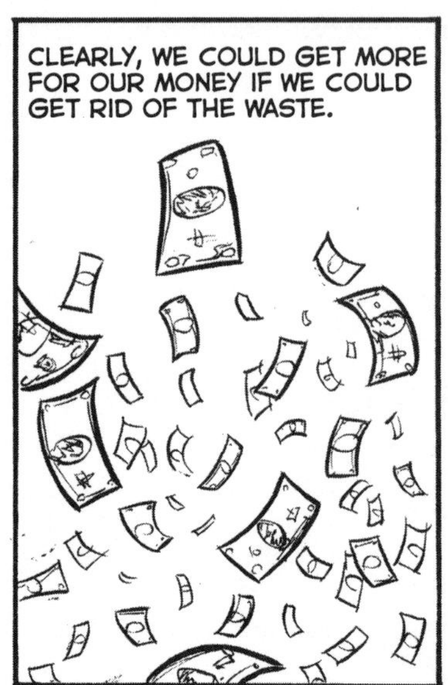
CLEARLY, WE COULD GET MORE FOR OUR MONEY IF WE COULD GET RID OF THE WASTE.

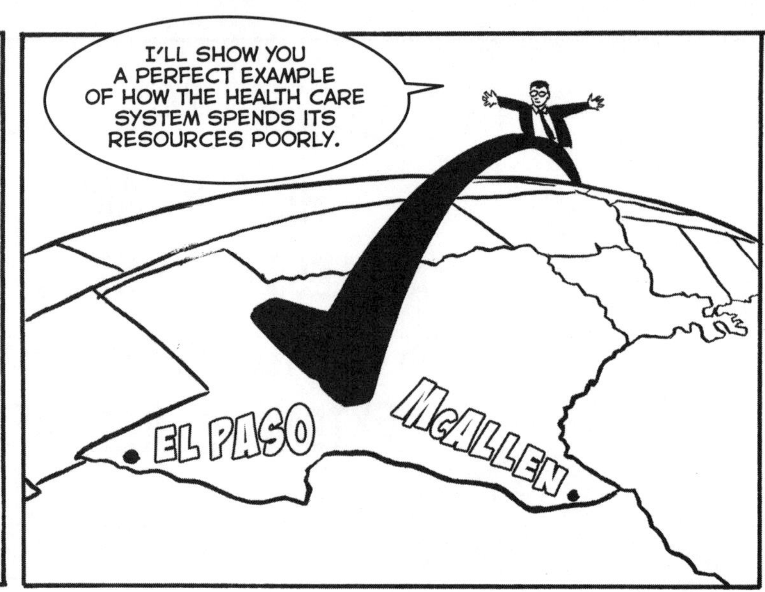
I'LL SHOW YOU A PERFECT EXAMPLE OF HOW THE HEALTH CARE SYSTEM SPENDS ITS RESOURCES POORLY.
EL PASO
McALLEN

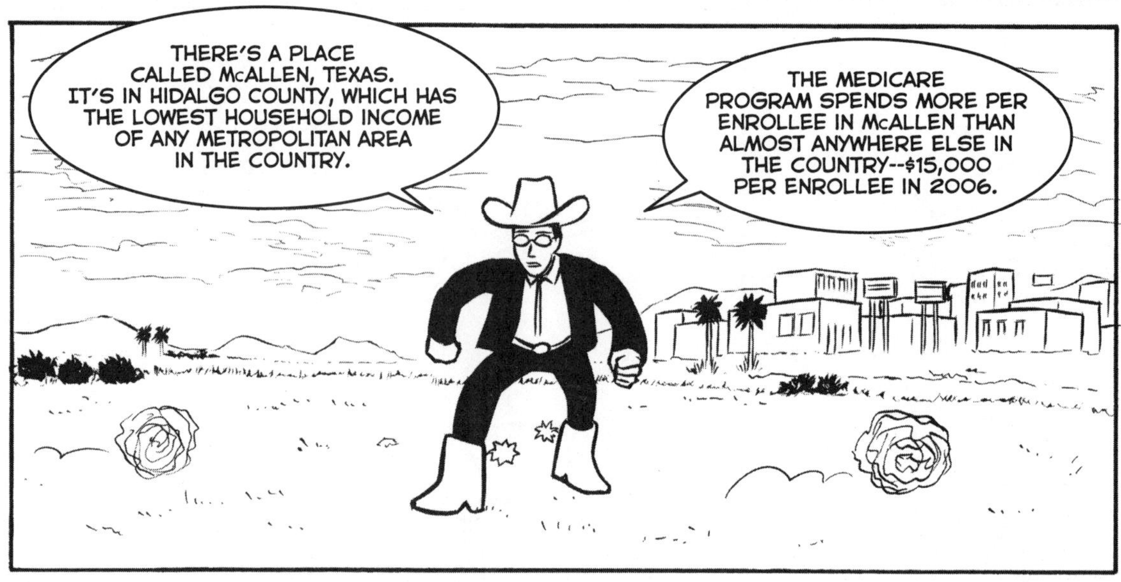
THERE'S A PLACE CALLED McALLEN, TEXAS. IT'S IN HIDALGO COUNTY, WHICH HAS THE LOWEST HOUSEHOLD INCOME OF ANY METROPOLITAN AREA IN THE COUNTRY.
THE MEDICARE PROGRAM SPENDS MORE PER ENROLLEE IN McALLEN THAN ALMOST ANYWHERE ELSE IN THE COUNTRY--$15,000 PER ENROLLEE IN 2006.

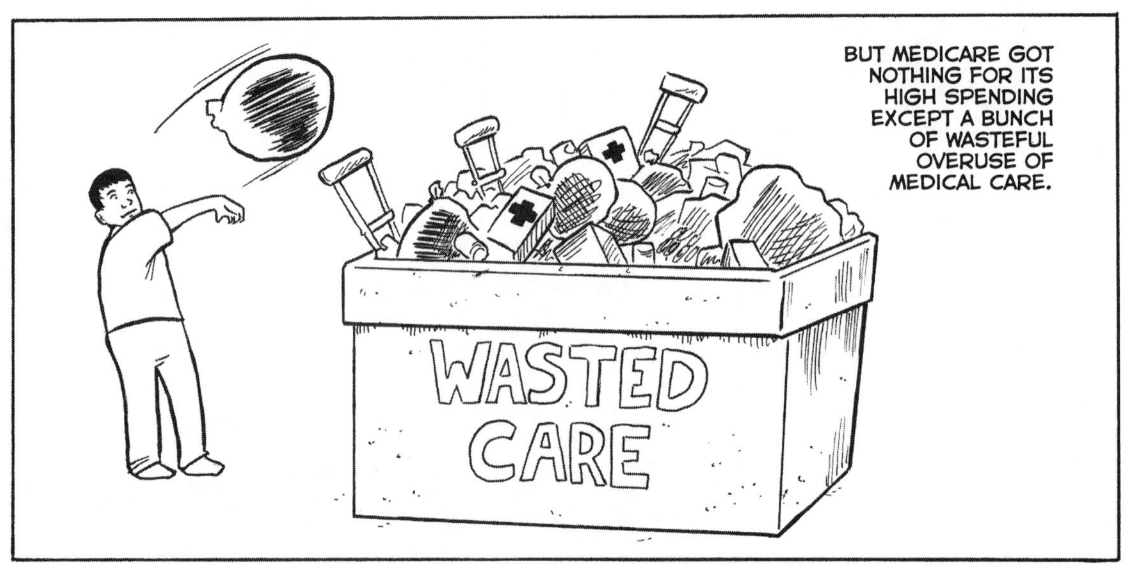
BUT MEDICARE GOT NOTHING FOR ITS HIGH SPENDING EXCEPT A BUNCH OF WASTEFUL OVERUSE OF MEDICAL CARE.
WASTED CARE

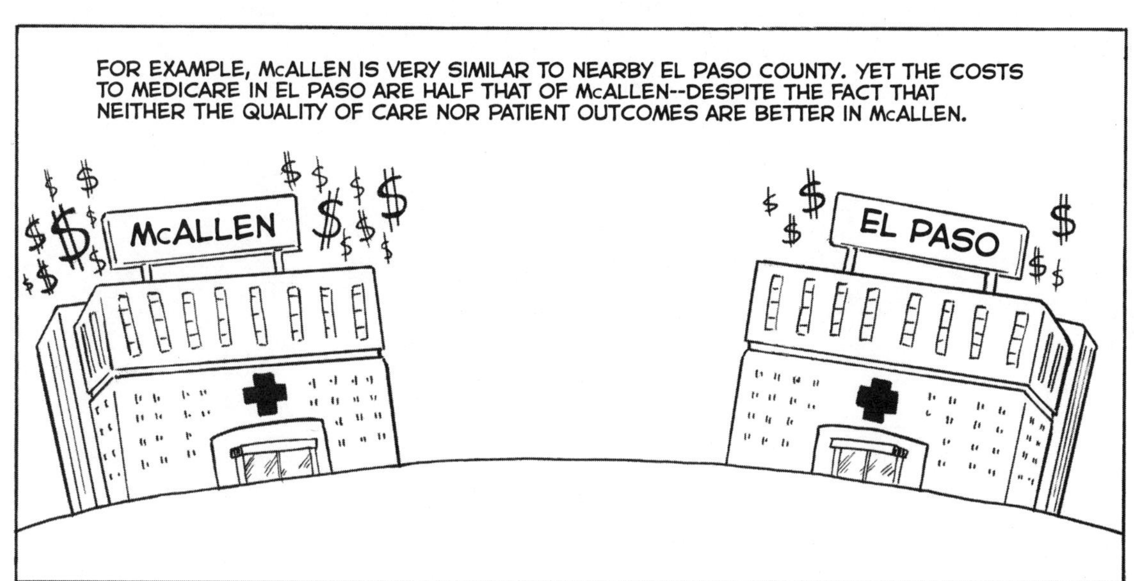
FOR EXAMPLE, McALLEN IS VERY SIMILAR TO NEARBY EL PASO COUNTY. YET THE COSTS TO MEDICARE IN EL PASO ARE HALF THAT OF McALLEN--DESPITE THE FACT THAT NEITHER THE QUALITY OF CARE NOR PATIENT OUTCOMES ARE BETTER IN McALLEN.
McALLEN
EL PASO

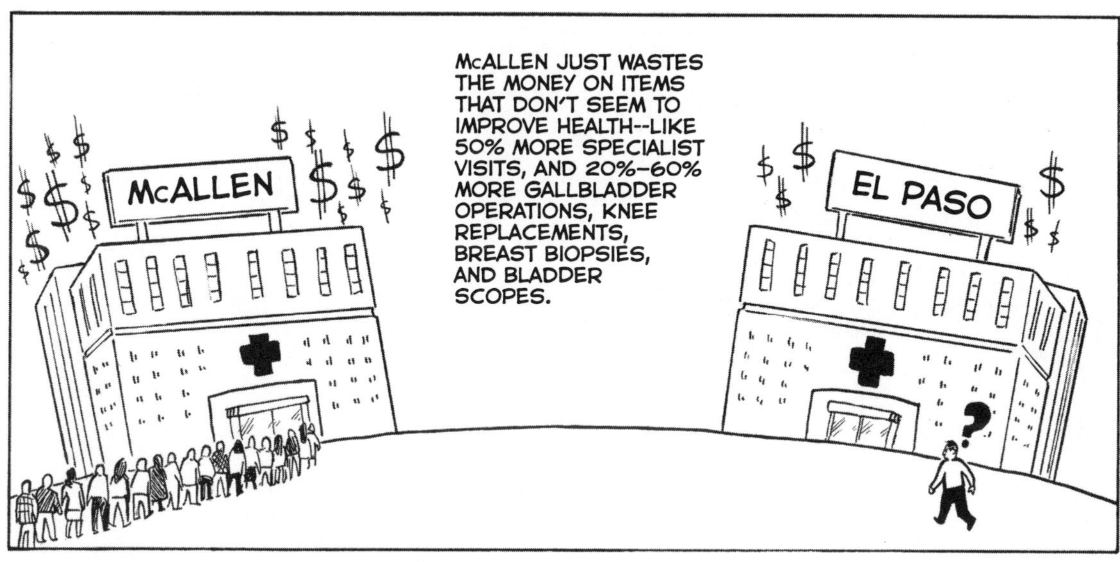
McALLEN JUST WASTES THE MONEY ON ITEMS THAT DON'T SEEM TO IMPROVE HEALTH--LIKE 50% MORE SPECIALIST VISITS, AND 20%–60% MORE GALLBLADDER OPERATIONS, KNEE REPLACEMENTS, BREAST BIOPSIES, AND BLADDER SCOPES.
McALLEN
EL PASO

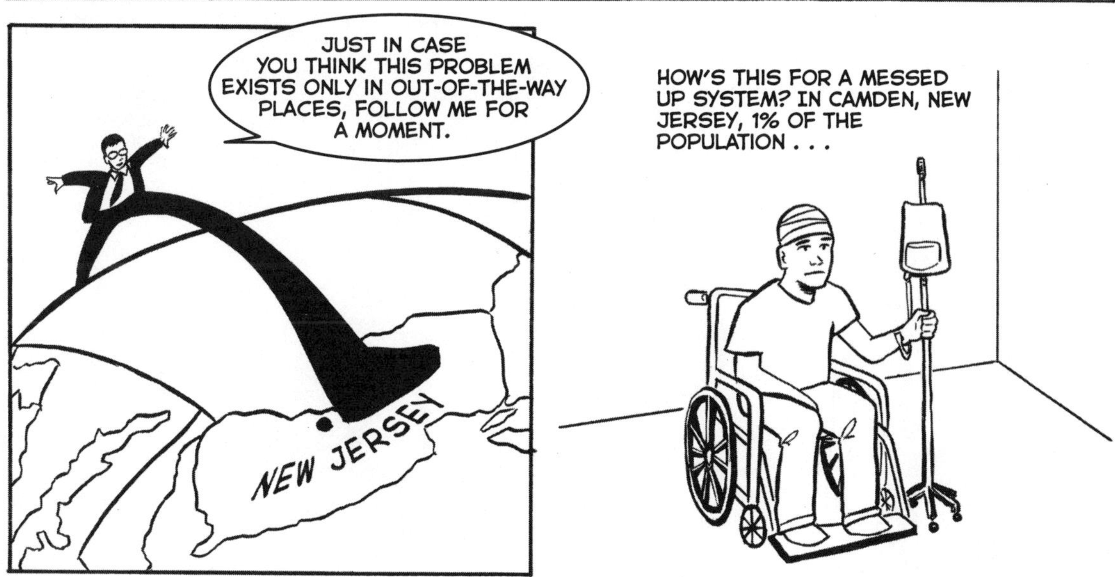
JUST IN CASE YOU THINK THIS PROBLEM EXISTS ONLY IN OUT-OF-THE-WAY PLACES, FOLLOW ME FOR A MOMENT.
NEW JERSEY
HOW'S THIS FOR A MESSED UP SYSTEM? IN CAMDEN, NEW JERSEY, 1% OF THE POPULATION . . .

. . . ACCOUNTS FOR MORE THAN 30% OF THE CITY'S HEALTH EXPENDITURES.

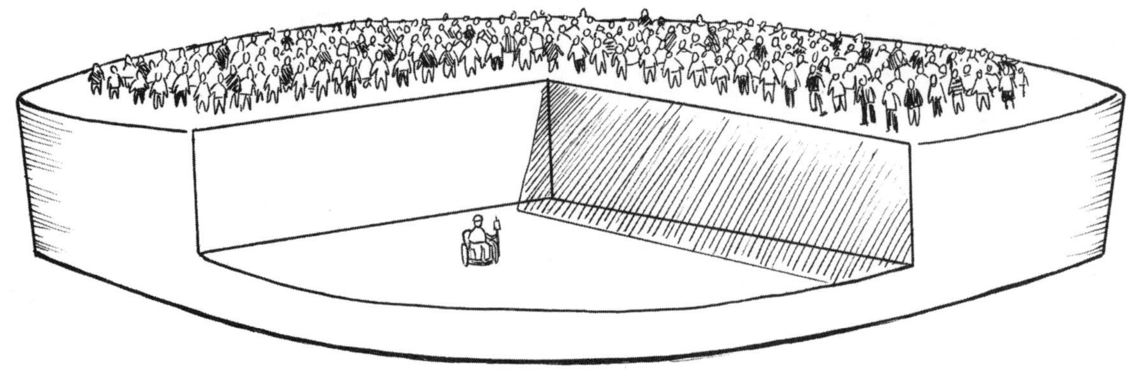

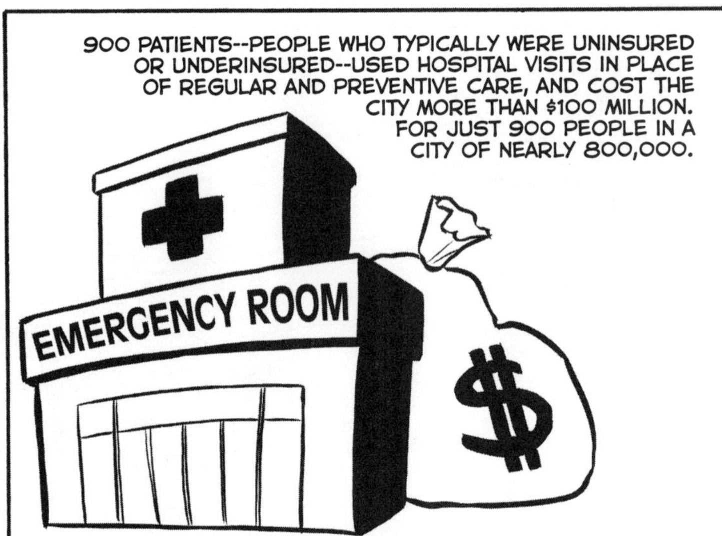

900 PATIENTS--PEOPLE WHO TYPICALLY WERE UNINSURED OR UNDERINSURED--USED HOSPITAL VISITS IN PLACE OF REGULAR AND PREVENTIVE CARE, AND COST THE CITY MORE THAN $100 MILLION. FOR JUST 900 PEOPLE IN A CITY OF NEARLY 800,000.
EMERGENCY ROOM
$

BUT, WAIT, THERE'S MORE! THE COST FOR TREATING ONE PARTICULAR PATIENT IN CAMDEN GREW TO MORE THAN $3 MILLION OVER SIX YEARS. AND ANOTHER PATIENT HAD 324 HOSPITAL ADMISSIONS IN THE SAME PERIOD.

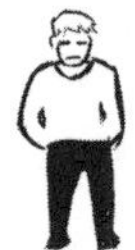

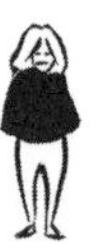

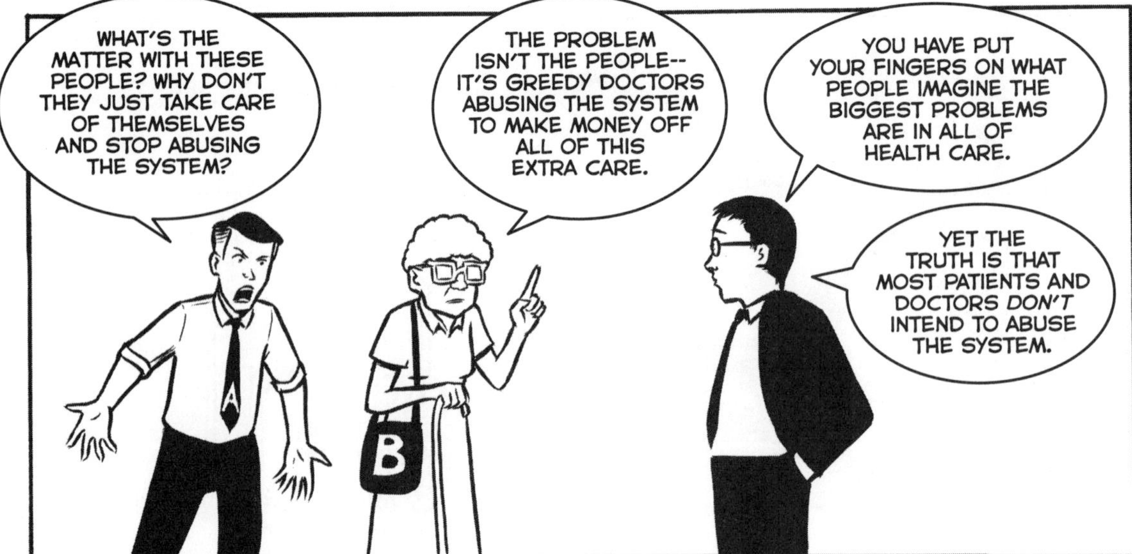

WHAT'S THE MATTER WITH THESE PEOPLE? WHY DON'T THEY JUST TAKE CARE OF THEMSELVES AND STOP ABUSING THE SYSTEM?
THE PROBLEM ISN'T THE PEOPLE-- IT'S GREEDY DOCTORS ABUSING THE SYSTEM TO MAKE MONEY OFF ALL OF THIS EXTRA CARE.
YOU HAVE PUT YOUR FINGERS ON WHAT PEOPLE IMAGINE THE BIGGEST PROBLEMS ARE IN ALL OF HEALTH CARE.
YET THE TRUTH IS THAT MOST PATIENTS AND DOCTORS *DON'T* INTEND TO ABUSE THE SYSTEM.
A
B

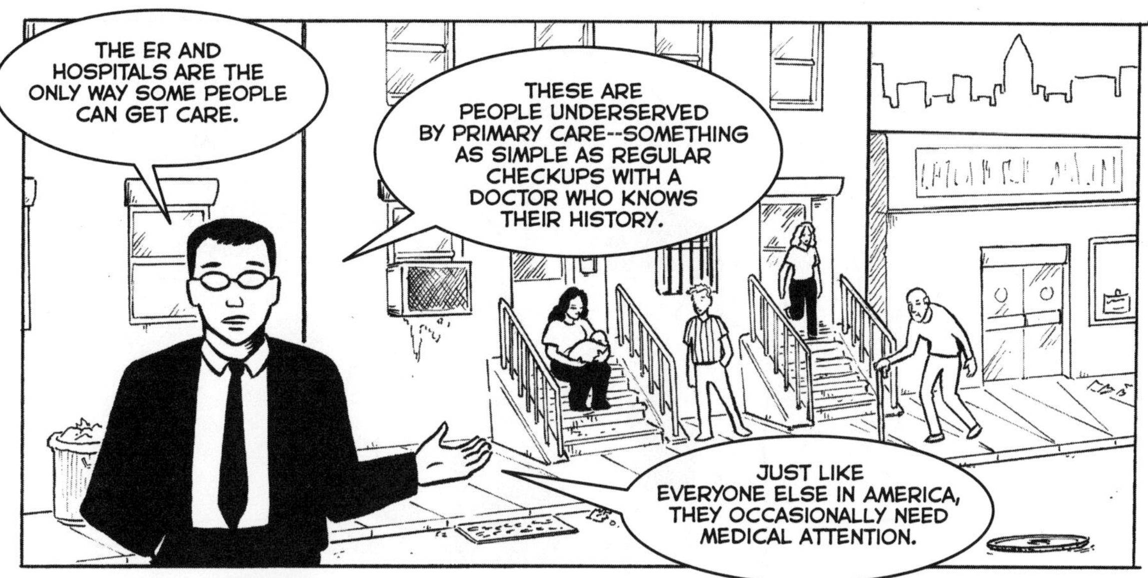
THE ER AND HOSPITALS ARE THE ONLY WAY SOME PEOPLE CAN GET CARE.
THESE ARE PEOPLE UNDERSERVED BY PRIMARY CARE--SOMETHING AS SIMPLE AS REGULAR CHECKUPS WITH A DOCTOR WHO KNOWS THEIR HISTORY.
JUST LIKE EVERYONE ELSE IN AMERICA, THEY OCCASIONALLY NEED MEDICAL ATTENTION.

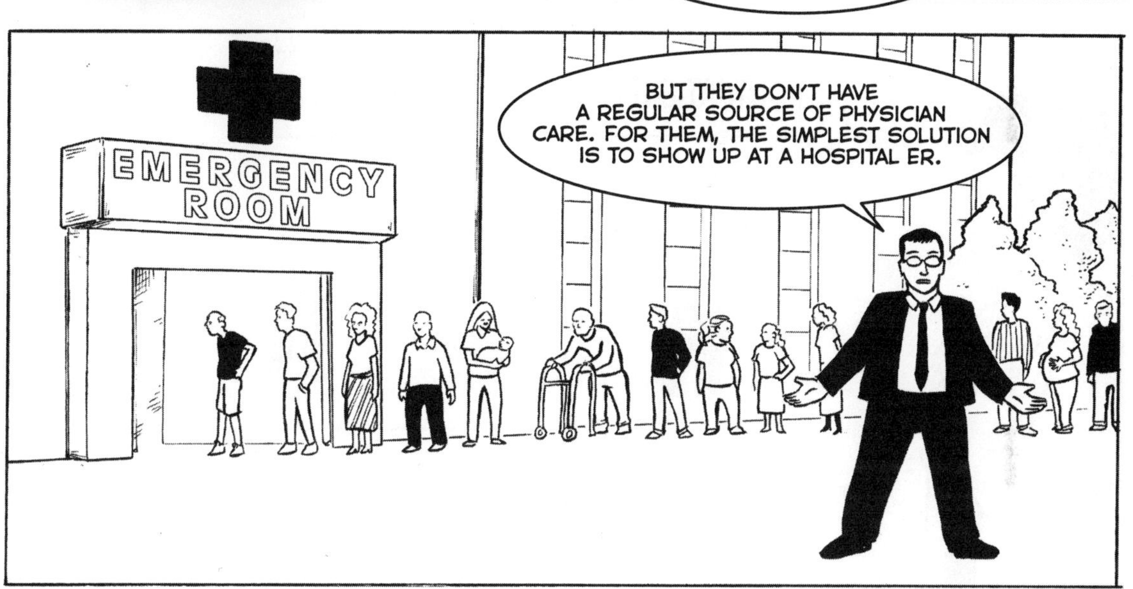
EMERGENCY ROOM
BUT THEY DON'T HAVE A REGULAR SOURCE OF PHYSICIAN CARE. FOR THEM, THE SIMPLEST SOLUTION IS TO SHOW UP AT A HOSPITAL ER.

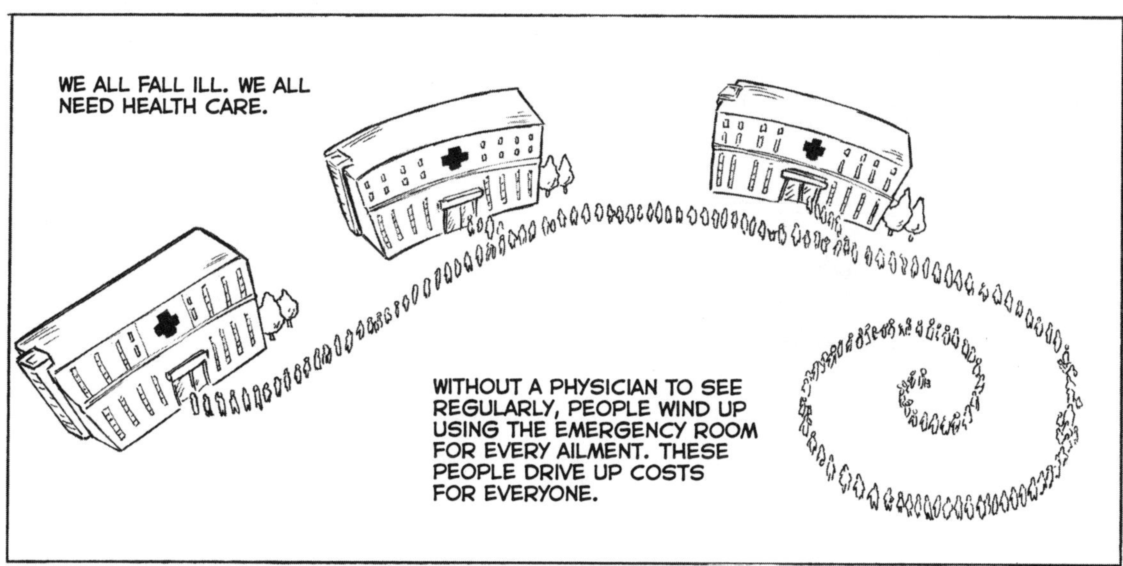
WE ALL FALL ILL. WE ALL NEED HEALTH CARE.
WITHOUT A PHYSICIAN TO SEE REGULARLY, PEOPLE WIND UP USING THE EMERGENCY ROOM FOR EVERY AILMENT. THESE PEOPLE DRIVE UP COSTS FOR EVERYONE.

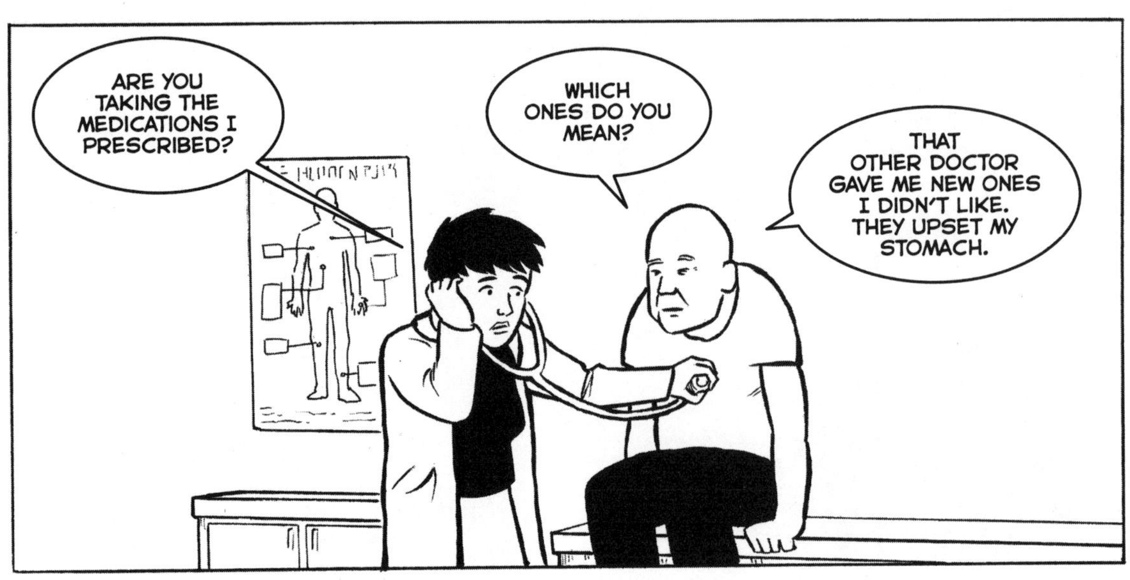
ARE YOU TAKING THE MEDICATIONS I PRESCRIBED?
WHICH ONES DO YOU MEAN?
THAT OTHER DOCTOR GAVE ME NEW ONES I DIDN'T LIKE. THEY UPSET MY STOMACH.

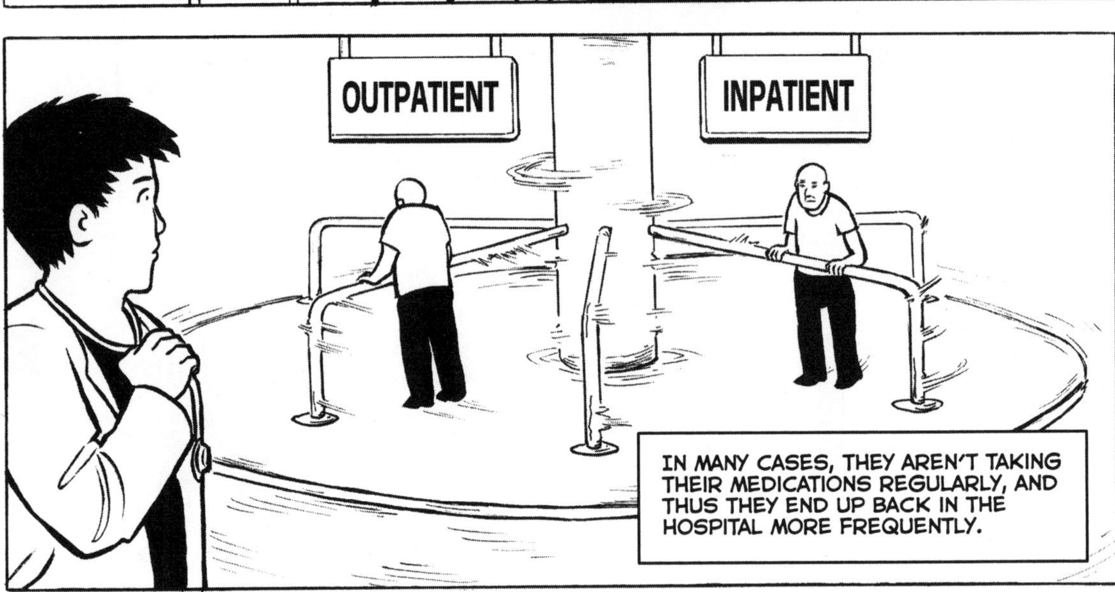
OUTPATIENT
INPATIENT
IN MANY CASES, THEY AREN'T TAKING THEIR MEDICATIONS REGULARLY, AND THUS THEY END UP BACK IN THE HOSPITAL MORE FREQUENTLY.

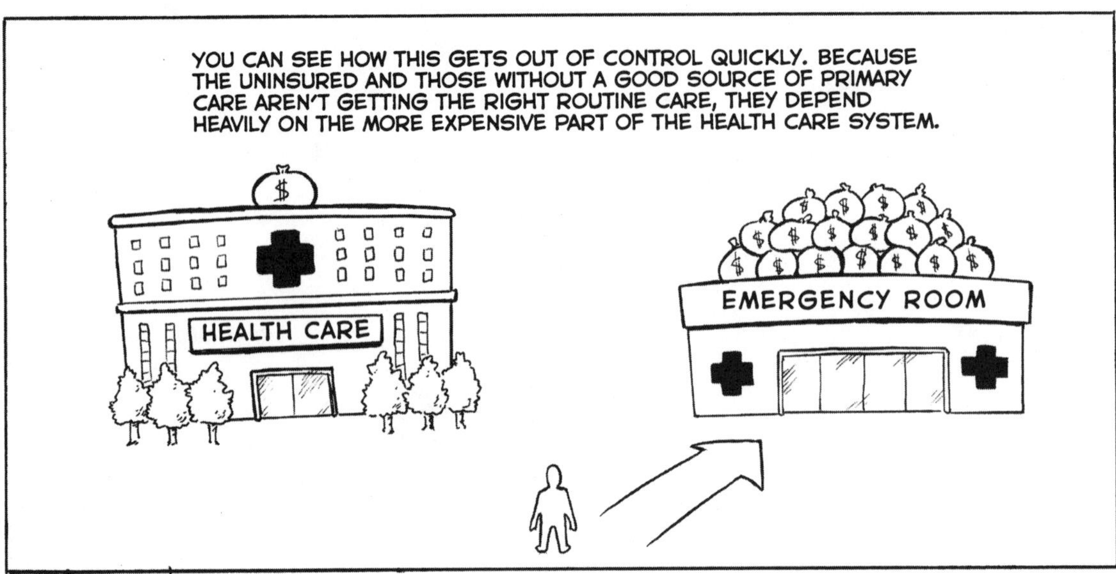
YOU CAN SEE HOW THIS GETS OUT OF CONTROL QUICKLY. BECAUSE THE UNINSURED AND THOSE WITHOUT A GOOD SOURCE OF PRIMARY CARE AREN'T GETTING THE RIGHT ROUTINE CARE, THEY DEPEND HEAVILY ON THE MORE EXPENSIVE PART OF THE HEALTH CARE SYSTEM.
HEALTH CARE
EMERGENCY ROOM

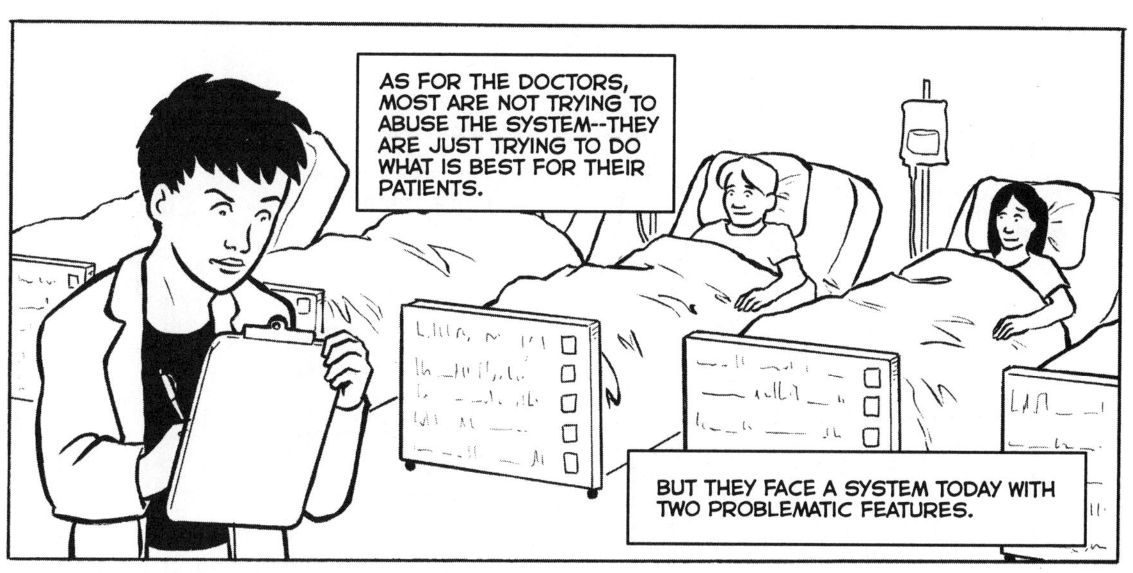
AS FOR THE DOCTORS, MOST ARE NOT TRYING TO ABUSE THE SYSTEM--THEY ARE JUST TRYING TO DO WHAT IS BEST FOR THEIR PATIENTS.
BUT THEY FACE A SYSTEM TODAY WITH TWO PROBLEMATIC FEATURES.

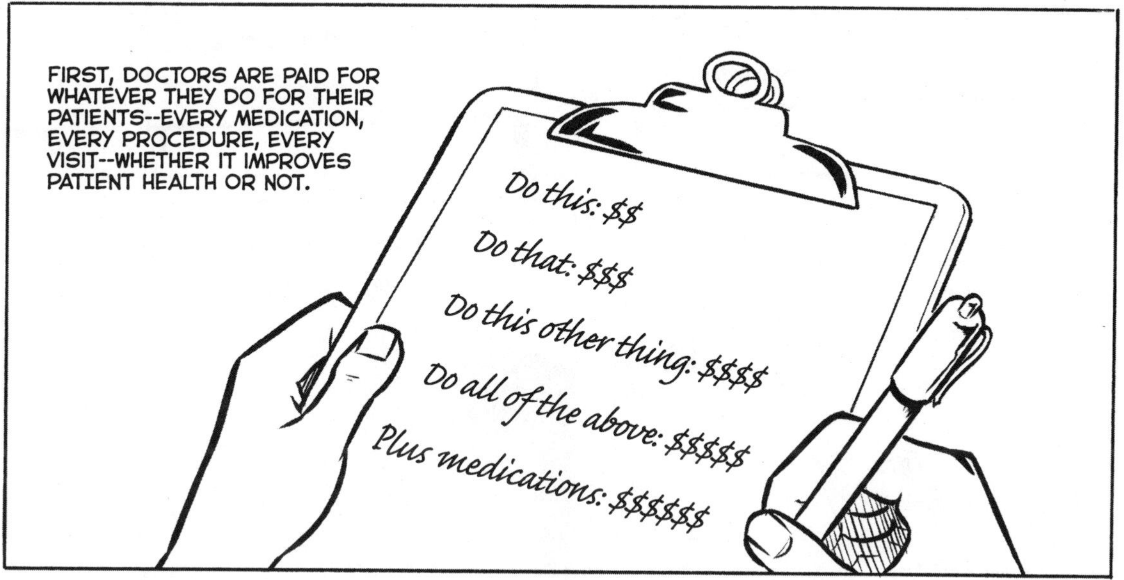
FIRST, DOCTORS ARE PAID FOR WHATEVER THEY DO FOR THEIR PATIENTS--EVERY MEDICATION, EVERY PROCEDURE, EVERY VISIT--WHETHER IT IMPROVES PATIENT HEALTH OR NOT.
Do this: $$
Do that: $$$
Do this other thing: $$$$
Do all of the above: $$$$$
Plus medications: $$$$$$

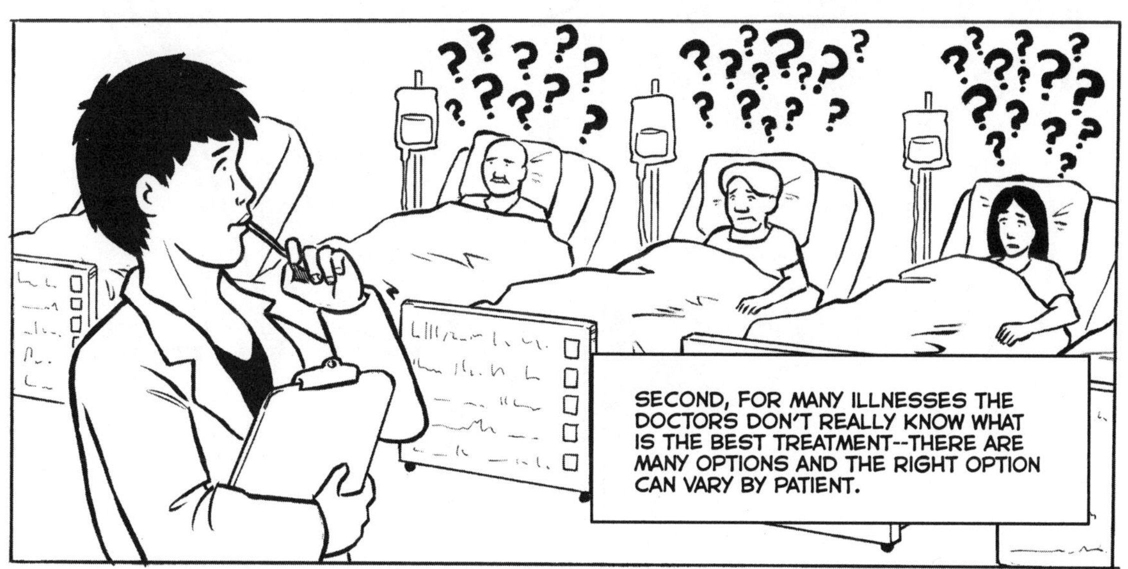
SECOND, FOR MANY ILLNESSES THE DOCTORS DON'T REALLY KNOW WHAT IS THE BEST TREATMENT--THERE ARE MANY OPTIONS AND THE RIGHT OPTION CAN VARY BY PATIENT.

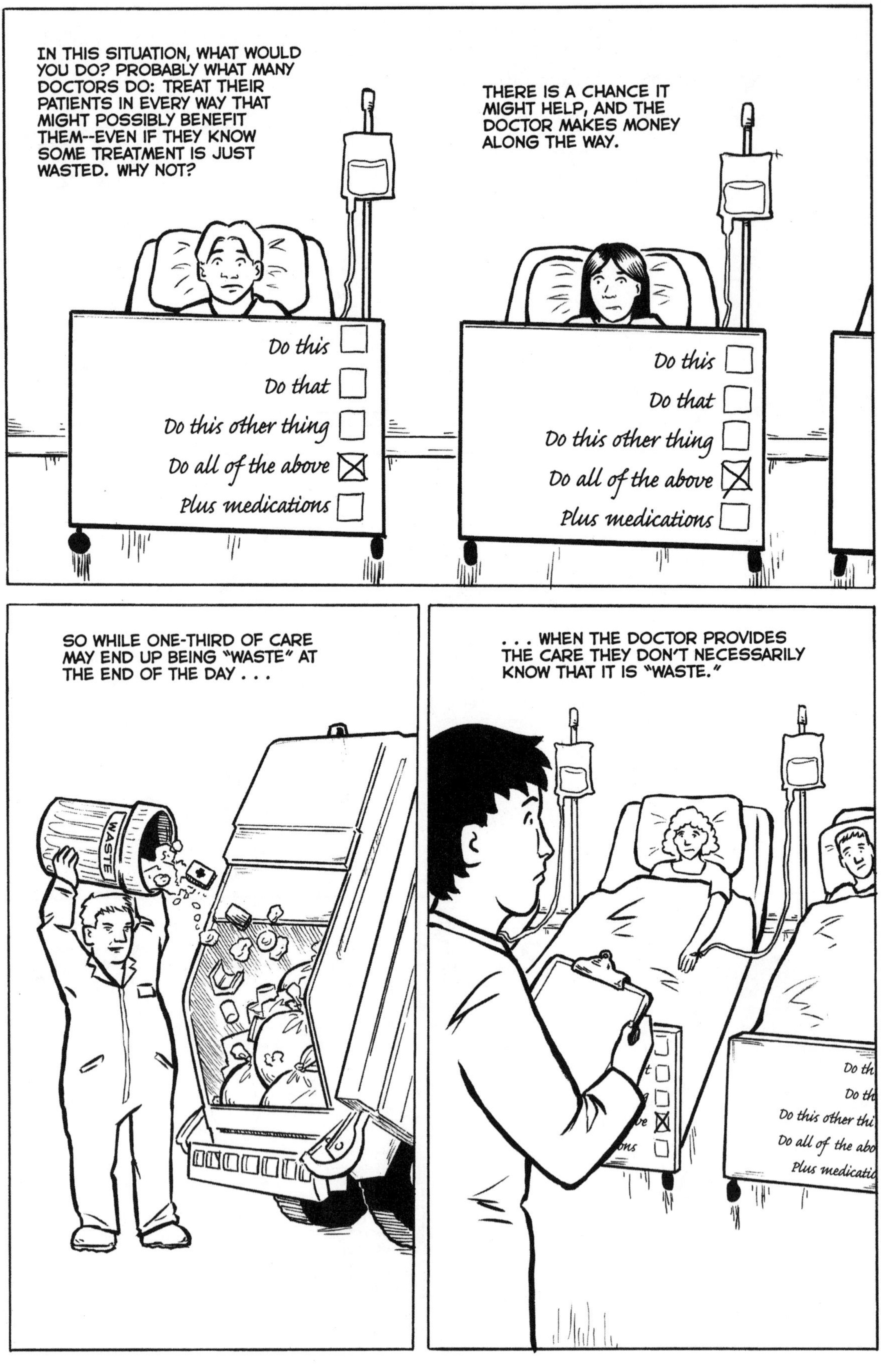

IN THIS SITUATION, WHAT WOULD YOU DO? PROBABLY WHAT MANY DOCTORS DO: TREAT THEIR PATIENTS IN EVERY WAY THAT MIGHT POSSIBLY BENEFIT THEM--EVEN IF THEY KNOW SOME TREATMENT IS JUST WASTED. WHY NOT?

Do this
Do that
Do this other thing
Do all of the above ☒
Plus medications

THERE IS A CHANCE IT MIGHT HELP, AND THE DOCTOR MAKES MONEY ALONG THE WAY.

Do this
Do that
Do this other thing
Do all of the above ☒
Plus medications

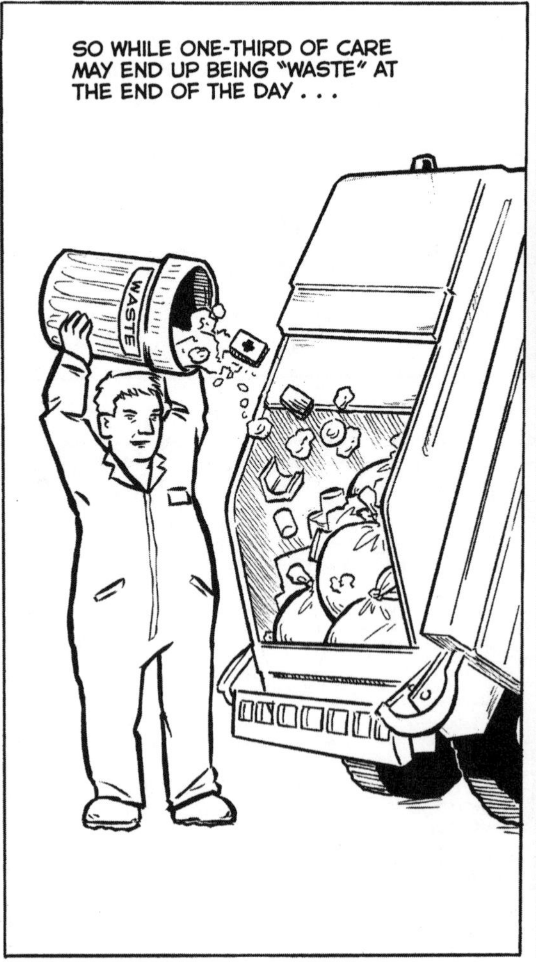

SO WHILE ONE-THIRD OF CARE MAY END UP BEING "WASTE" AT THE END OF THE DAY . . .

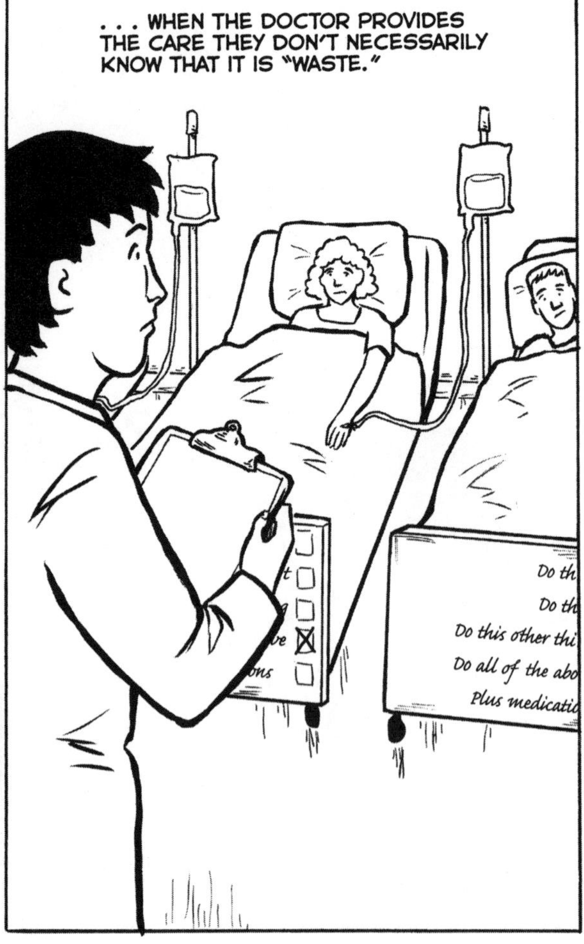

. . . WHEN THE DOCTOR PROVIDES THE CARE THEY DON'T NECESSARILY KNOW THAT IT IS "WASTE."

CHAPTER 4 WE THE PEOPLE...NEED TO BE INSURED

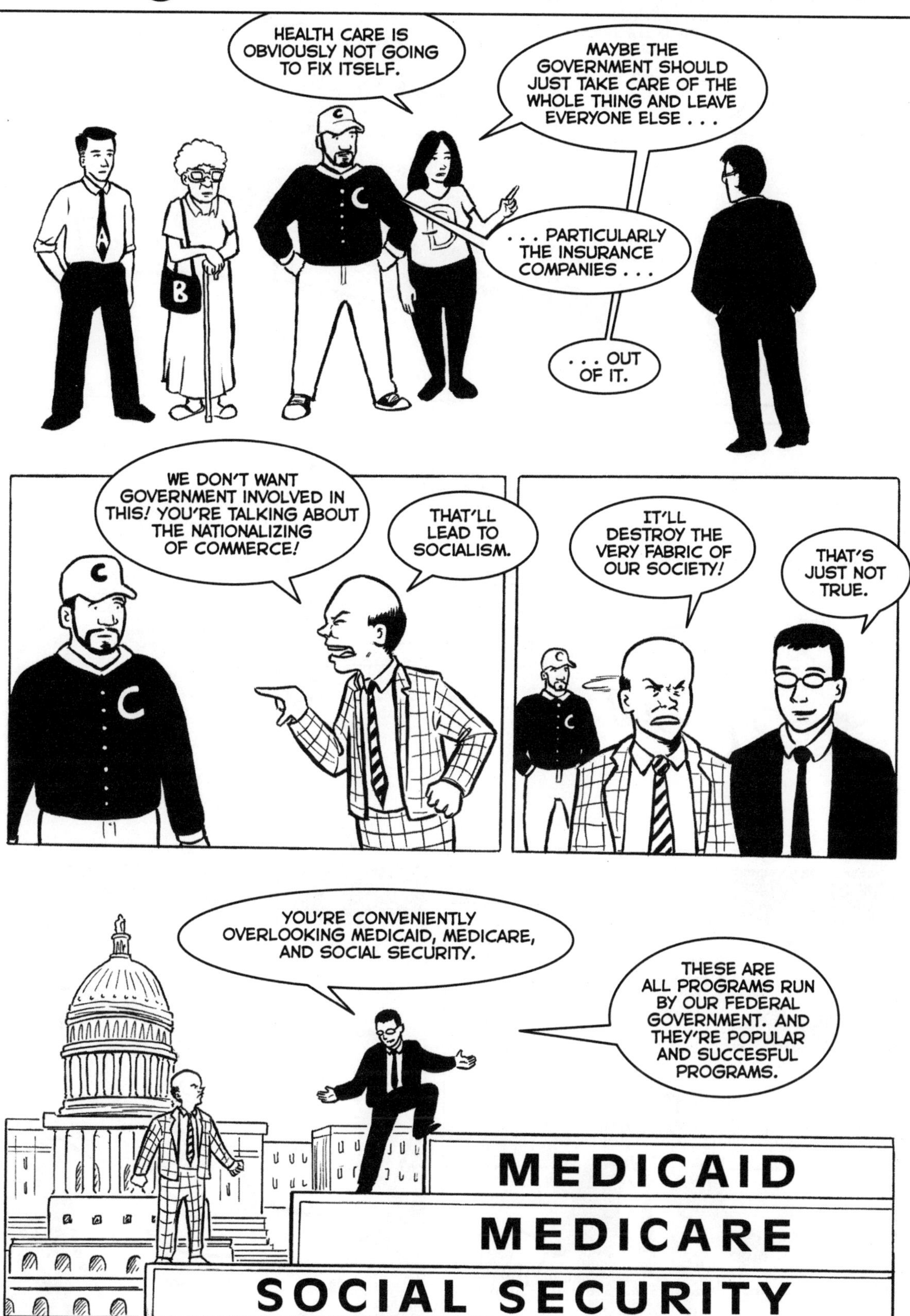

HEALTH CARE IS OBVIOUSLY NOT GOING TO FIX ITSELF.
MAYBE THE GOVERNMENT SHOULD JUST TAKE CARE OF THE WHOLE THING AND LEAVE EVERYONE ELSE . . .
. . . PARTICULARLY THE INSURANCE COMPANIES . . .
. . . OUT OF IT.
WE DON'T WANT GOVERNMENT INVOLVED IN THIS! YOU'RE TALKING ABOUT THE NATIONALIZING OF COMMERCE!
THAT'LL LEAD TO SOCIALISM.
IT'LL DESTROY THE VERY FABRIC OF OUR SOCIETY!
THAT'S JUST NOT TRUE.
YOU'RE CONVENIENTLY OVERLOOKING MEDICAID, MEDICARE, AND SOCIAL SECURITY.
THESE ARE ALL PROGRAMS RUN BY OUR FEDERAL GOVERNMENT. AND THEY'RE POPULAR AND SUCCESFUL PROGRAMS.
MEDICAID
MEDICARE
SOCIAL SECURITY

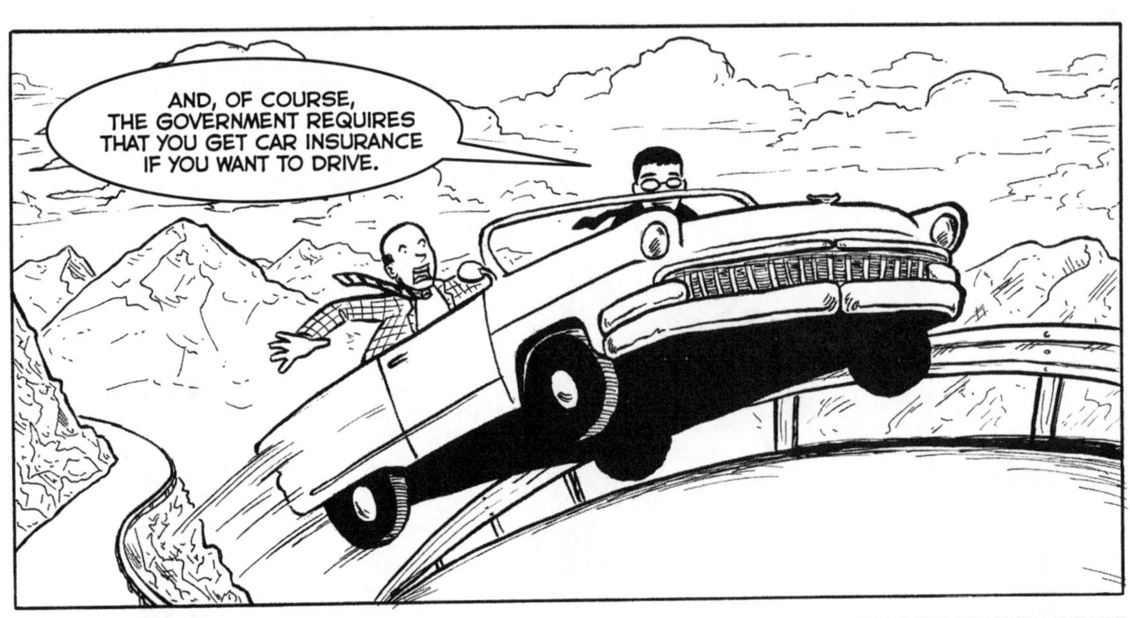
AND, OF COURSE, THE GOVERNMENT REQUIRES THAT YOU GET CAR INSURANCE IF YOU WANT TO DRIVE.

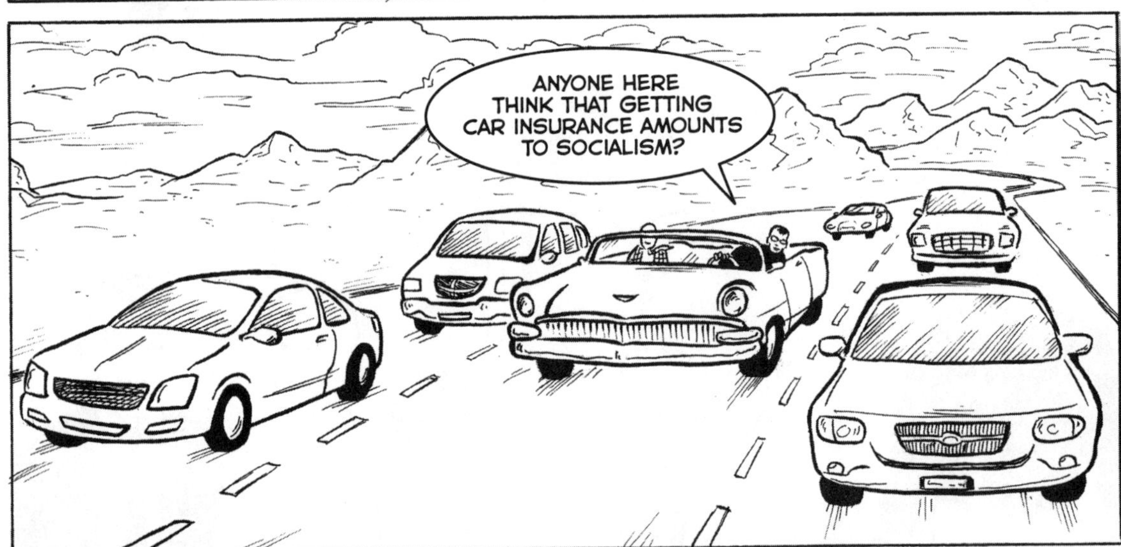
ANYONE HERE THINK THAT GETTING CAR INSURANCE AMOUNTS TO SOCIALISM?

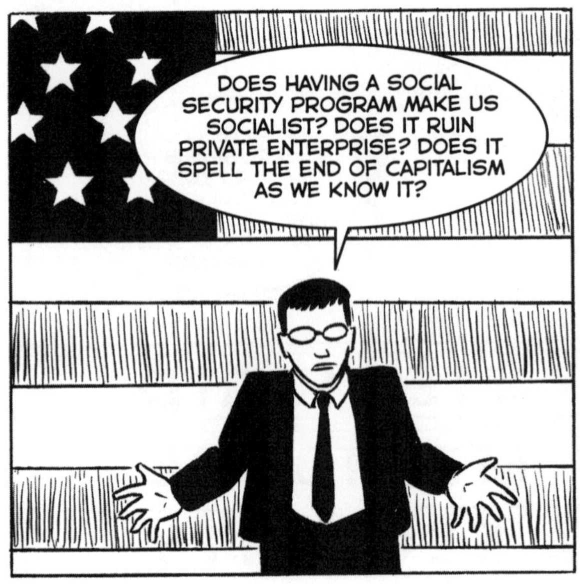
DOES HAVING A SOCIAL SECURITY PROGRAM MAKE US SOCIALIST? DOES IT RUIN PRIVATE ENTERPRISE? DOES IT SPELL THE END OF CAPITALISM AS WE KNOW IT?

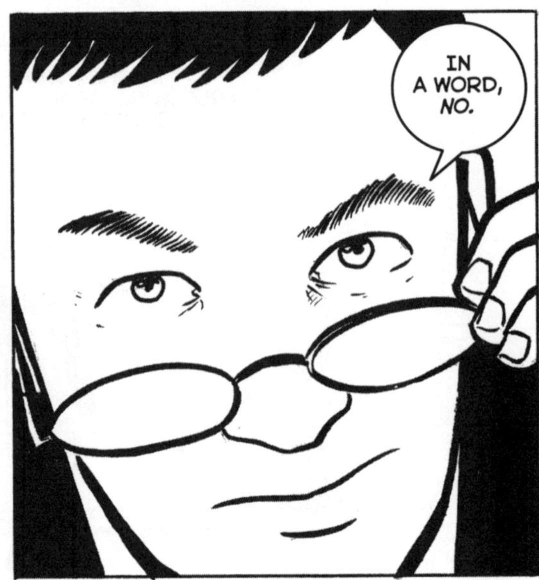
IN A WORD, *NO.*

TAKING THE LEAD IN MAKING SURE AMERICANS CAN GET HEALTH CARE IS EXACTLY THE SORT OF PROBLEM OUR REPUBLICAN FORM OF GOVERNMENT IS SUPPOSED TO SOLVE. TO DO NOTHING IS THE EQUIVALENT OF TREADING WATER . . . WHICH ONLY MEANS THAT MORE PEOPLE WILL DROWN THE LONGER WE DELAY.

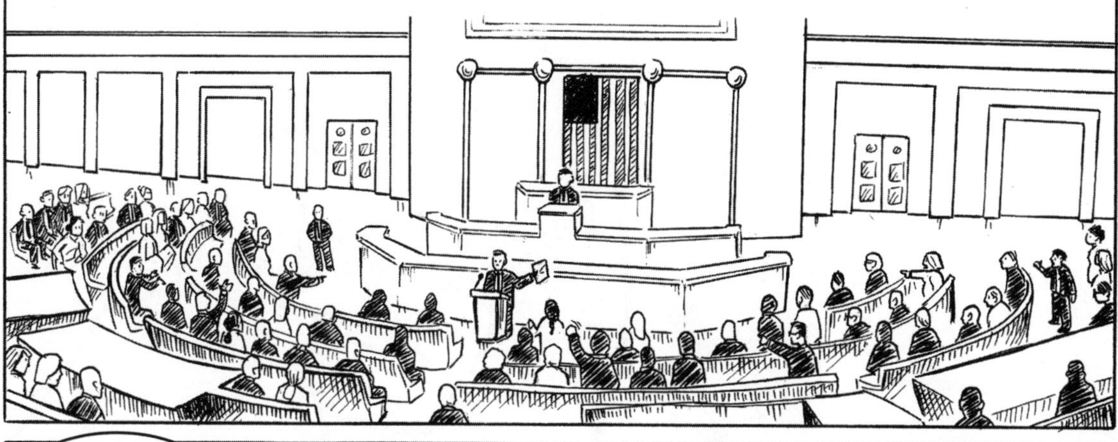

IT'S UP TO THE GOVERNMENT TO HANDLE THE PROBLEMS OF THE UNINSURED.

BUT WE CAN'T LEAN ON THE GOVERNMENT TO SOLVE ALL OUR PROBLEMS--THAT'S NOT THE AMERICAN WAY!

THIS IS THE DEBATE OVER HEALTH CARE THAT HAS PARALYZED OUR NATION'S EFFORTS TO FIX IT. FOR 60 YEARS, WE HAVE BEEN STUCK BETWEEN THOSE WHO THINK GOVERNMENT SHOULD DO **MORE** AND THOSE WHO THINK GOVERNMENT SHOULD DO **LESS.**

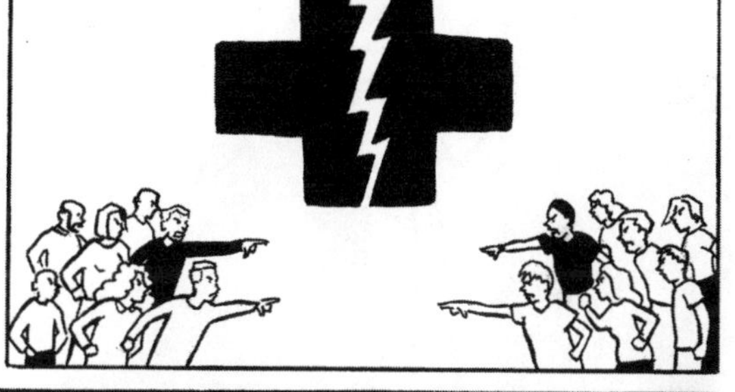

MANY ON THE LEFT HAVE LONG ADVOCATED FOR A SINGLE-PAYER PROGRAM--GET RID OF PRIVATE INSURANCE AND HAVE GOVERNMENT TAKE OVER THE SYSTEM, PAID FOR BY TAXES ON BUSINESSES.

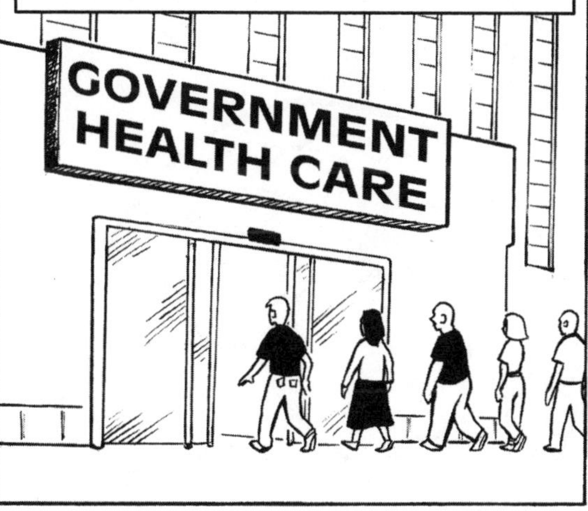

MANY ON THE RIGHT HAVE ADVOCATED A SYSTEM WHERE WE NO LONGER HAVE GOVERNMENT PROVIDE ANY INSURANCE, BUT RATHER HAVE INDIVIDUALS CHOOSE FROM PRIVATE INSURANCE COMPANIES.

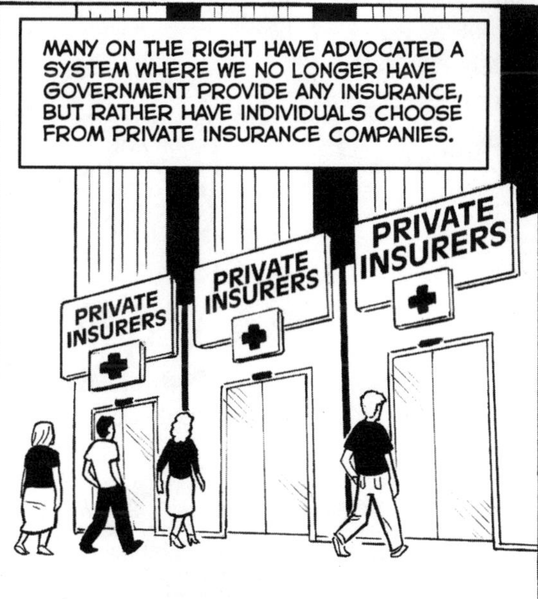

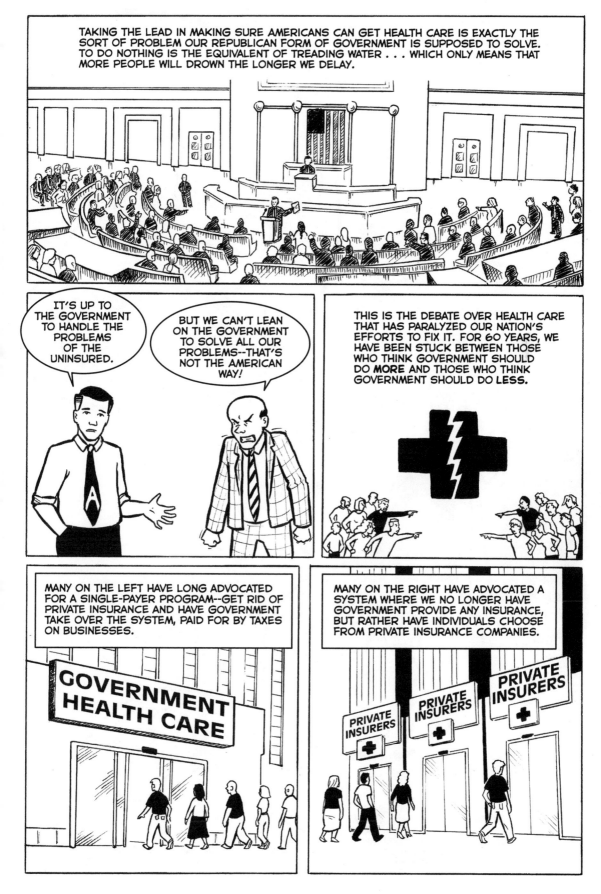

BOTH APPROACHES FACE PROBLEMS.

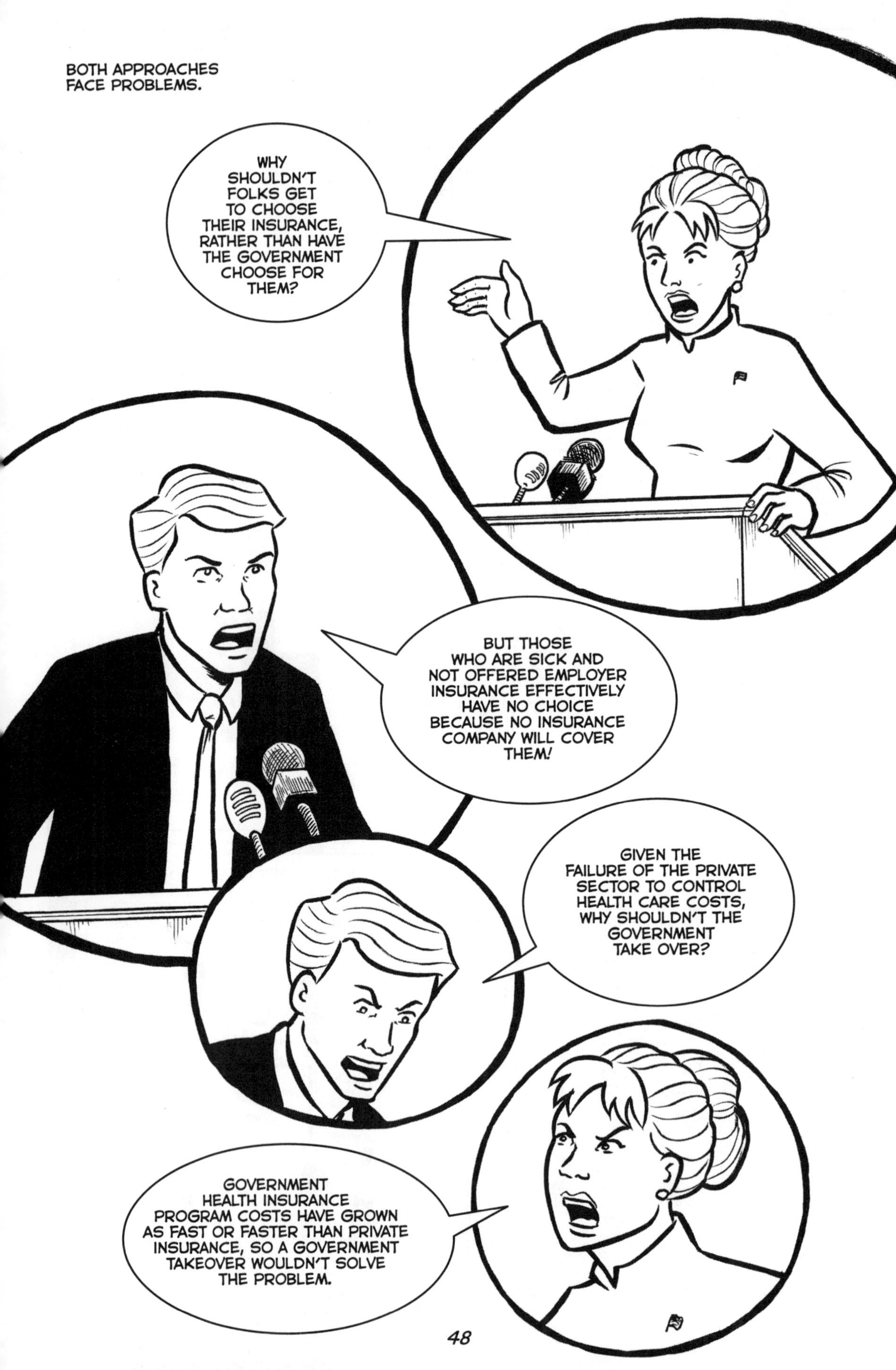

WHY SHOULDN'T FOLKS GET TO CHOOSE THEIR INSURANCE, RATHER THAN HAVE THE GOVERNMENT CHOOSE FOR THEM?
BUT THOSE WHO ARE SICK AND NOT OFFERED EMPLOYER INSURANCE EFFECTIVELY HAVE NO CHOICE BECAUSE NO INSURANCE COMPANY WILL COVER THEM!
GIVEN THE FAILURE OF THE PRIVATE SECTOR TO CONTROL HEALTH CARE COSTS, WHY SHOULDN'T THE GOVERNMENT TAKE OVER?
GOVERNMENT HEALTH INSURANCE PROGRAM COSTS HAVE GROWN AS FAST OR FASTER THAN PRIVATE INSURANCE, SO A GOVERNMENT TAKEOVER WOULDN'T SOLVE THE PROBLEM.

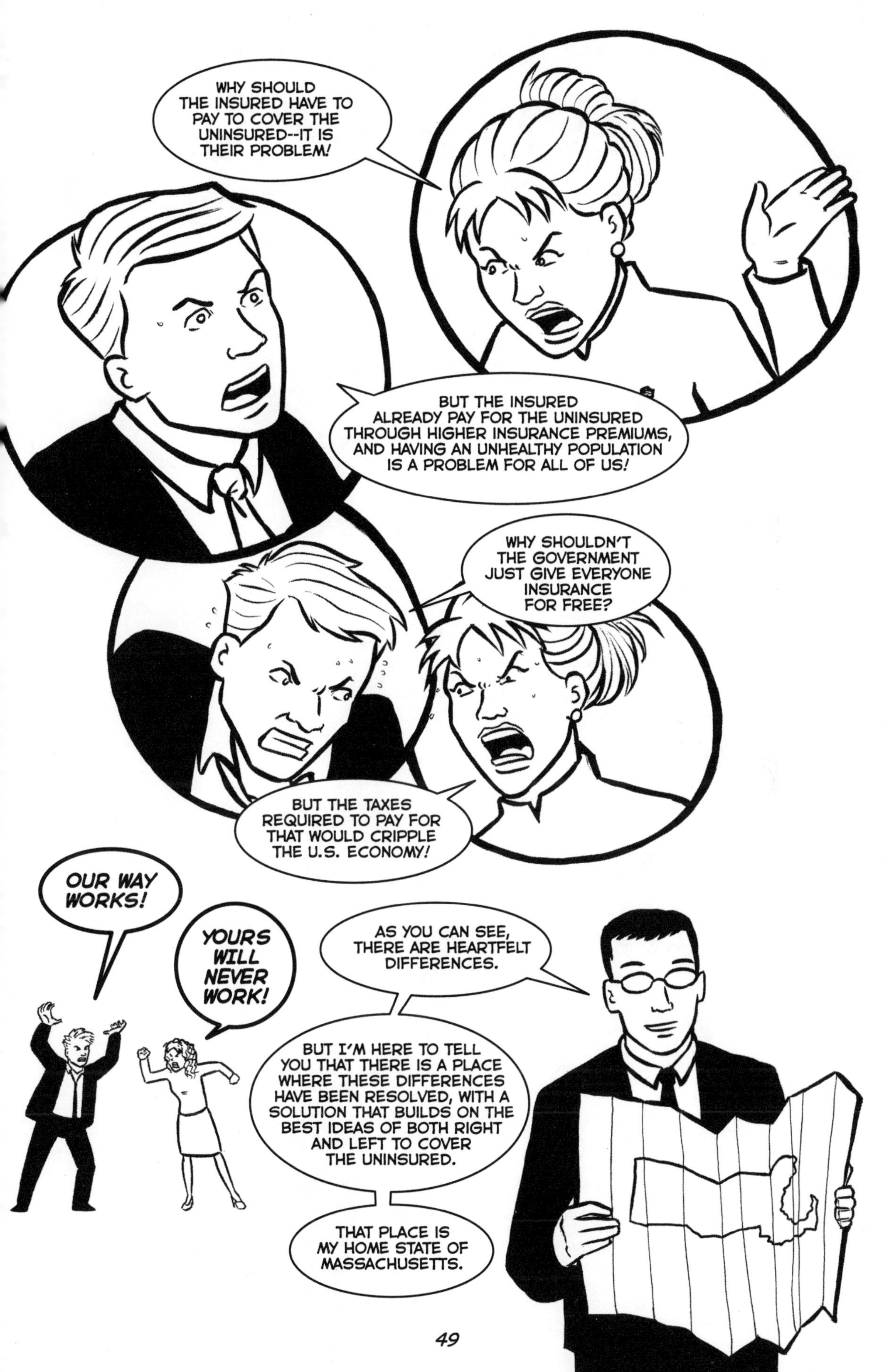
WHY SHOULD THE INSURED HAVE TO PAY TO COVER THE UNINSURED--IT IS THEIR PROBLEM!
BUT THE INSURED ALREADY PAY FOR THE UNINSURED THROUGH HIGHER INSURANCE PREMIUMS, AND HAVING AN UNHEALTHY POPULATION IS A PROBLEM FOR ALL OF US!
WHY SHOULDN'T THE GOVERNMENT JUST GIVE EVERYONE INSURANCE FOR FREE?
BUT THE TAXES REQUIRED TO PAY FOR THAT WOULD CRIPPLE THE U.S. ECONOMY!
OUR WAY WORKS!
YOURS WILL NEVER WORK!
AS YOU CAN SEE, THERE ARE HEARTFELT DIFFERENCES.
BUT I'M HERE TO TELL YOU THAT THERE IS A PLACE WHERE THESE DIFFERENCES HAVE BEEN RESOLVED, WITH A SOLUTION THAT BUILDS ON THE BEST IDEAS OF BOTH RIGHT AND LEFT TO COVER THE UNINSURED.
THAT PLACE IS MY HOME STATE OF MASSACHUSETTS.

CHAPTER 5 MAKING IT WORK IN MASSACHUSETTS

IN 2006, MASSACHUSETTS WAS THE SITE OF "THE MEDICAL SHOT HEARD 'ROUND THE COUNTRY."

THE STATE DECIDED TO MAKE SOME CHANGES THAT WOULD ADDRESS THE CORE ISSUE OF CARING FOR THE UNINSURED.

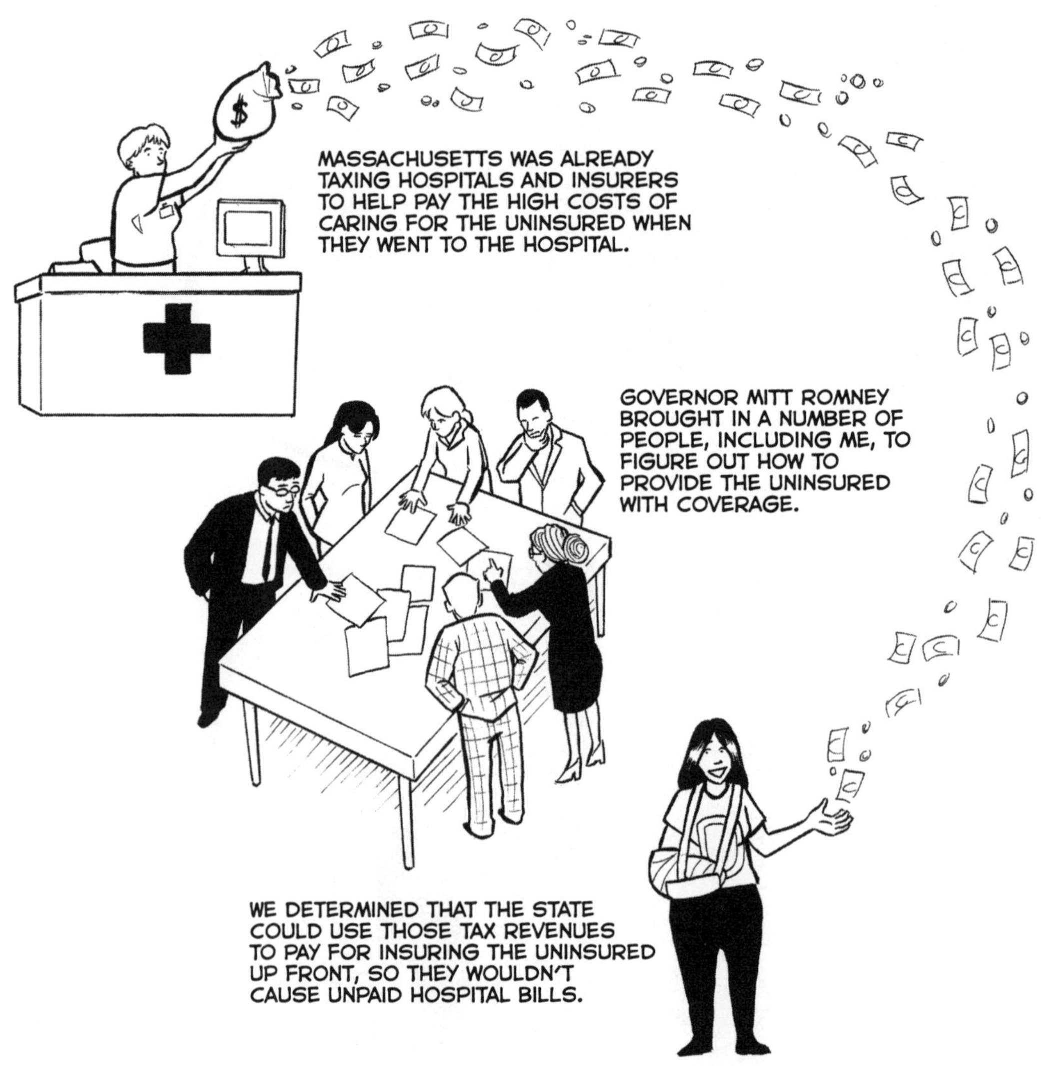
MASSACHUSETTS WAS ALREADY TAXING HOSPITALS AND INSURERS TO HELP PAY THE HIGH COSTS OF CARING FOR THE UNINSURED WHEN THEY WENT TO THE HOSPITAL.
GOVERNOR MITT ROMNEY BROUGHT IN A NUMBER OF PEOPLE, INCLUDING ME, TO FIGURE OUT HOW TO PROVIDE THE UNINSURED WITH COVERAGE.
WE DETERMINED THAT THE STATE COULD USE THOSE TAX REVENUES TO PAY FOR INSURING THE UNINSURED UP FRONT, SO THEY WOULDN'T CAUSE UNPAID HOSPITAL BILLS.

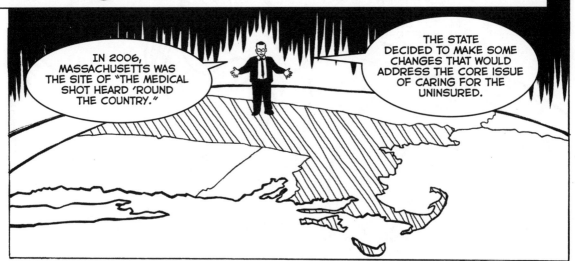

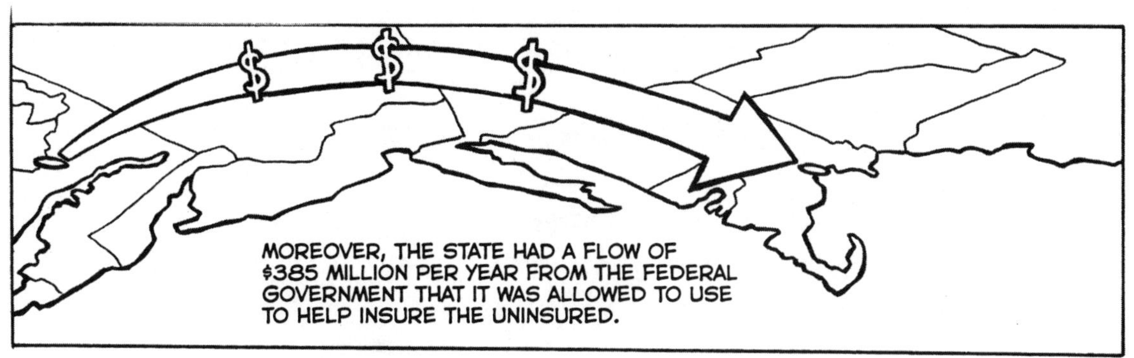
MOREOVER, THE STATE HAD A FLOW OF
$385 MILLION PER YEAR FROM THE FEDERAL
GOVERNMENT THAT IT WAS ALLOWED TO USE
TO HELP INSURE THE UNINSURED.

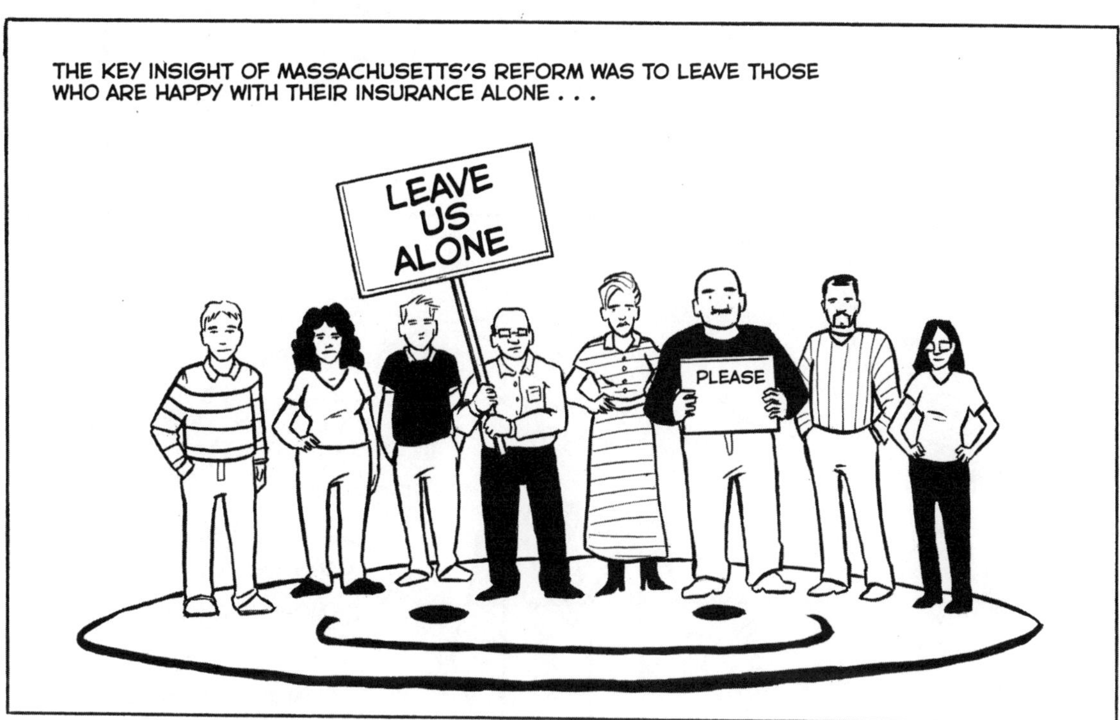
THE KEY INSIGHT OF MASSACHUSETTS'S REFORM WAS TO LEAVE THOSE
WHO ARE HAPPY WITH THEIR INSURANCE ALONE . . .
LEAVE US ALONE
PLEASE

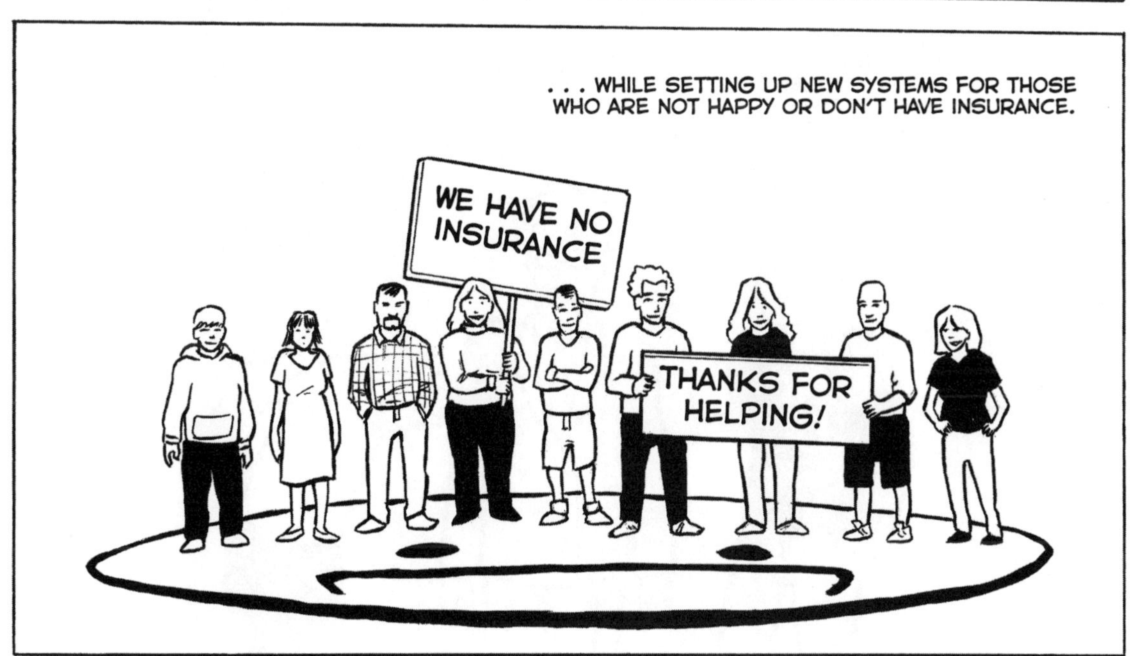
. . . WHILE SETTING UP NEW SYSTEMS FOR THOSE
WHO ARE NOT HAPPY OR DON'T HAVE INSURANCE.
WE HAVE NO INSURANCE
THANKS FOR HELPING!

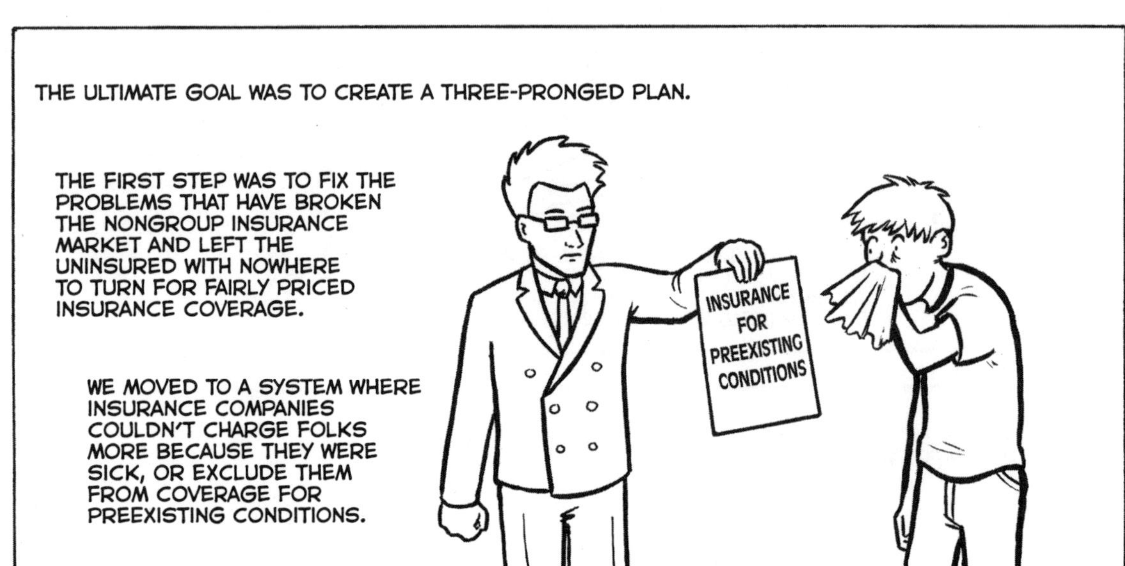
THE ULTIMATE GOAL WAS TO CREATE A THREE-PRONGED PLAN.
THE FIRST STEP WAS TO FIX THE PROBLEMS THAT HAVE BROKEN THE NONGROUP INSURANCE MARKET AND LEFT THE UNINSURED WITH NOWHERE TO TURN FOR FAIRLY PRICED INSURANCE COVERAGE.
INSURANCE FOR PREEXISTING CONDITIONS
WE MOVED TO A SYSTEM WHERE INSURANCE COMPANIES COULDN'T CHARGE FOLKS MORE BECAUSE THEY WERE SICK, OR EXCLUDE THEM FROM COVERAGE FOR PREEXISTING CONDITIONS.

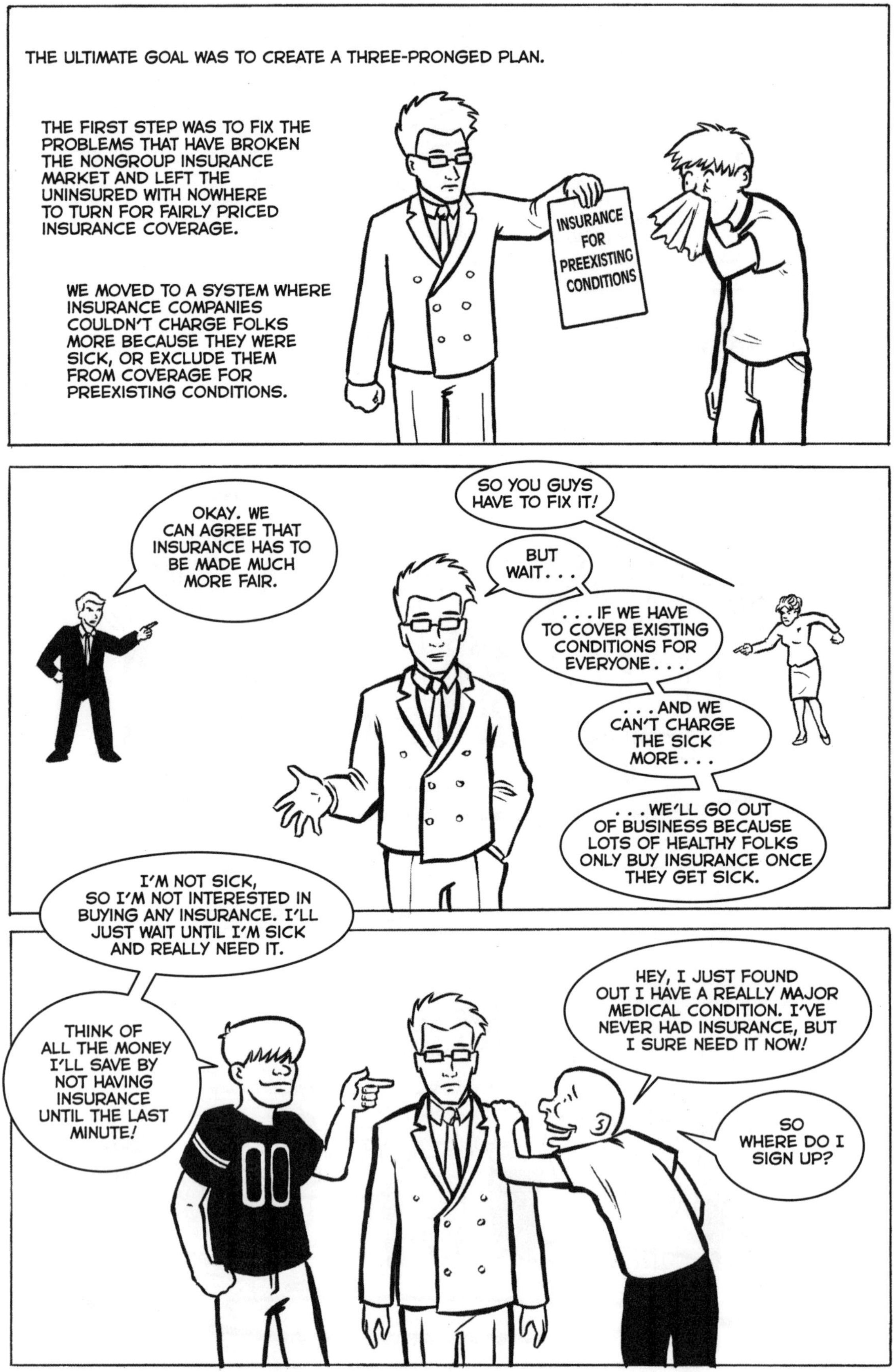

OKAY. WE CAN AGREE THAT INSURANCE HAS TO BE MADE MUCH MORE FAIR.

SO YOU GUYS HAVE TO FIX IT!

BUT WAIT. . .

. . . IF WE HAVE TO COVER EXISTING CONDITIONS FOR EVERYONE . . .

. . . AND WE CAN'T CHARGE THE SICK MORE . . .

. . . WE'LL GO OUT OF BUSINESS BECAUSE LOTS OF HEALTHY FOLKS ONLY BUY INSURANCE ONCE THEY GET SICK.

I'M NOT SICK, SO I'M NOT INTERESTED IN BUYING ANY INSURANCE. I'LL JUST WAIT UNTIL I'M SICK AND REALLY NEED IT.

THINK OF ALL THE MONEY I'LL SAVE BY NOT HAVING INSURANCE UNTIL THE LAST MINUTE!

HEY, I JUST FOUND OUT I HAVE A REALLY MAJOR MEDICAL CONDITION. I'VE NEVER HAD INSURANCE, BUT I SURE NEED IT NOW!

SO WHERE DO I SIGN UP?

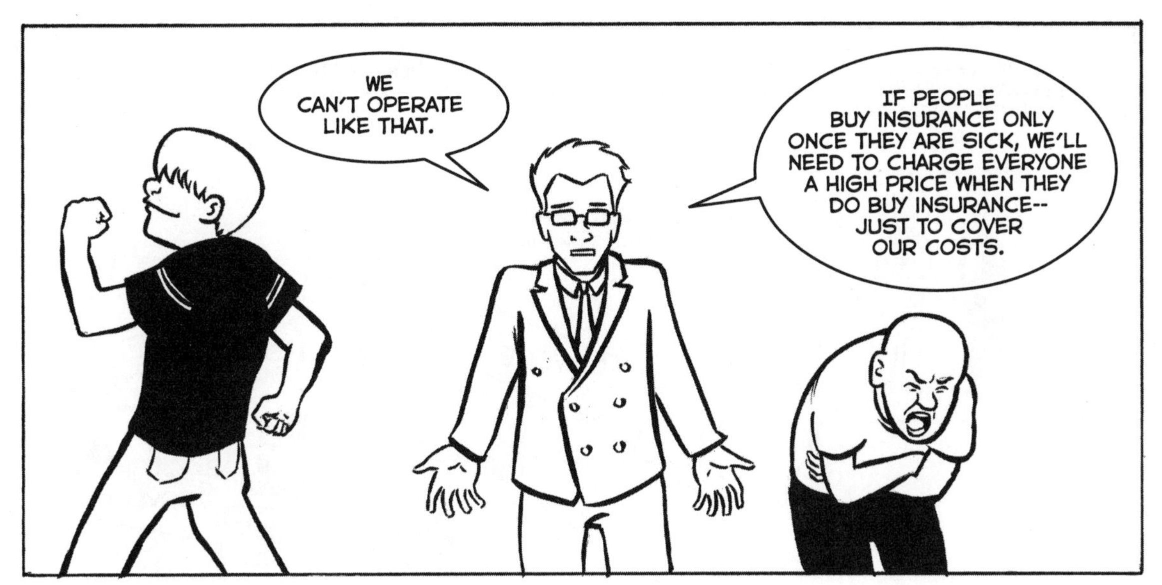
WE CAN'T OPERATE LIKE THAT.
IF PEOPLE BUY INSURANCE ONLY ONCE THEY ARE SICK, WE'LL NEED TO CHARGE EVERYONE A HIGH PRICE WHEN THEY DO BUY INSURANCE-- JUST TO COVER OUR COSTS.

SO IF YOU DON'T LET US DISCRIMINATE AGAINST THE SICK, WE'LL JUST CHARGE EVERYONE LIKE THEY ARE *SICK*.

ACROSS THE BOARD
HIKES
EFFECTIVE IMMEDIATELY

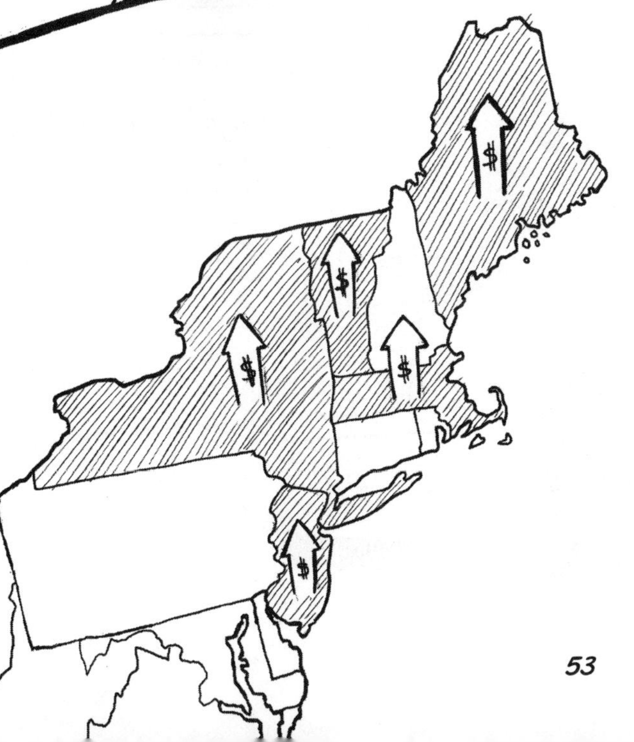

THIS IS NOT JUST A THEORETICAL POINT. FIVE STATES TRIED TO TELL INSURERS THAT THEY COULDN'T CHARGE THE SICK MORE OR REJECT COVERAGE FOR PREEXISTING CONDITIONS.

THOSE FIVE STATES BECAME FIVE OF THE MOST EXPENSIVE PLACES IN THE NATION TO BUY NONGROUP COVERAGE.

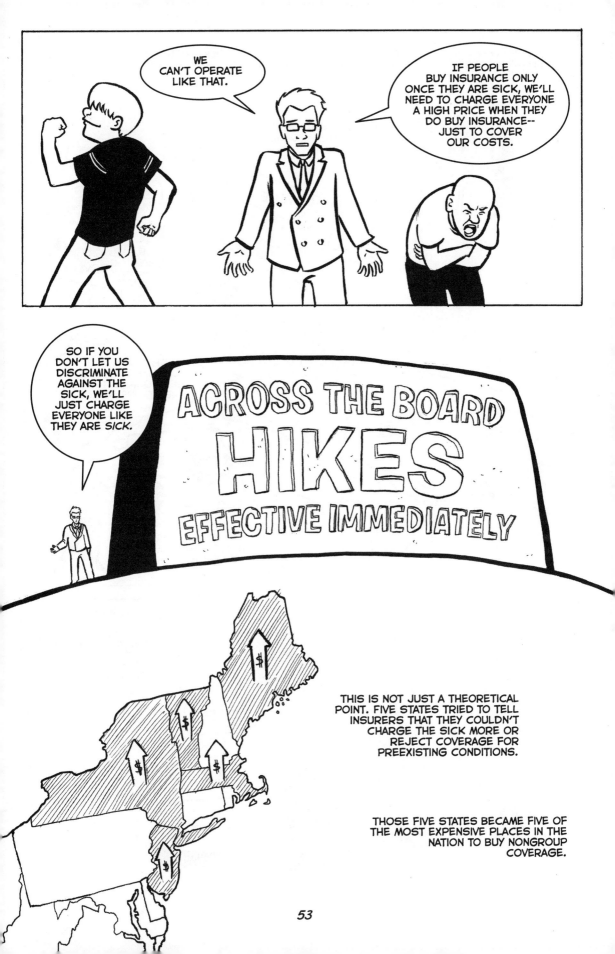

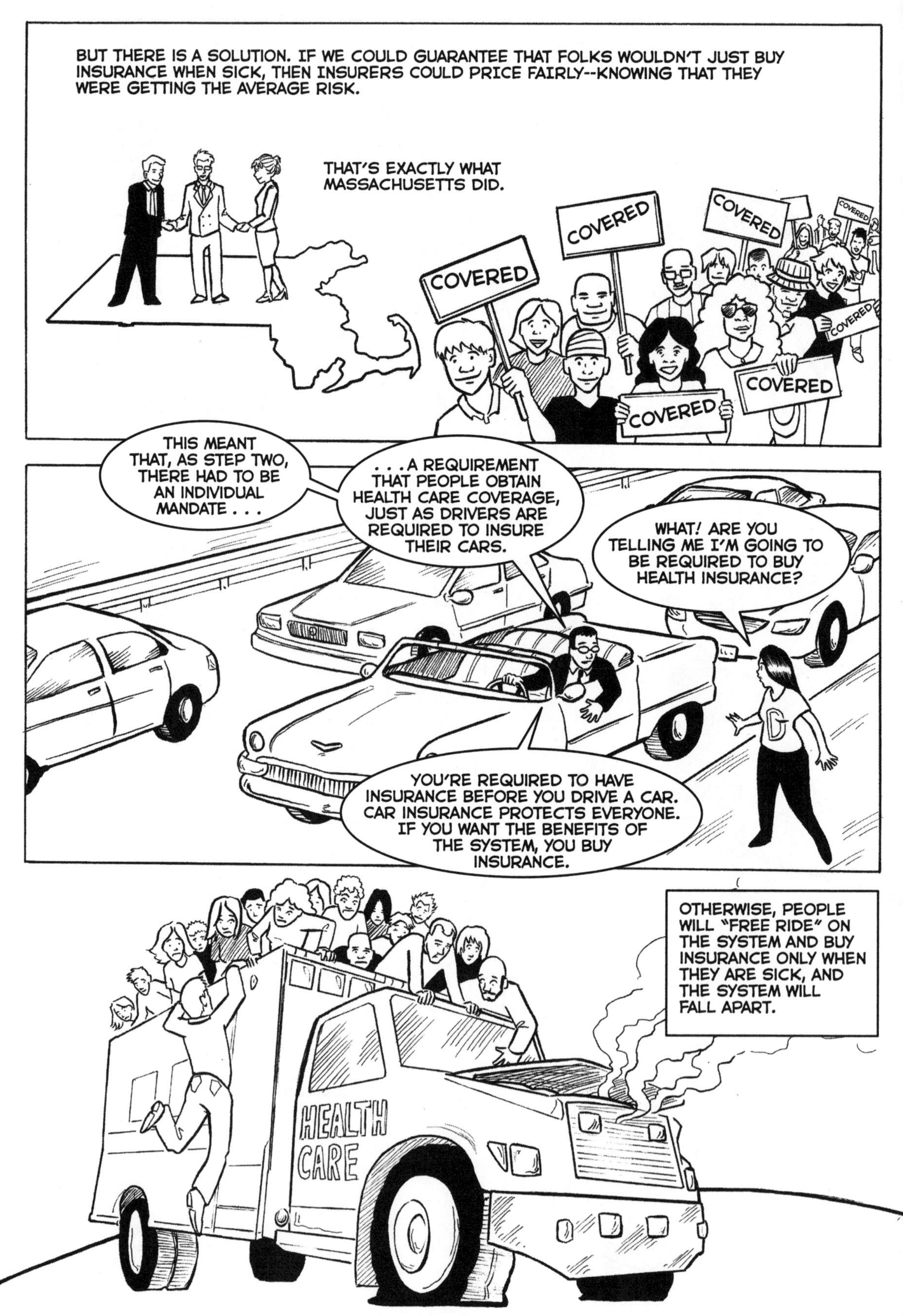
BUT THERE IS A SOLUTION. IF WE COULD GUARANTEE THAT FOLKS WOULDN'T JUST BUY INSURANCE WHEN SICK, THEN INSURERS COULD PRICE FAIRLY--KNOWING THAT THEY WERE GETTING THE AVERAGE RISK.
THAT'S EXACTLY WHAT MASSACHUSETTS DID.
COVERED
COVERED
COVERED
COVERED
COVERED
COVERED
COVERED
COVERED
THIS MEANT THAT, AS STEP TWO, THERE HAD TO BE AN INDIVIDUAL MANDATE . . .
. . . A REQUIREMENT THAT PEOPLE OBTAIN HEALTH CARE COVERAGE, JUST AS DRIVERS ARE REQUIRED TO INSURE THEIR CARS.
WHAT! ARE YOU TELLING ME I'M GOING TO BE REQUIRED TO BUY HEALTH INSURANCE?
YOU'RE REQUIRED TO HAVE INSURANCE BEFORE YOU DRIVE A CAR. CAR INSURANCE PROTECTS EVERYONE. IF YOU WANT THE BENEFITS OF THE SYSTEM, YOU BUY INSURANCE.
OTHERWISE, PEOPLE WILL "FREE RIDE" ON THE SYSTEM AND BUY INSURANCE ONLY WHEN THEY ARE SICK, AND THE SYSTEM WILL FALL APART.
HEALTH CARE

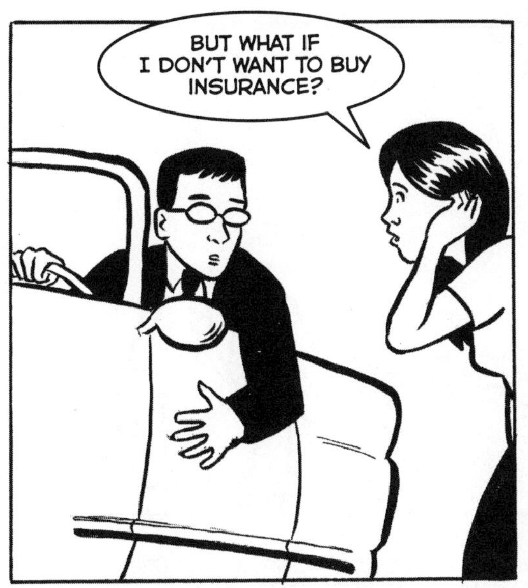
BUT WHAT IF I DON'T WANT TO BUY INSURANCE?

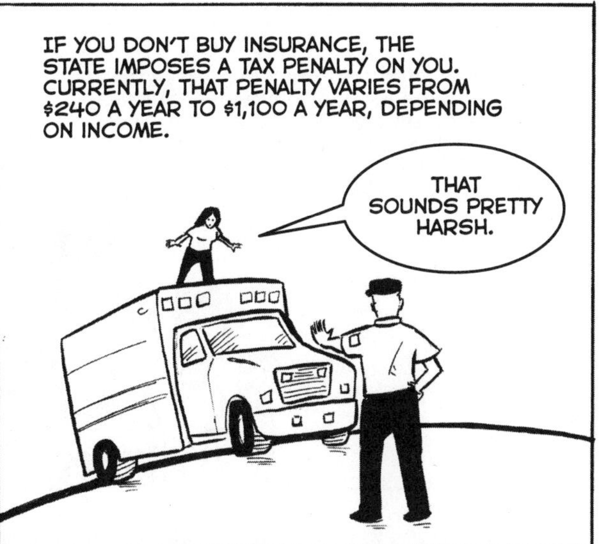
IF YOU DON'T BUY INSURANCE, THE STATE IMPOSES A TAX PENALTY ON YOU. CURRENTLY, THAT PENALTY VARIES FROM $240 A YEAR TO $1,100 A YEAR, DEPENDING ON INCOME.
THAT SOUNDS PRETTY HARSH.

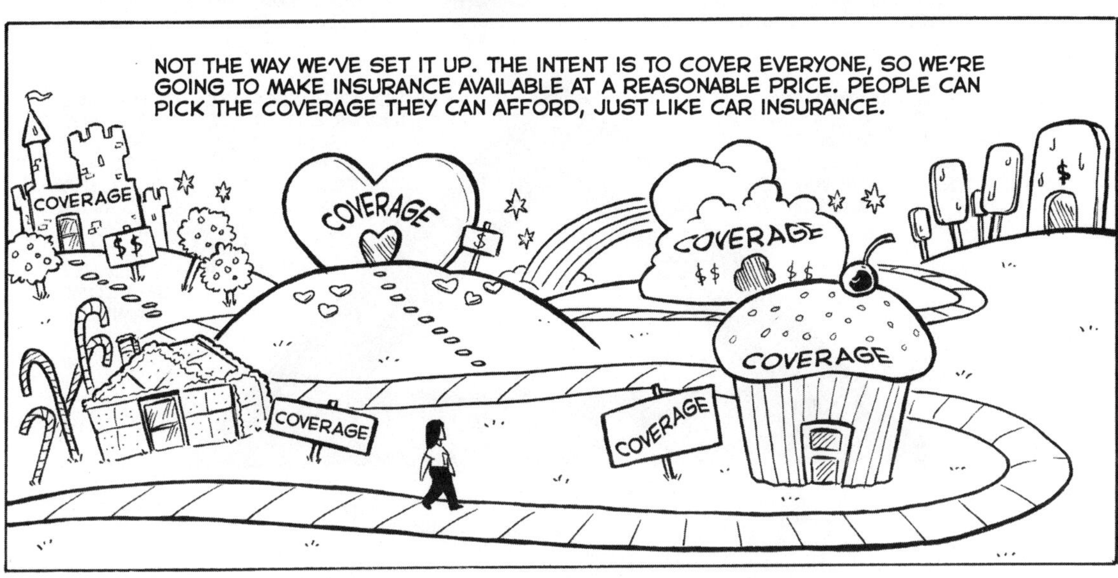
NOT THE WAY WE'VE SET IT UP. THE INTENT IS TO COVER EVERYONE, SO WE'RE GOING TO MAKE INSURANCE AVAILABLE AT A REASONABLE PRICE. PEOPLE CAN PICK THE COVERAGE THEY CAN AFFORD, JUST LIKE CAR INSURANCE.
COVERAGE
$$
COVERAGE
$
COVERAGE
$$ $$
COVERAGE
$
COVERAGE
COVERAGE

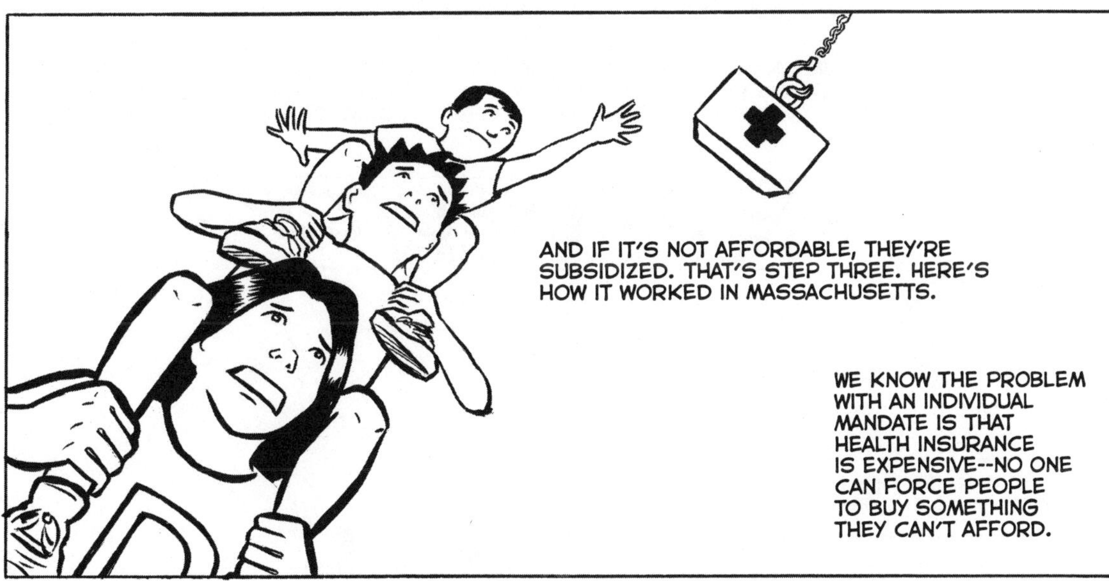
AND IF IT'S NOT AFFORDABLE, THEY'RE SUBSIDIZED. THAT'S STEP THREE. HERE'S HOW IT WORKED IN MASSACHUSETTS.
WE KNOW THE PROBLEM WITH AN INDIVIDUAL MANDATE IS THAT HEALTH INSURANCE IS EXPENSIVE--NO ONE CAN FORCE PEOPLE TO BUY SOMETHING THEY CAN'T AFFORD.

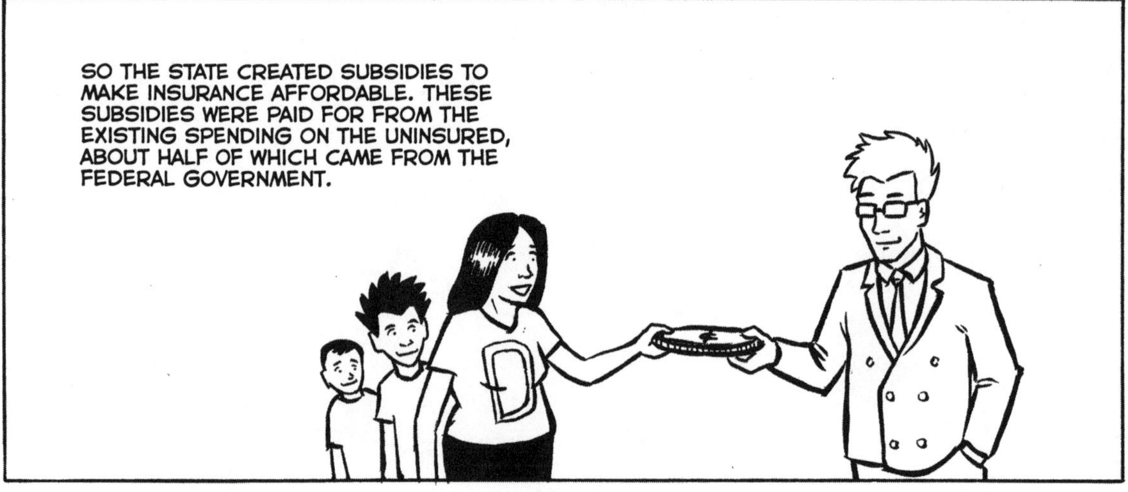

SO THE STATE CREATED SUBSIDIES TO MAKE INSURANCE AFFORDABLE. THESE SUBSIDIES WERE PAID FOR FROM THE EXISTING SPENDING ON THE UNINSURED, ABOUT HALF OF WHICH CAME FROM THE FEDERAL GOVERNMENT.

CHILDREN WERE COVERED FOR FREE BY THE STATE'S MEDICAID PROGRAM. ADULTS WHOSE INCOME WAS BELOW 300% OF THE FEDERAL POVERTY LINE HAD THEIR INSURANCE HEAVILY SUBSIDIZED.

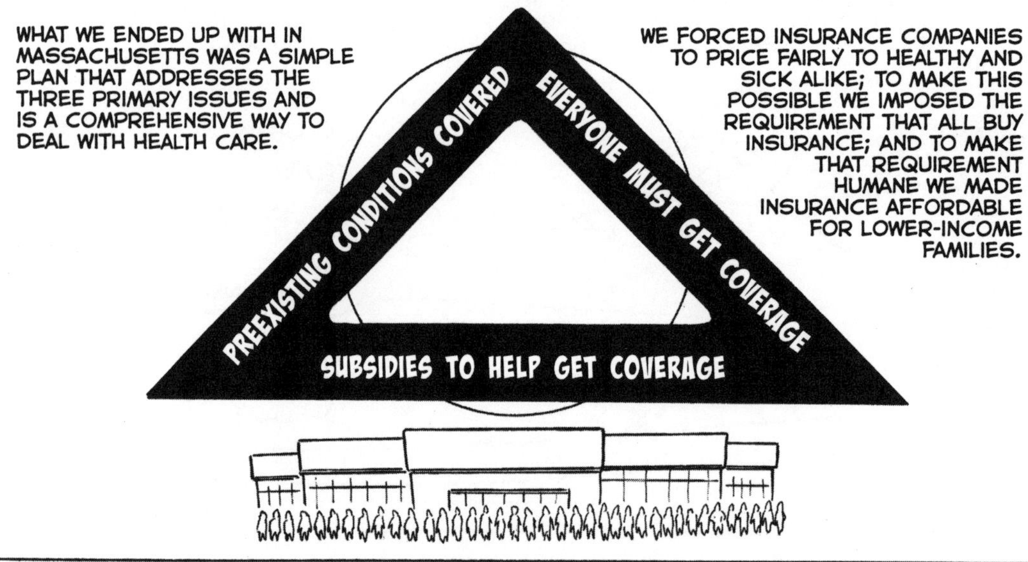

WHAT WE ENDED UP WITH IN MASSACHUSETTS WAS A SIMPLE PLAN THAT ADDRESSES THE THREE PRIMARY ISSUES AND IS A COMPREHENSIVE WAY TO DEAL WITH HEALTH CARE.
PREEXISTING CONDITIONS COVERED
EVERYONE MUST GET COVERAGE
SUBSIDIES TO HELP GET COVERAGE
WE FORCED INSURANCE COMPANIES TO PRICE FAIRLY TO HEALTHY AND SICK ALIKE; TO MAKE THIS POSSIBLE WE IMPOSED THE REQUIREMENT THAT ALL BUY INSURANCE; AND TO MAKE THAT REQUIREMENT HUMANE WE MADE INSURANCE AFFORDABLE FOR LOWER-INCOME FAMILIES.

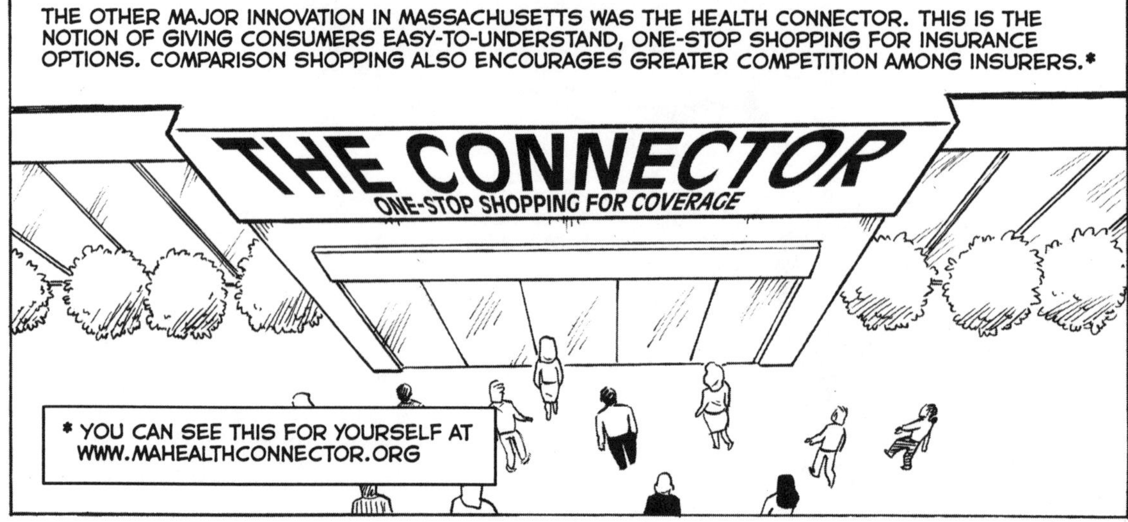

THE OTHER MAJOR INNOVATION IN MASSACHUSETTS WAS THE HEALTH CONNECTOR. THIS IS THE NOTION OF GIVING CONSUMERS EASY-TO-UNDERSTAND, ONE-STOP SHOPPING FOR INSURANCE OPTIONS. COMPARISON SHOPPING ALSO ENCOURAGES GREATER COMPETITION AMONG INSURERS.*
THE CONNECTOR
ONE-STOP SHOPPING FOR COVERAGE
* YOU CAN SEE THIS FOR YOURSELF AT WWW.MAHEALTHCONNECTOR.ORG

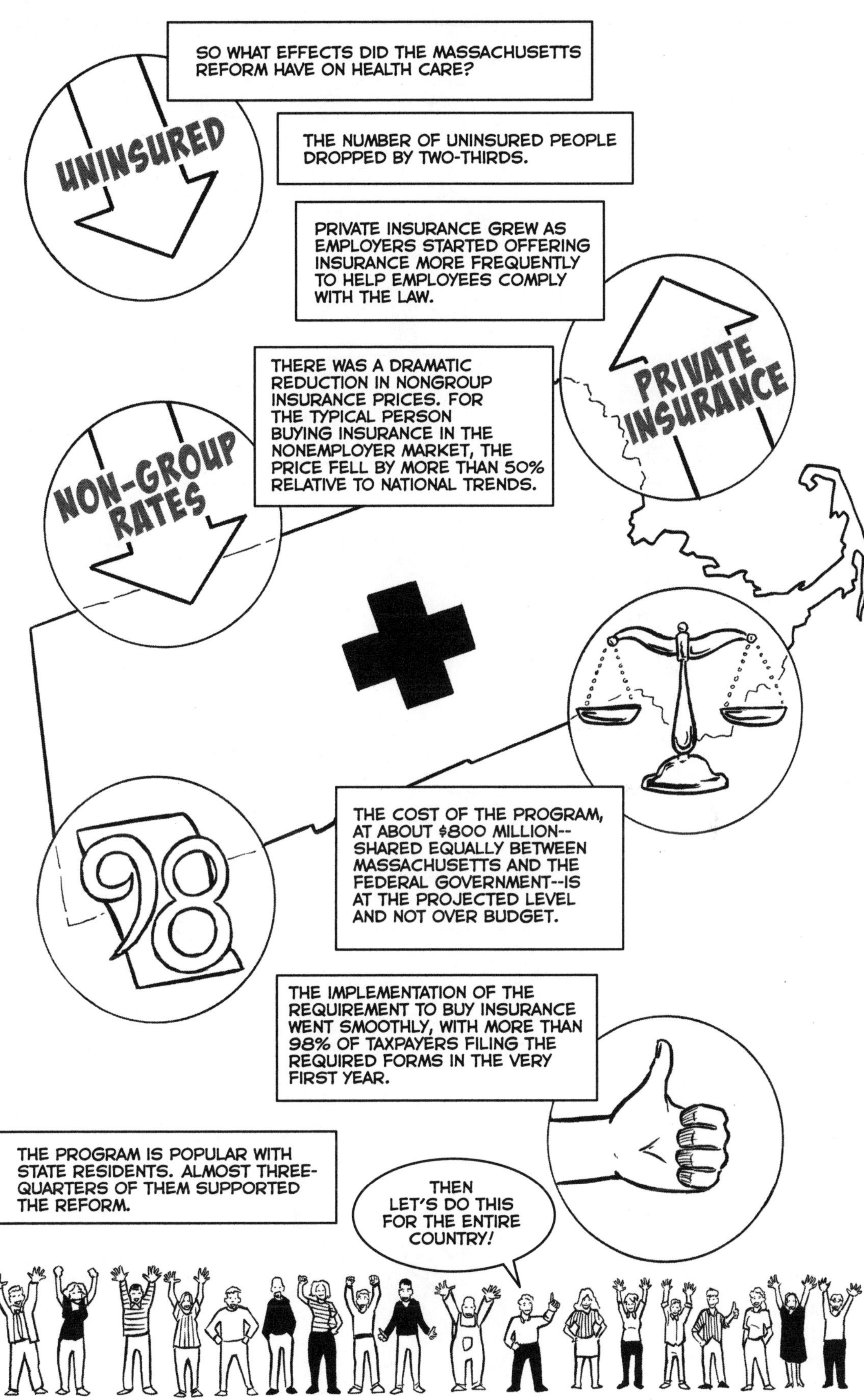
SO WHAT EFFECTS DID THE MASSACHUSETTS REFORM HAVE ON HEALTH CARE?
UNINSURED
THE NUMBER OF UNINSURED PEOPLE DROPPED BY TWO-THIRDS.
PRIVATE INSURANCE GREW AS EMPLOYERS STARTED OFFERING INSURANCE MORE FREQUENTLY TO HELP EMPLOYEES COMPLY WITH THE LAW.
PRIVATE INSURANCE
THERE WAS A DRAMATIC REDUCTION IN NONGROUP INSURANCE PRICES. FOR THE TYPICAL PERSON BUYING INSURANCE IN THE NONEMPLOYER MARKET, THE PRICE FELL BY MORE THAN 50% RELATIVE TO NATIONAL TRENDS.
NON-GROUP RATES
THE COST OF THE PROGRAM, AT ABOUT $800 MILLION--SHARED EQUALLY BETWEEN MASSACHUSETTS AND THE FEDERAL GOVERNMENT--IS AT THE PROJECTED LEVEL AND NOT OVER BUDGET.
98
THE IMPLEMENTATION OF THE REQUIREMENT TO BUY INSURANCE WENT SMOOTHLY, WITH MORE THAN 98% OF TAXPAYERS FILING THE REQUIRED FORMS IN THE VERY FIRST YEAR.
THE PROGRAM IS POPULAR WITH STATE RESIDENTS. ALMOST THREE-QUARTERS OF THEM SUPPORTED THE REFORM.
THEN LET'S DO THIS FOR THE ENTIRE COUNTRY!

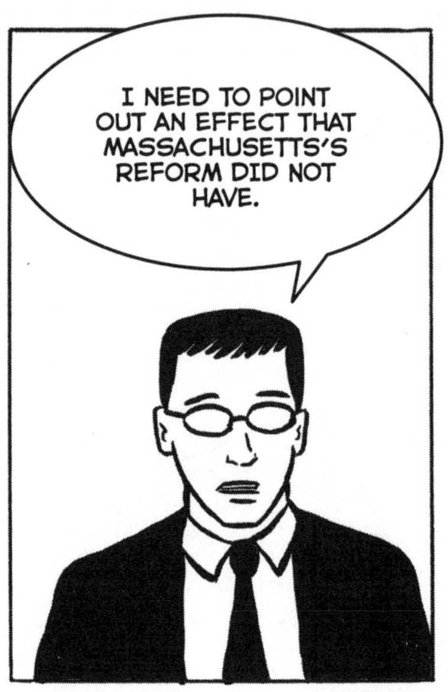
I NEED TO POINT OUT AN EFFECT THAT MASSACHUSETTS'S REFORM DID NOT HAVE.

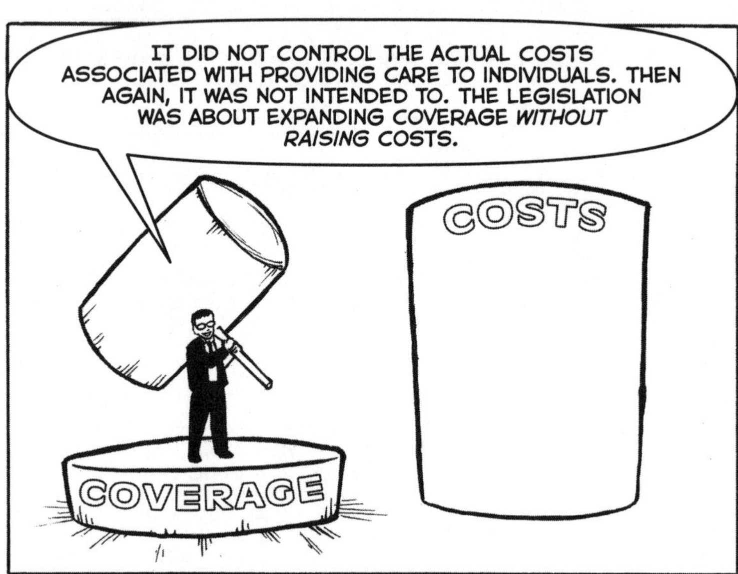
IT DID NOT CONTROL THE ACTUAL COSTS ASSOCIATED WITH PROVIDING CARE TO INDIVIDUALS. THEN AGAIN, IT WAS NOT INTENDED TO. THE LEGISLATION WAS ABOUT EXPANDING COVERAGE *WITHOUT RAISING* COSTS.
COSTS
COVERAGE

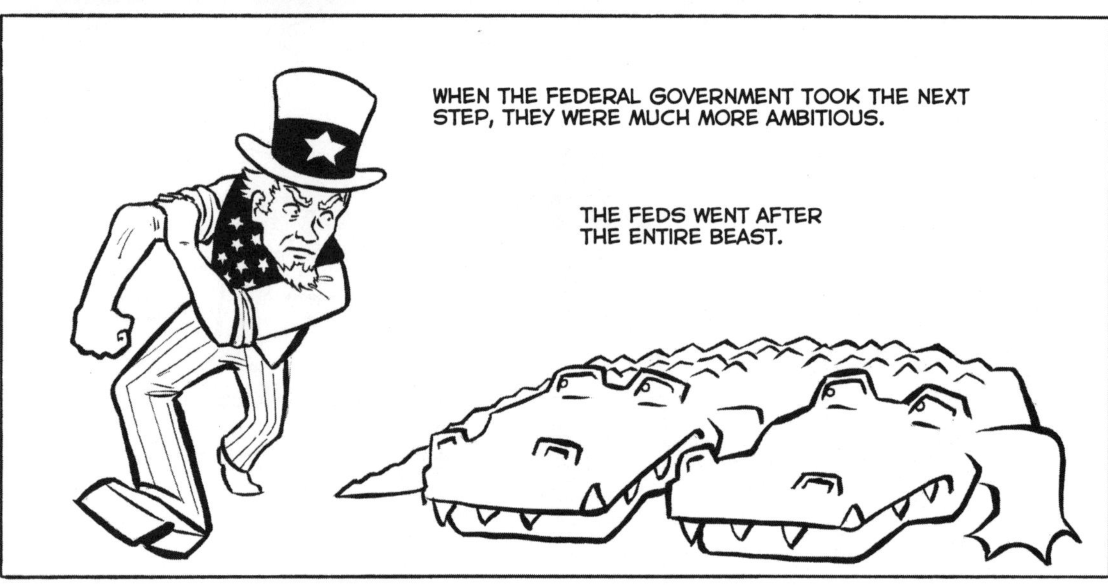
WHEN THE FEDERAL GOVERNMENT TOOK THE NEXT STEP, THEY WERE MUCH MORE AMBITIOUS.
THE FEDS WENT AFTER THE ENTIRE BEAST.

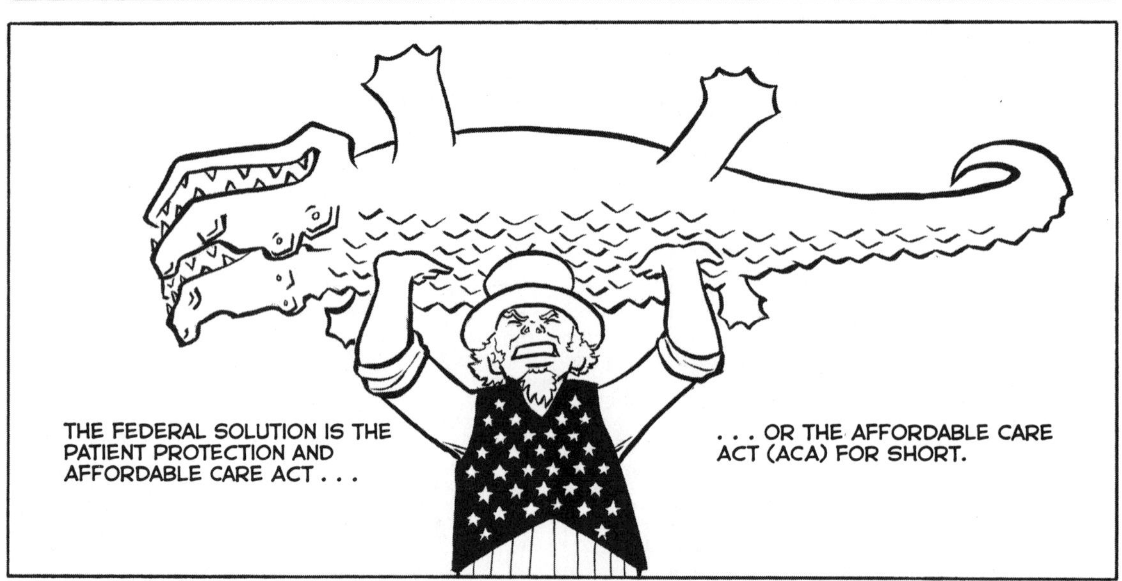
THE FEDERAL SOLUTION IS THE PATIENT PROTECTION AND AFFORDABLE CARE ACT . . .
. . . OR THE AFFORDABLE CARE ACT (ACA) FOR SHORT.

CHAPTER 6 THE AFFORDABLE CARE ACT, A.K.A. ACA

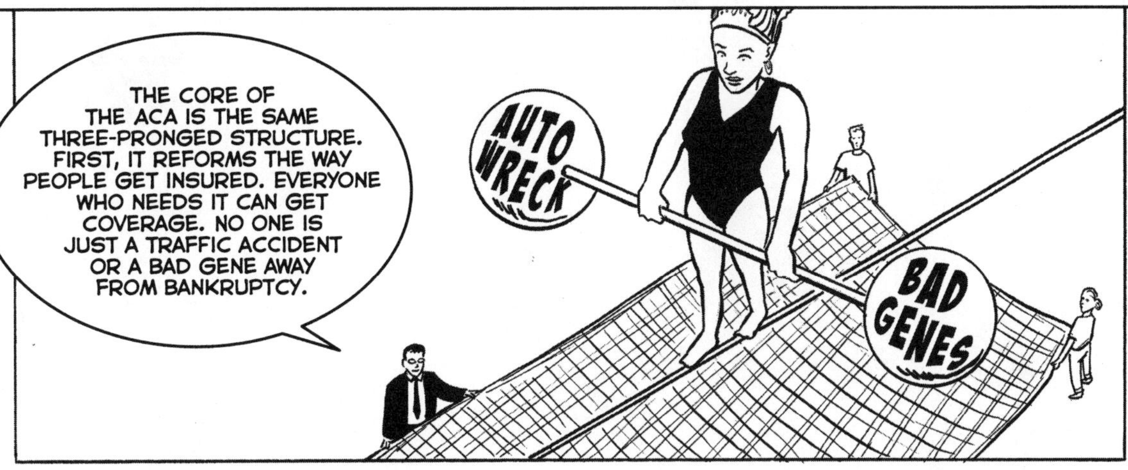

THE CORE OF THE ACA IS THE SAME THREE-PRONGED STRUCTURE. FIRST, IT REFORMS THE WAY PEOPLE GET INSURED. EVERYONE WHO NEEDS IT CAN GET COVERAGE. NO ONE IS JUST A TRAFFIC ACCIDENT OR A BAD GENE AWAY FROM BANKRUPTCY.
AUTO WRECK
BAD GENES

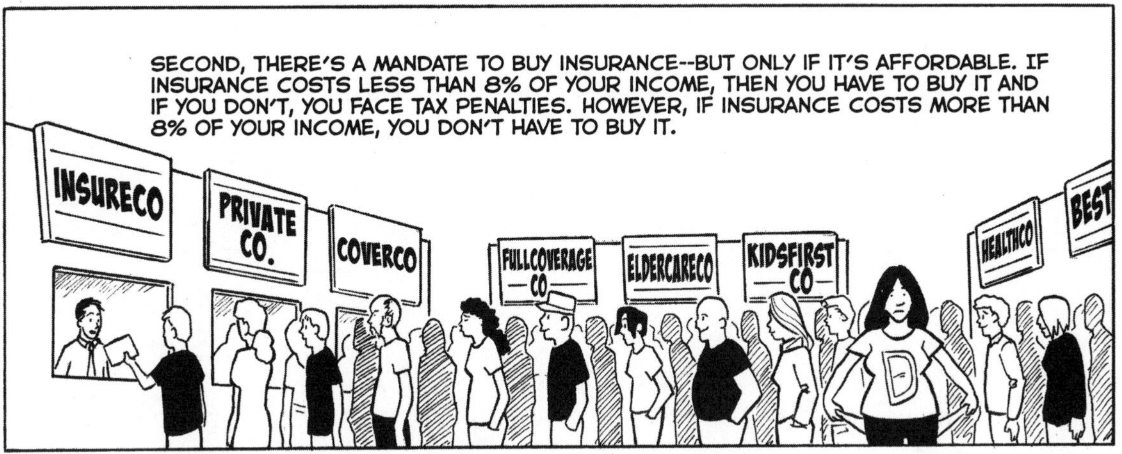

SECOND, THERE'S A MANDATE TO BUY INSURANCE--BUT ONLY IF IT'S AFFORDABLE. IF INSURANCE COSTS LESS THAN 8% OF YOUR INCOME, THEN YOU HAVE TO BUY IT AND IF YOU DON'T, YOU FACE TAX PENALTIES. HOWEVER, IF INSURANCE COSTS MORE THAN 8% OF YOUR INCOME, YOU DON'T HAVE TO BUY IT.
INSURECO
PRIVATE CO.
COVERCO
FULLCOVERAGE CO
ELDERCARECO
KIDSFIRST CO
HEALTHCO
BEST
D

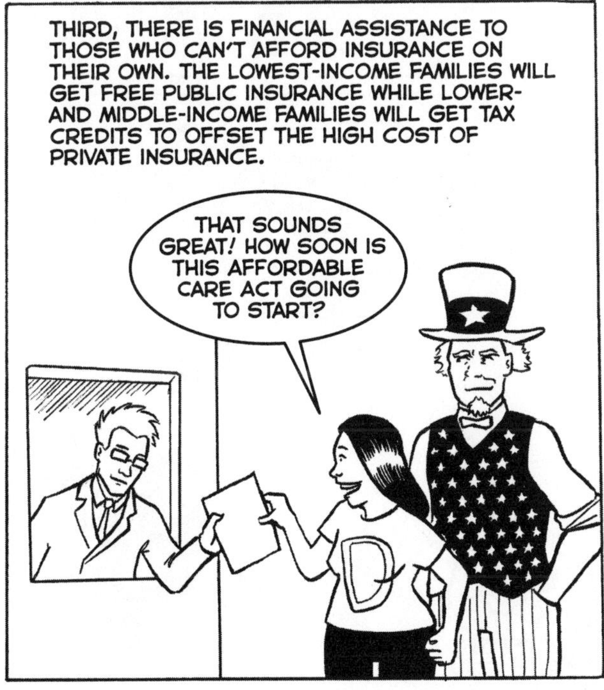

THIRD, THERE IS FINANCIAL ASSISTANCE TO THOSE WHO CAN'T AFFORD INSURANCE ON THEIR OWN. THE LOWEST-INCOME FAMILIES WILL GET FREE PUBLIC INSURANCE WHILE LOWER- AND MIDDLE-INCOME FAMILIES WILL GET TAX CREDITS TO OFFSET THE HIGH COST OF PRIVATE INSURANCE.
THAT SOUNDS GREAT! HOW SOON IS THIS AFFORDABLE CARE ACT GOING TO START?
D

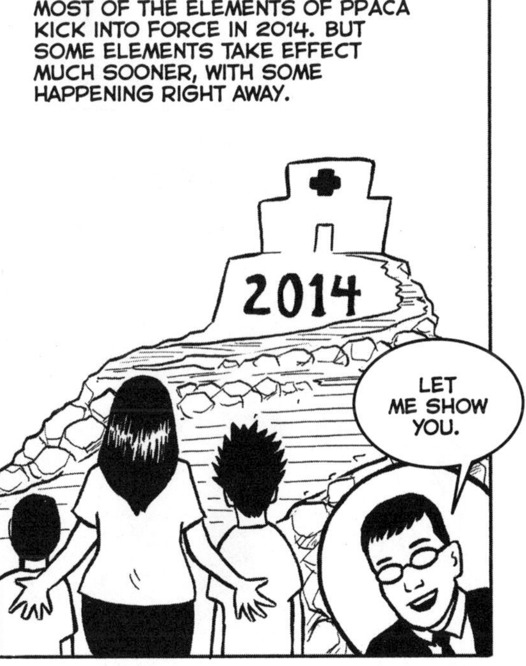

MOST OF THE ELEMENTS OF PPACA KICK INTO FORCE IN 2014. BUT SOME ELEMENTS TAKE EFFECT MUCH SOONER, WITH SOME HAPPENING RIGHT AWAY.
2014
LET ME SHOW YOU.

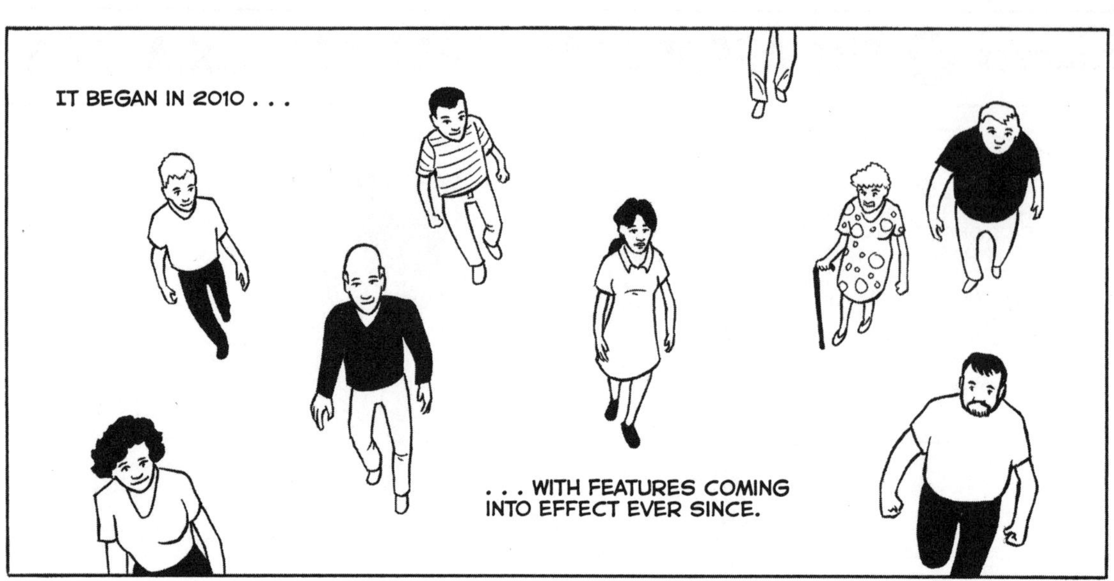
IT BEGAN IN 2010 . . .
. . . WITH FEATURES COMING INTO EFFECT EVER SINCE.

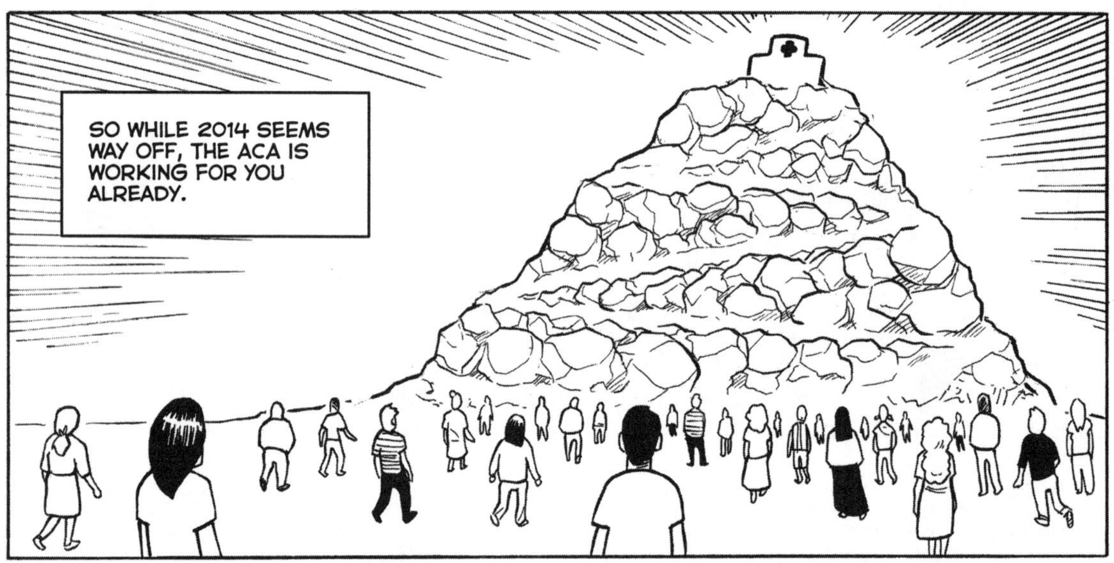
SO WHILE 2014 SEEMS WAY OFF, THE ACA IS WORKING FOR YOU ALREADY.

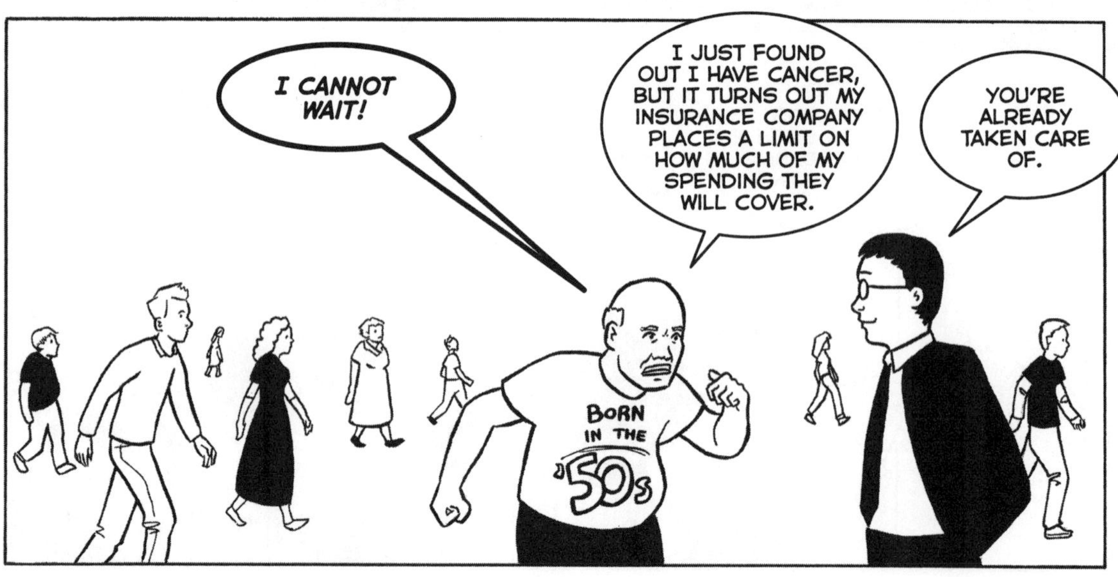
I CANNOT WAIT!
I JUST FOUND OUT I HAVE CANCER, BUT IT TURNS OUT MY INSURANCE COMPANY PLACES A LIMIT ON HOW MUCH OF MY SPENDING THEY WILL COVER.
YOU'RE ALREADY TAKEN CARE OF.
BORN IN THE 50s

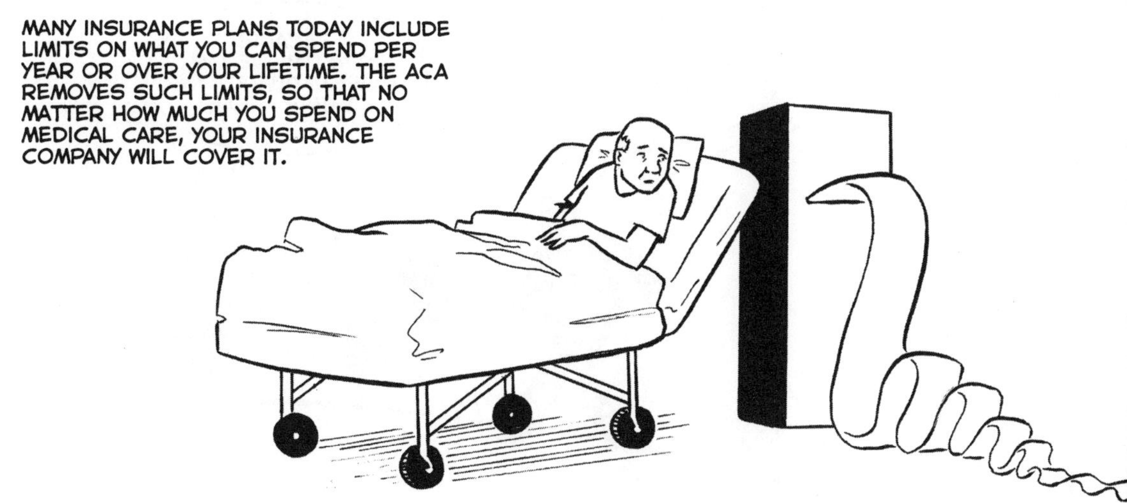
MANY INSURANCE PLANS TODAY INCLUDE LIMITS ON WHAT YOU CAN SPEND PER YEAR OR OVER YOUR LIFETIME. THE ACA REMOVES SUCH LIMITS, SO THAT NO MATTER HOW MUCH YOU SPEND ON MEDICAL CARE, YOUR INSURANCE COMPANY WILL COVER IT.

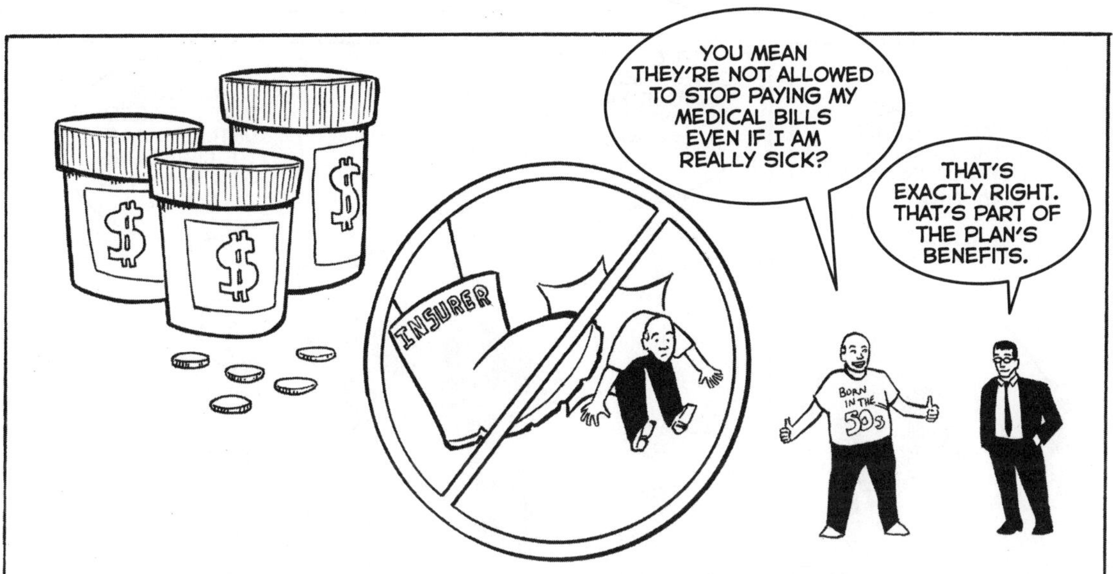
YOU MEAN THEY'RE NOT ALLOWED TO STOP PAYING MY MEDICAL BILLS EVEN IF I AM REALLY SICK?
THAT'S EXACTLY RIGHT. THAT'S PART OF THE PLAN'S BENEFITS.
INSURER
BORN IN THE 50s

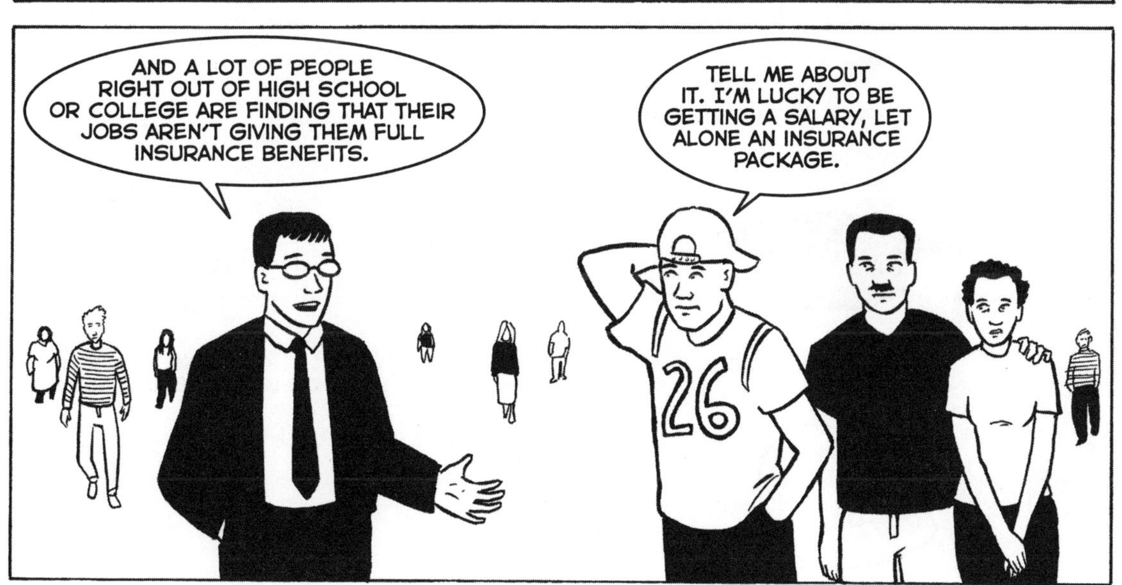
AND A LOT OF PEOPLE RIGHT OUT OF HIGH SCHOOL OR COLLEGE ARE FINDING THAT THEIR JOBS AREN'T GIVING THEM FULL INSURANCE BENEFITS.
TELL ME ABOUT IT. I'M LUCKY TO BE GETTING A SALARY, LET ALONE AN INSURANCE PACKAGE.
26

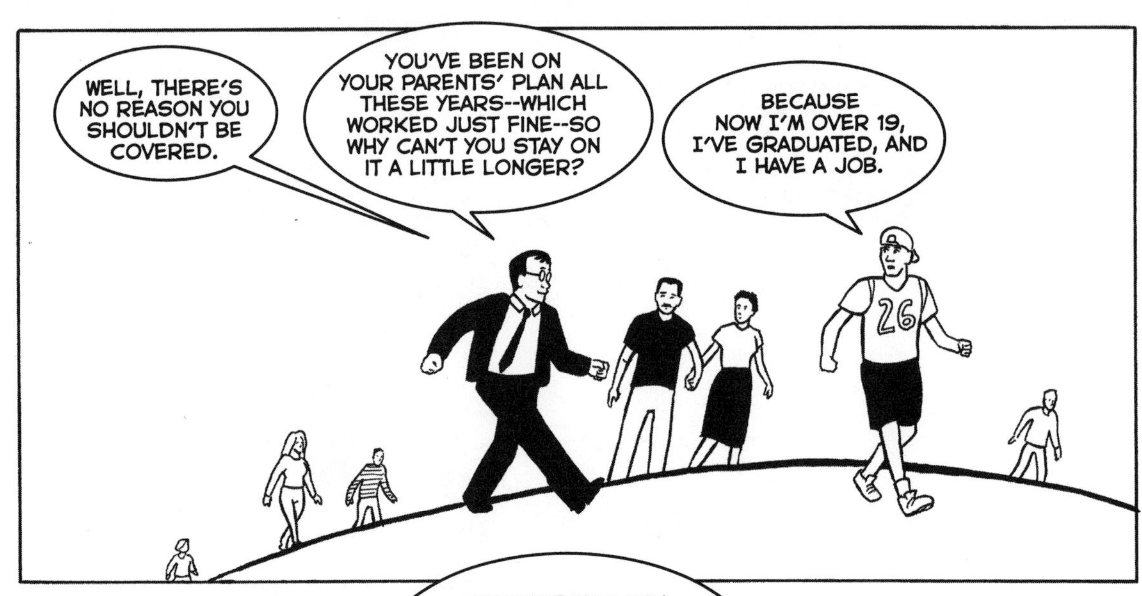
WELL, THERE'S NO REASON YOU SHOULDN'T BE COVERED.
YOU'VE BEEN ON YOUR PARENTS' PLAN ALL THESE YEARS--WHICH WORKED JUST FINE--SO WHY CAN'T YOU STAY ON IT A LITTLE LONGER?
BECAUSE NOW I'M OVER 19, I'VE GRADUATED, AND I HAVE A JOB.

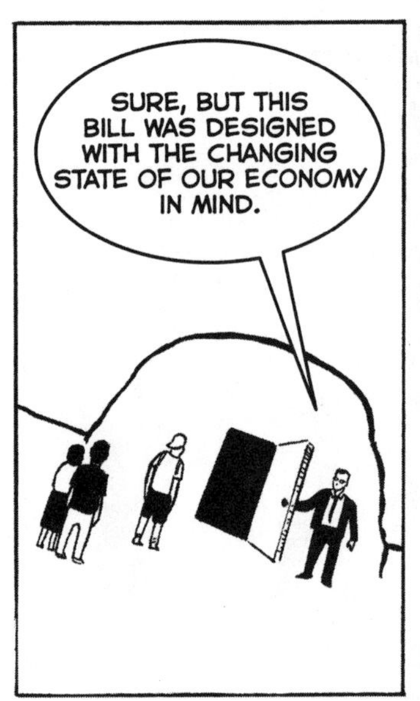
SURE, BUT THIS BILL WAS DESIGNED WITH THE CHANGING STATE OF OUR ECONOMY IN MIND.

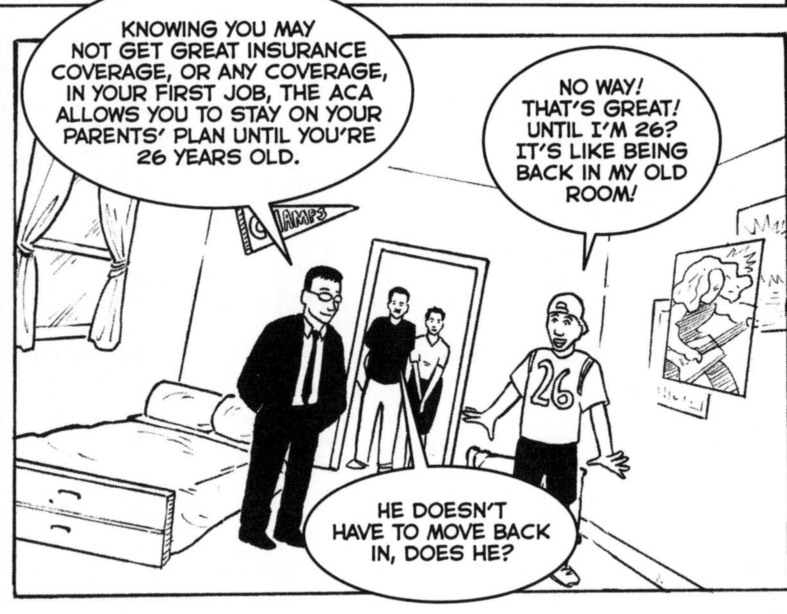
KNOWING YOU MAY NOT GET GREAT INSURANCE COVERAGE, OR ANY COVERAGE, IN YOUR FIRST JOB, THE ACA ALLOWS YOU TO STAY ON YOUR PARENTS' PLAN UNTIL YOU'RE 26 YEARS OLD.
NO WAY! THAT'S GREAT! UNTIL I'M 26? IT'S LIKE BEING BACK IN MY OLD ROOM!
HE DOESN'T HAVE TO MOVE BACK IN, DOES HE?

NO--HE CAN BE PART OF THE PLAN WHETHER:

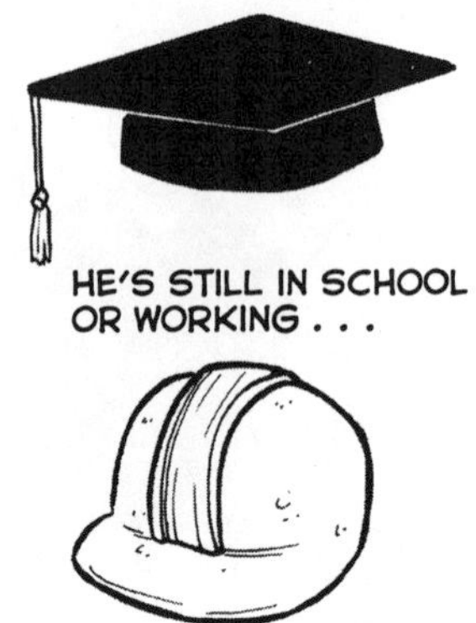

HE'S STILL IN SCHOOL OR WORKING . . .

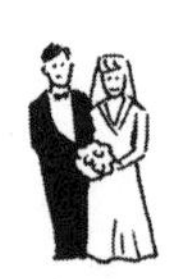

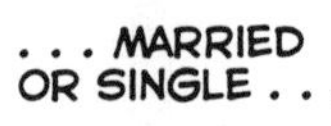

. . . MARRIED OR SINGLE . . .

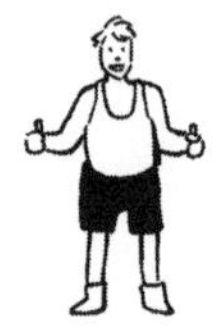

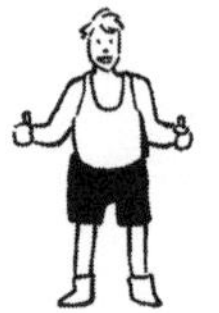

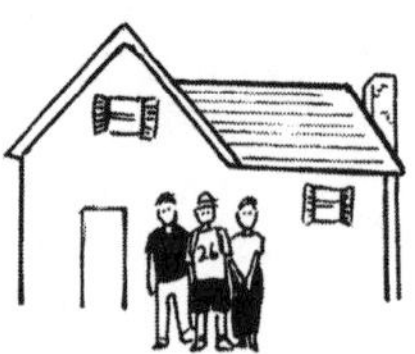

. . . OR LIVING WITH YOU OR SOMEWHERE ELSE.

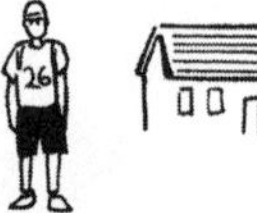

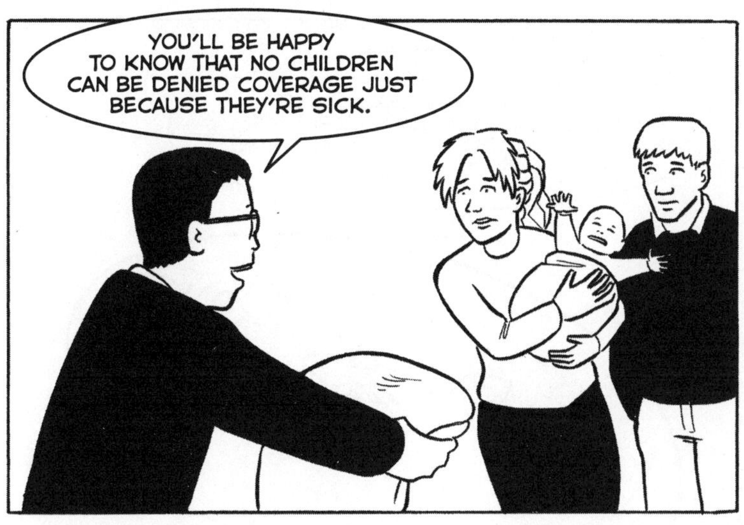
YOU'LL BE HAPPY TO KNOW THAT NO CHILDREN CAN BE DENIED COVERAGE JUST BECAUSE THEY'RE SICK.

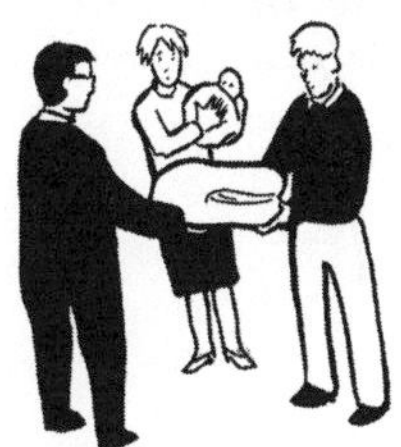
SO WE CAN GET COVERAGE FOR OUR DAUGHTER EVEN THOUGH SHE HAD A BIRTH DEFECT?

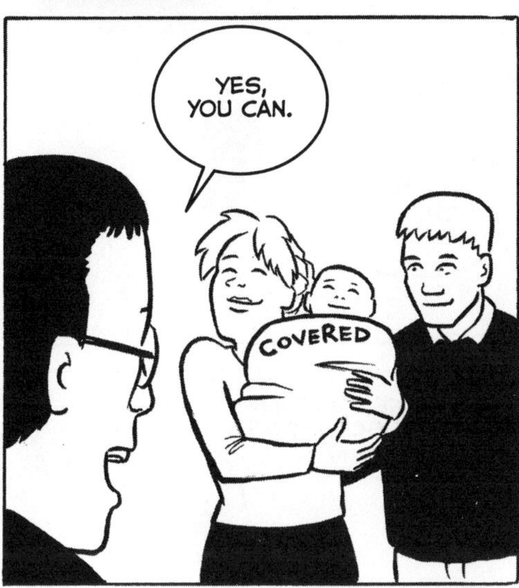
YES, YOU CAN.
COVERED

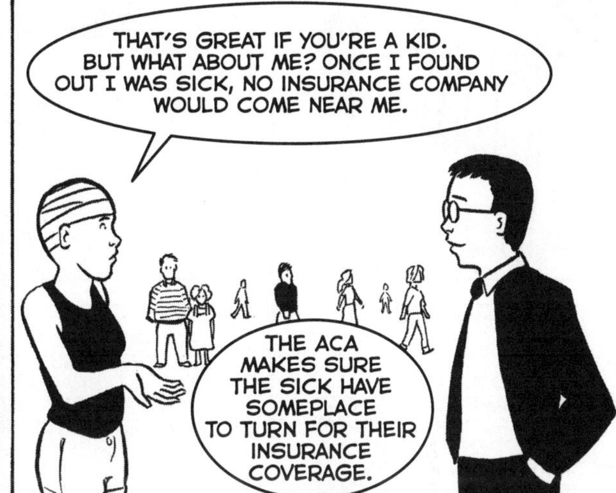
THAT'S GREAT IF YOU'RE A KID. BUT WHAT ABOUT ME? ONCE I FOUND OUT I WAS SICK, NO INSURANCE COMPANY WOULD COME NEAR ME.
THE ACA MAKES SURE THE SICK HAVE SOMEPLACE TO TURN FOR THEIR INSURANCE COVERAGE.

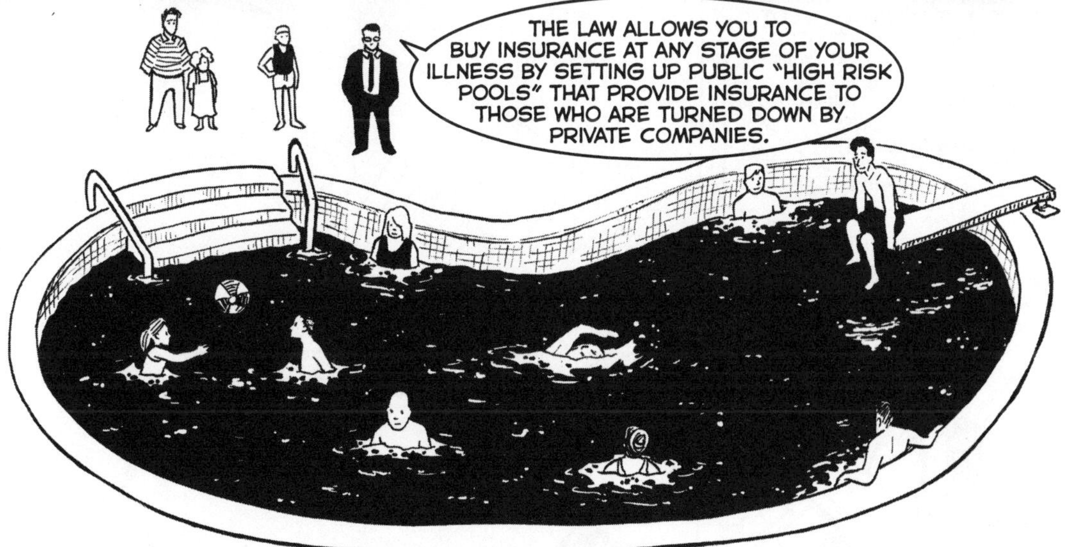
THE LAW ALLOWS YOU TO BUY INSURANCE AT ANY STAGE OF YOUR ILLNESS BY SETTING UP PUBLIC "HIGH RISK POOLS" THAT PROVIDE INSURANCE TO THOSE WHO ARE TURNED DOWN BY PRIVATE COMPANIES.
HIGH-RISK

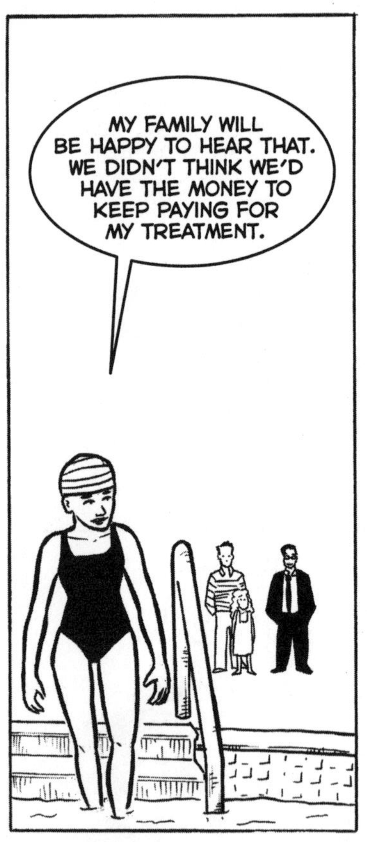
MY FAMILY WILL BE HAPPY TO HEAR THAT. WE DIDN'T THINK WE'D HAVE THE MONEY TO KEEP PAYING FOR MY TREATMENT.

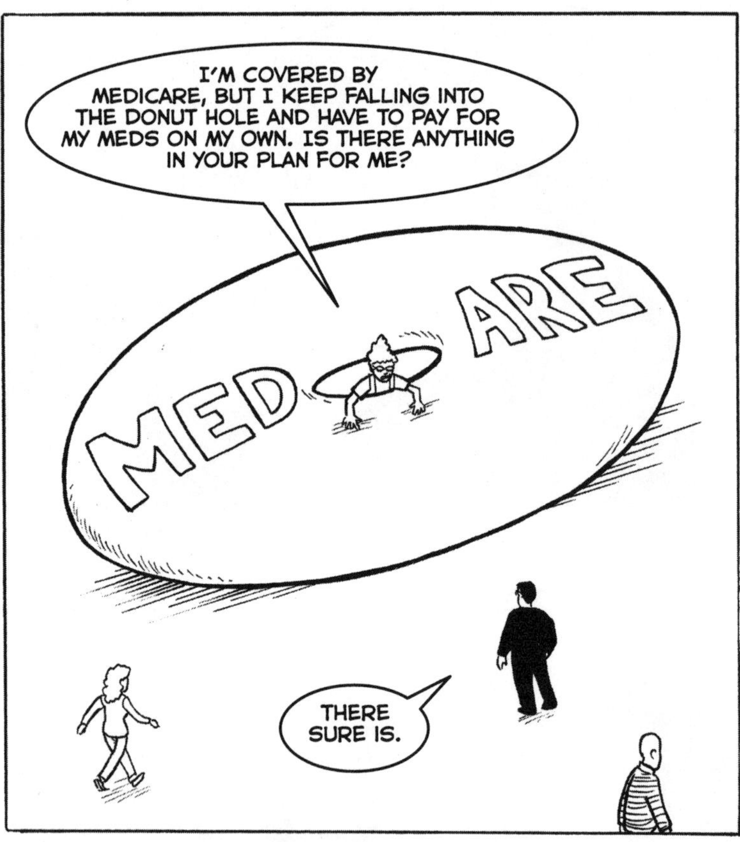
I'M COVERED BY MEDICARE, BUT I KEEP FALLING INTO THE DONUT HOLE AND HAVE TO PAY FOR MY MEDS ON MY OWN. IS THERE ANYTHING IN YOUR PLAN FOR ME?
MED ARE
THERE SURE IS.

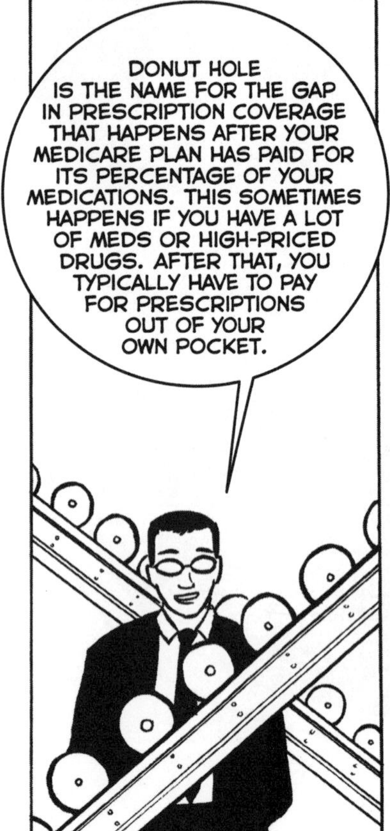
DONUT HOLE IS THE NAME FOR THE GAP IN PRESCRIPTION COVERAGE THAT HAPPENS AFTER YOUR MEDICARE PLAN HAS PAID FOR ITS PERCENTAGE OF YOUR MEDICATIONS. THIS SOMETIMES HAPPENS IF YOU HAVE A LOT OF MEDS OR HIGH-PRICED DRUGS. AFTER THAT, YOU TYPICALLY HAVE TO PAY FOR PRESCRIPTIONS OUT OF YOUR OWN POCKET.

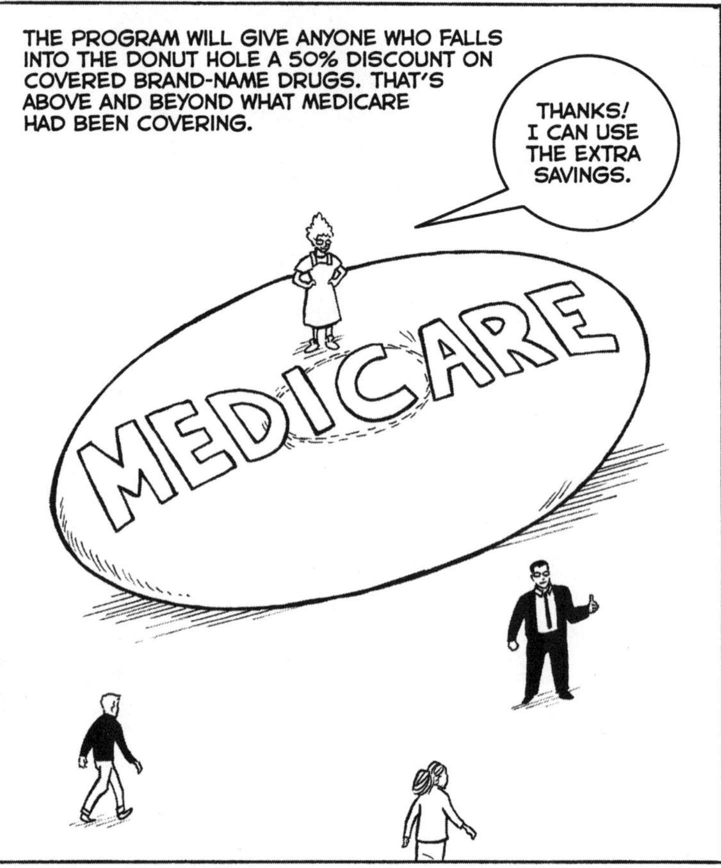
THE PROGRAM WILL GIVE ANYONE WHO FALLS INTO THE DONUT HOLE A 50% DISCOUNT ON COVERED BRAND-NAME DRUGS. THAT'S ABOVE AND BEYOND WHAT MEDICARE HAD BEEN COVERING.
THANKS! I CAN USE THE EXTRA SAVINGS.
MEDICARE

ONE WAY TO BETTER, CHEAPER HEALTH CARE INCLUDES PREVENTING INDIVIDUAL HEALTH PROBLEMS BEFORE THEY OCCUR. THE ACA MANDATES THAT PRIVATE INSURANCE COVER THOSE PREVENTIVE SERVICES--AT NO COST TO THE CONSUMER.

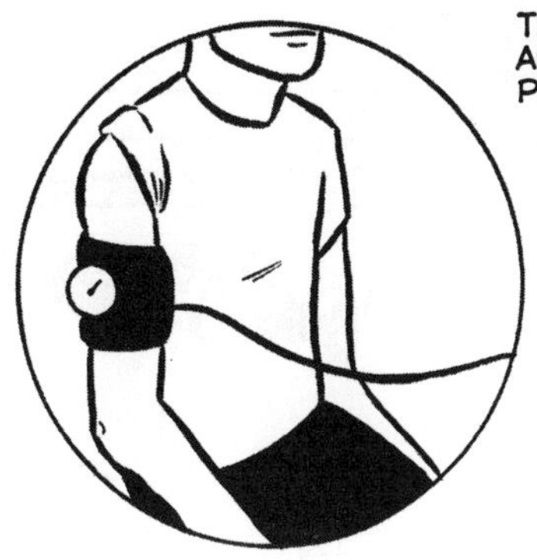

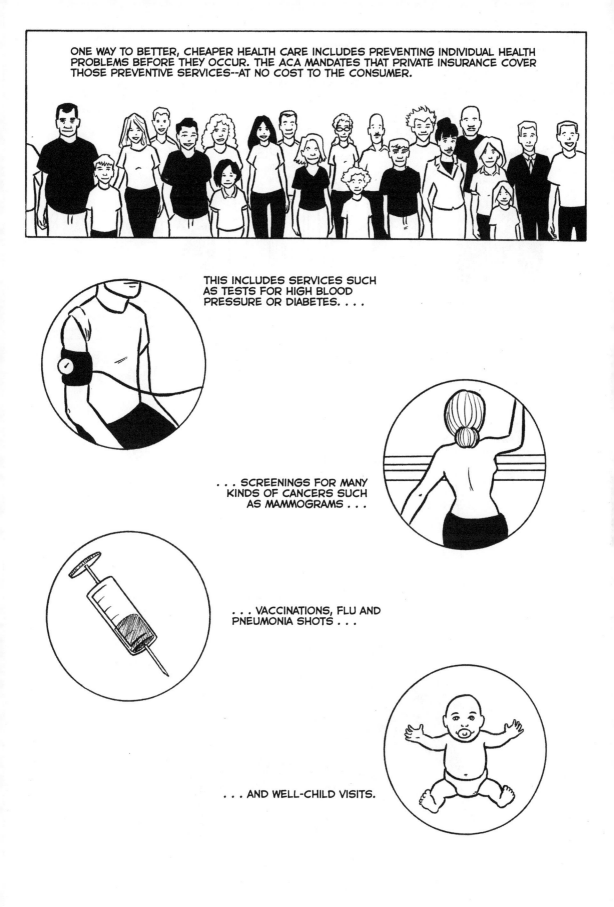

THIS INCLUDES SERVICES SUCH AS TESTS FOR HIGH BLOOD PRESSURE OR DIABETES. . . .

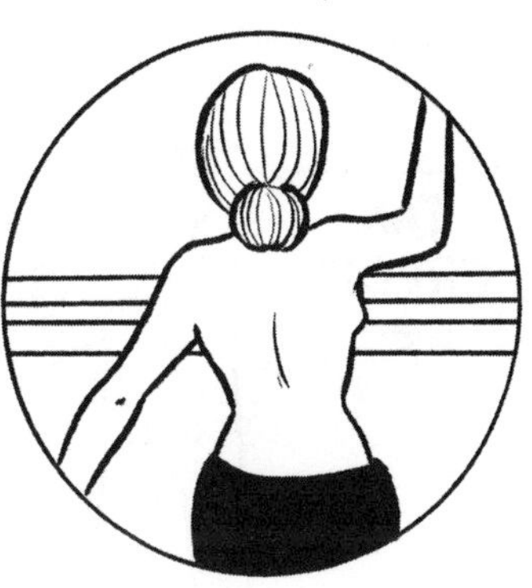

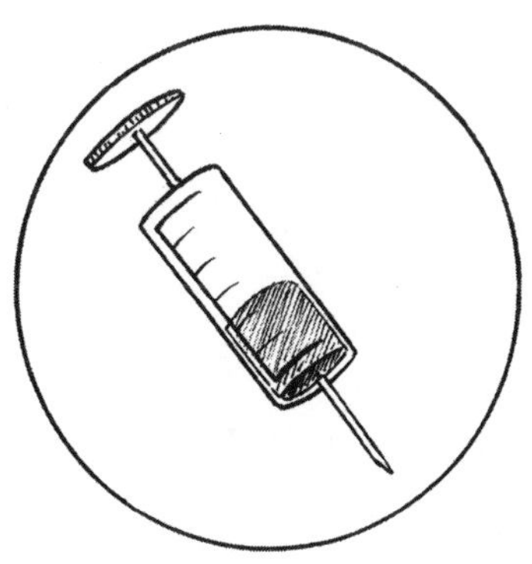

. . . SCREENINGS FOR MANY KINDS OF CANCERS SUCH AS MAMMOGRAMS . . .

. . . VACCINATIONS, FLU AND PNEUMONIA SHOTS . . .

. . . AND WELL-CHILD VISITS.

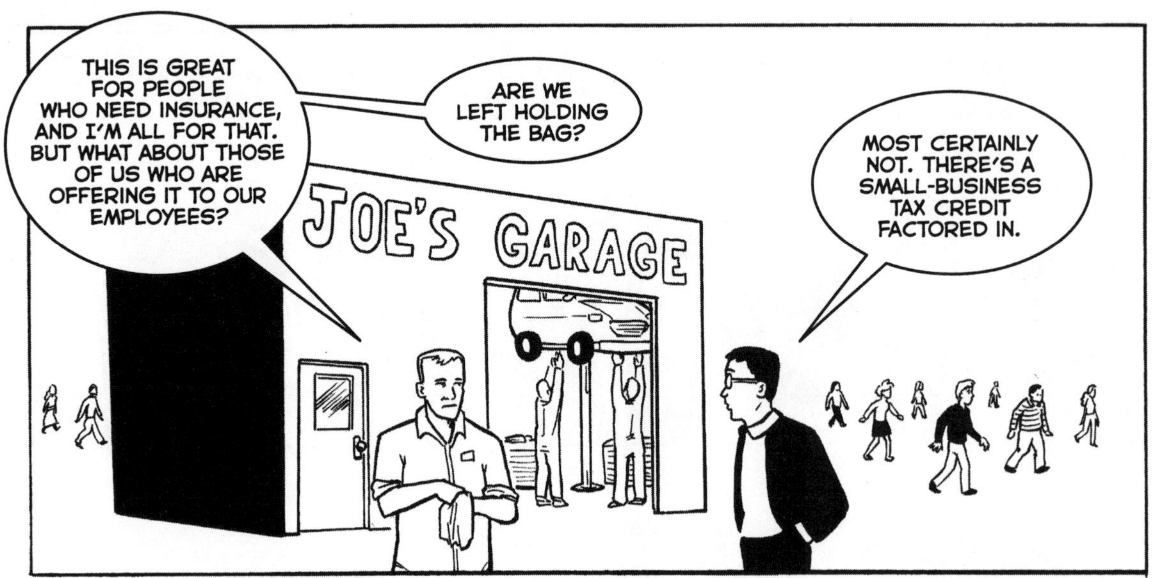
THIS IS GREAT FOR PEOPLE WHO NEED INSURANCE, AND I'M ALL FOR THAT. BUT WHAT ABOUT THOSE OF US WHO ARE OFFERING IT TO OUR EMPLOYEES?
ARE WE LEFT HOLDING THE BAG?
JOE'S GARAGE
MOST CERTAINLY NOT. THERE'S A SMALL-BUSINESS TAX CREDIT FACTORED IN.

IF YOU OWN A BUSINESS AND EMPLOY FEWER THAN 25 PEOPLE--AND YOU PROVIDE THEM HEALTH INSURANCE--YOU COULD QUALIFY FOR A TAX CREDIT THAT WOULD OFFSET THE COST OF YOUR INSURANCE.

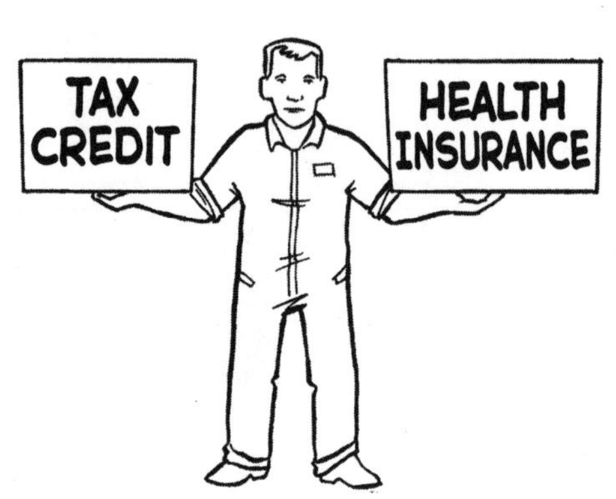
TAX CREDIT
HEALTH INSURANCE

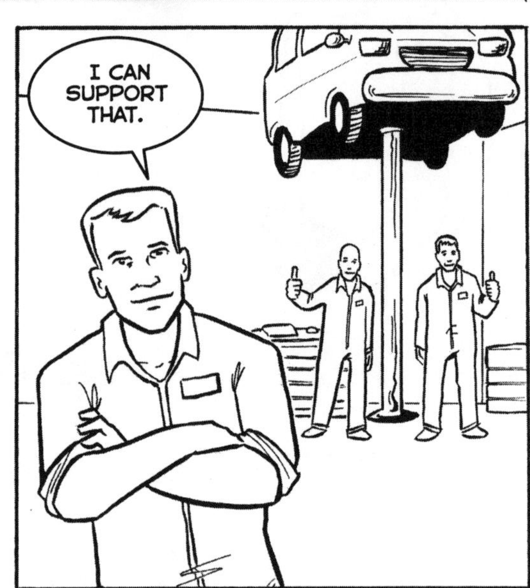
I CAN SUPPORT THAT.

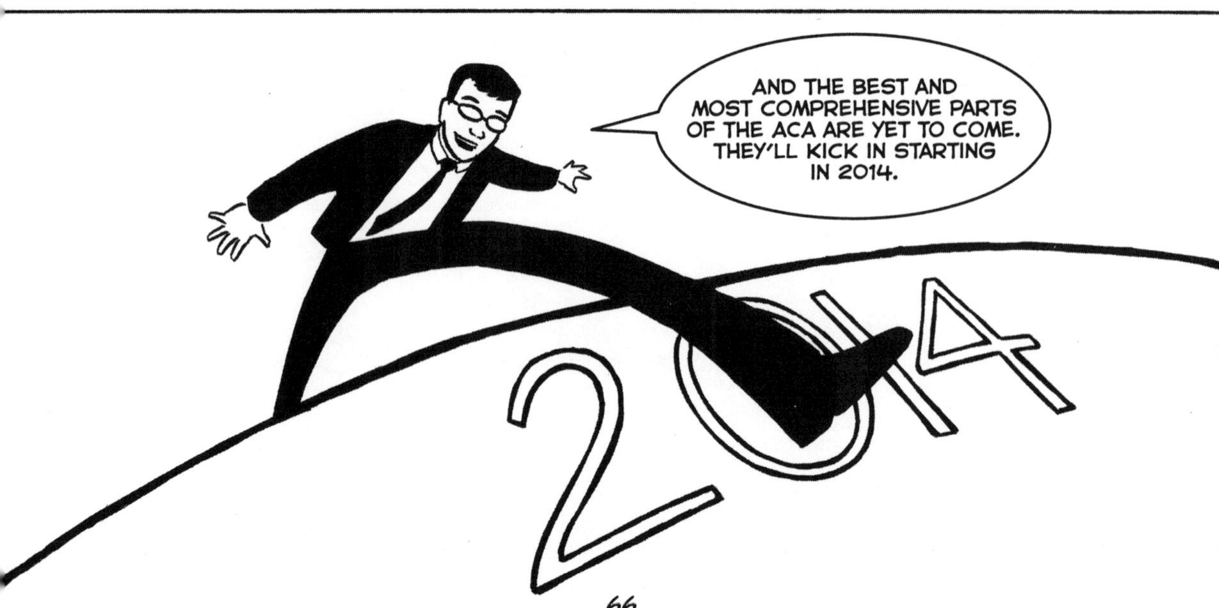
AND THE BEST AND MOST COMPREHENSIVE PARTS OF THE ACA ARE YET TO COME. THEY'LL KICK IN STARTING IN 2014.
2014

CHAPTER 7 DON'T WORRY, WE'VE GOT YOU COVERED

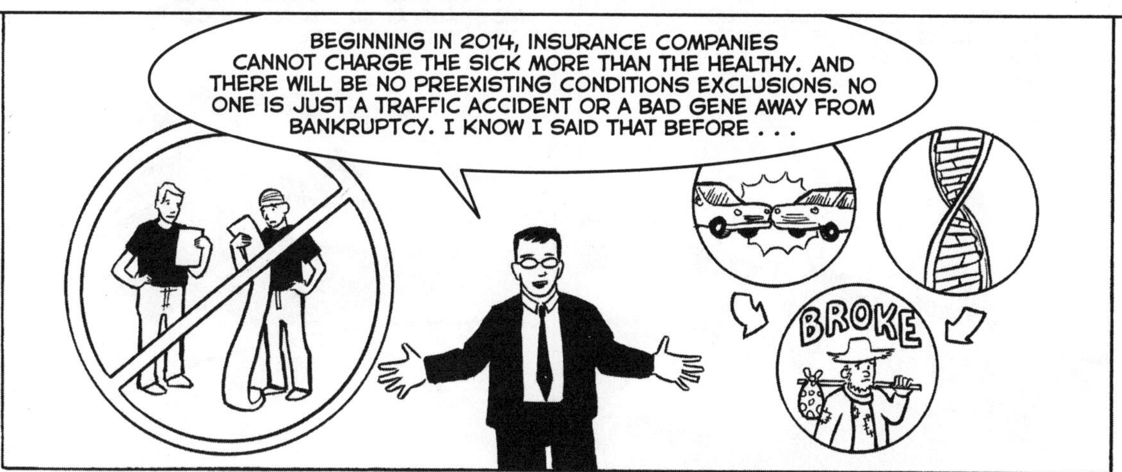

BEGINNING IN 2014, INSURANCE COMPANIES CANNOT CHARGE THE SICK MORE THAN THE HEALTHY. AND THERE WILL BE NO PREEXISTING CONDITIONS EXCLUSIONS. NO ONE IS JUST A TRAFFIC ACCIDENT OR A BAD GENE AWAY FROM BANKRUPTCY. I KNOW I SAID THAT BEFORE . . .
BROKE

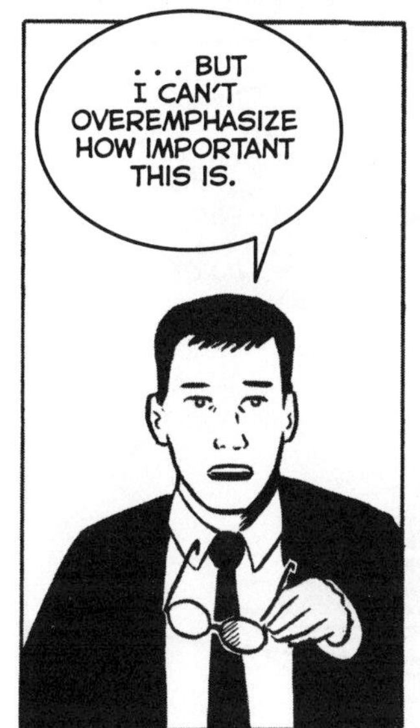

. . . BUT I CAN'T OVEREMPHASIZE HOW IMPORTANT THIS IS.

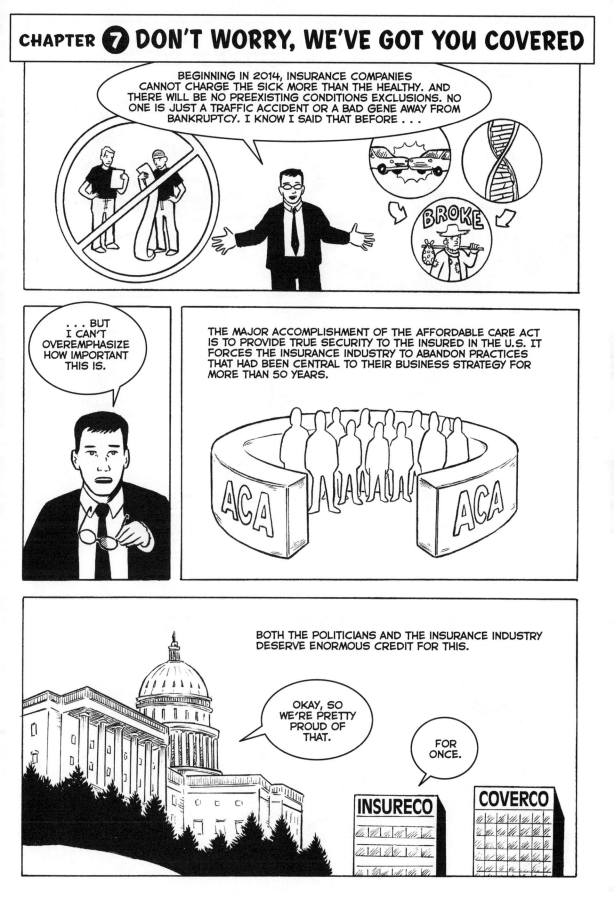

THE MAJOR ACCOMPLISHMENT OF THE AFFORDABLE CARE ACT IS TO PROVIDE TRUE SECURITY TO THE INSURED IN THE U.S. IT FORCES THE INSURANCE INDUSTRY TO ABANDON PRACTICES THAT HAD BEEN CENTRAL TO THEIR BUSINESS STRATEGY FOR MORE THAN 50 YEARS.

ACA
ACA

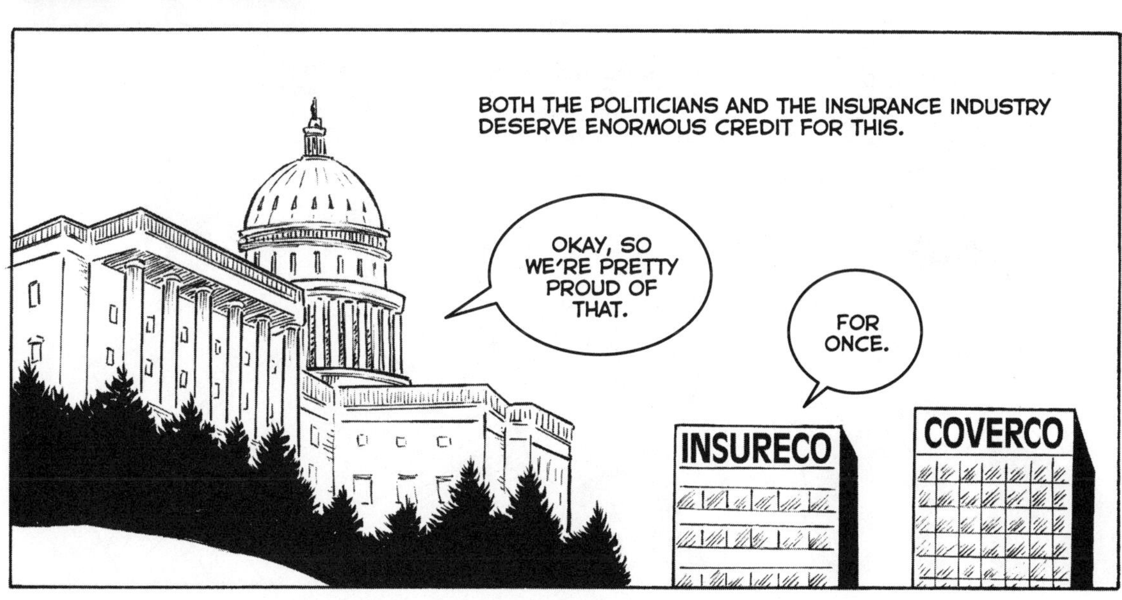

BOTH THE POLITICIANS AND THE INSURANCE INDUSTRY DESERVE ENORMOUS CREDIT FOR THIS.
OKAY, SO WE'RE PRETTY PROUD OF THAT.
FOR ONCE.
INSURECO
COVERCO

OF COURSE, AS WE DISCUSSED EARLIER, WE CAN'T GET FAIRLY PRICED INSURANCE WITHOUT ALSO HAVING AN INDIVIDUAL MANDATE.

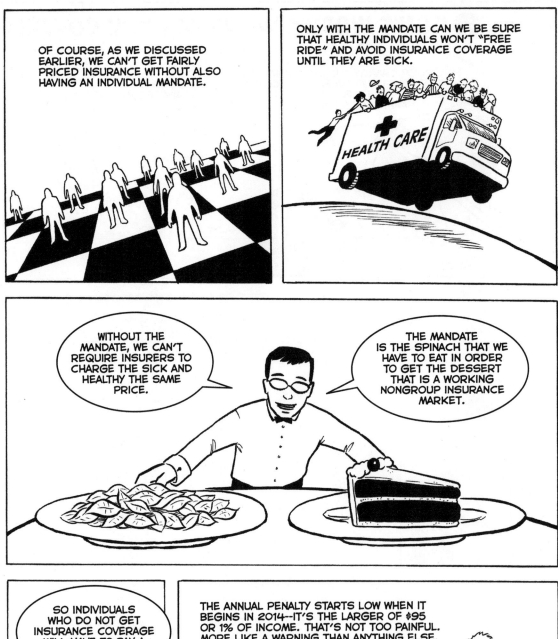

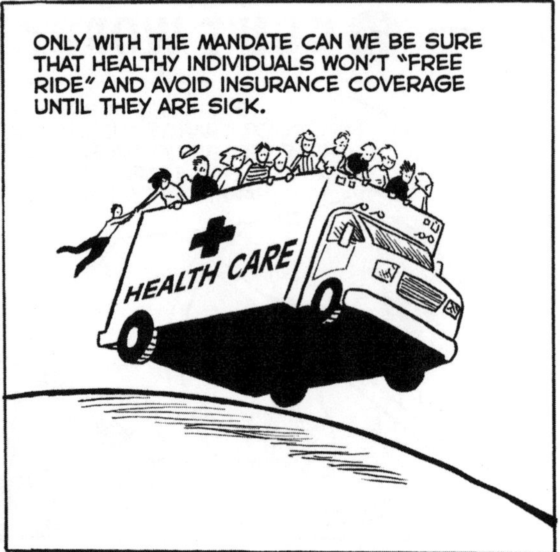

ONLY WITH THE MANDATE CAN WE BE SURE THAT HEALTHY INDIVIDUALS WON'T "FREE RIDE" AND AVOID INSURANCE COVERAGE UNTIL THEY ARE SICK.

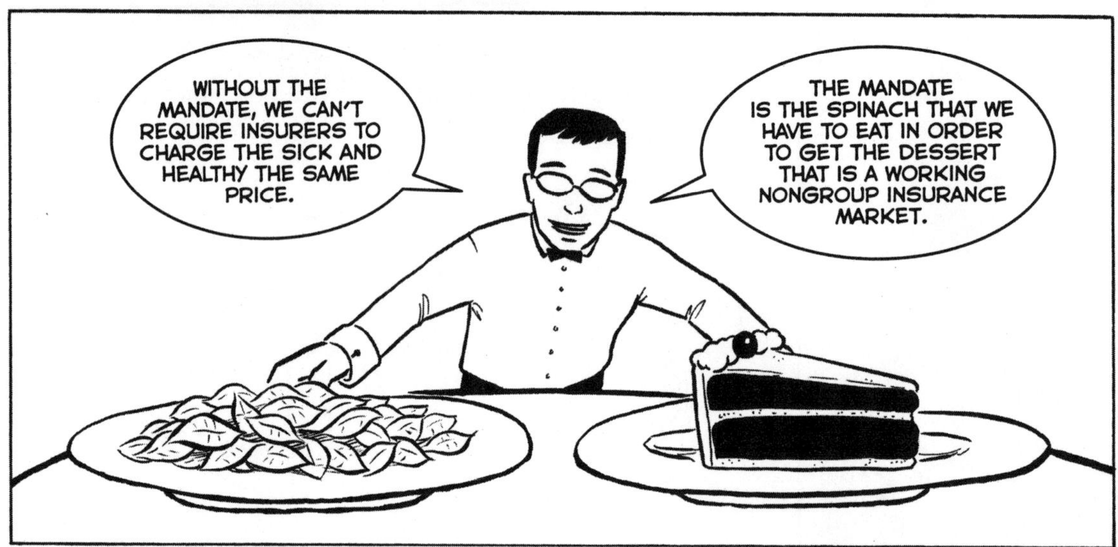
WITHOUT THE MANDATE, WE CAN'T REQUIRE INSURERS TO CHARGE THE SICK AND HEALTHY THE SAME PRICE.
THE MANDATE IS THE SPINACH THAT WE HAVE TO EAT IN ORDER TO GET THE DESSERT THAT IS A WORKING NONGROUP INSURANCE MARKET.

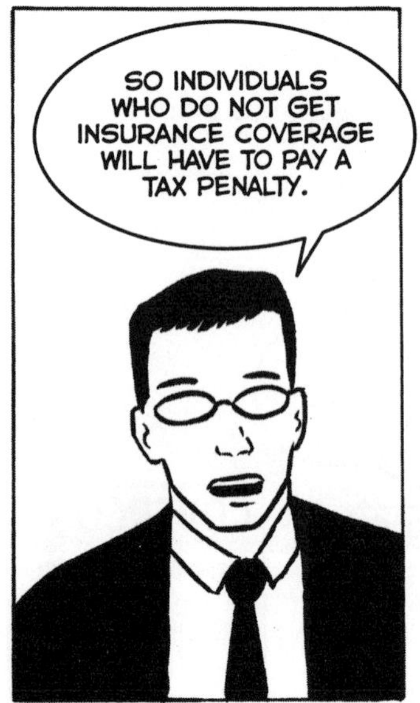
SO INDIVIDUALS WHO DO NOT GET INSURANCE COVERAGE WILL HAVE TO PAY A TAX PENALTY.

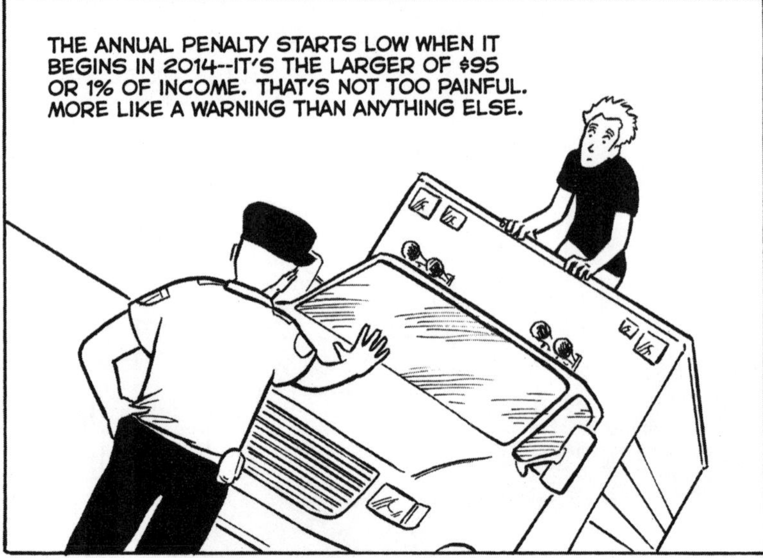
THE ANNUAL PENALTY STARTS LOW WHEN IT BEGINS IN 2014--IT'S THE LARGER OF $95 OR 1% OF INCOME. THAT'S NOT TOO PAINFUL. MORE LIKE A WARNING THAN ANYTHING ELSE.

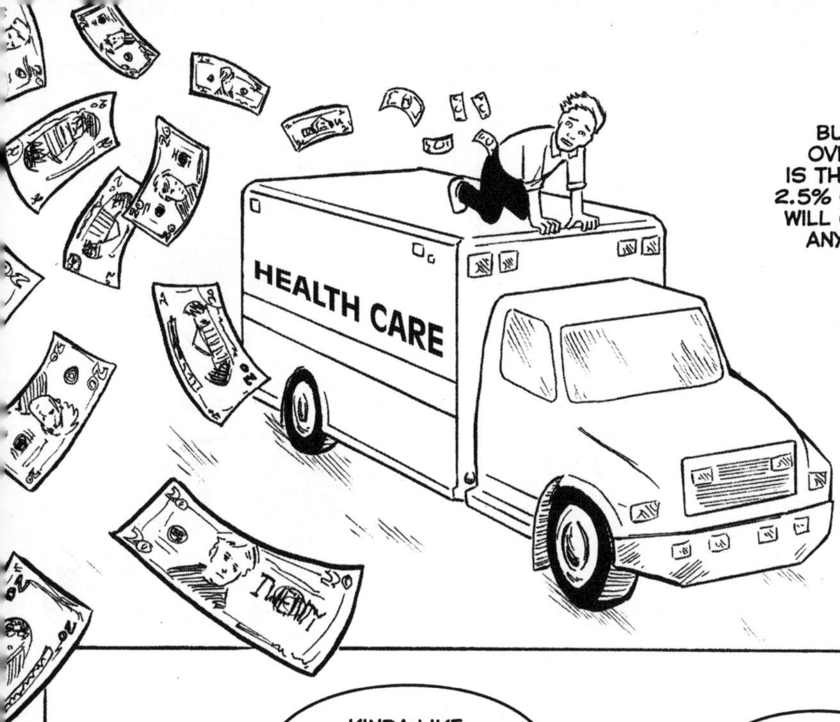

BUT THE PENALTY GROWS OVER TIME, SO BY 2016 IT IS THE LARGER OF $695 OR 2.5% OF YOUR INCOME. THAT WILL GET THE ATTENTION OF ANYONE WHO THINKS THEY CAN GET BY WITHOUT HEALTH INSURANCE.

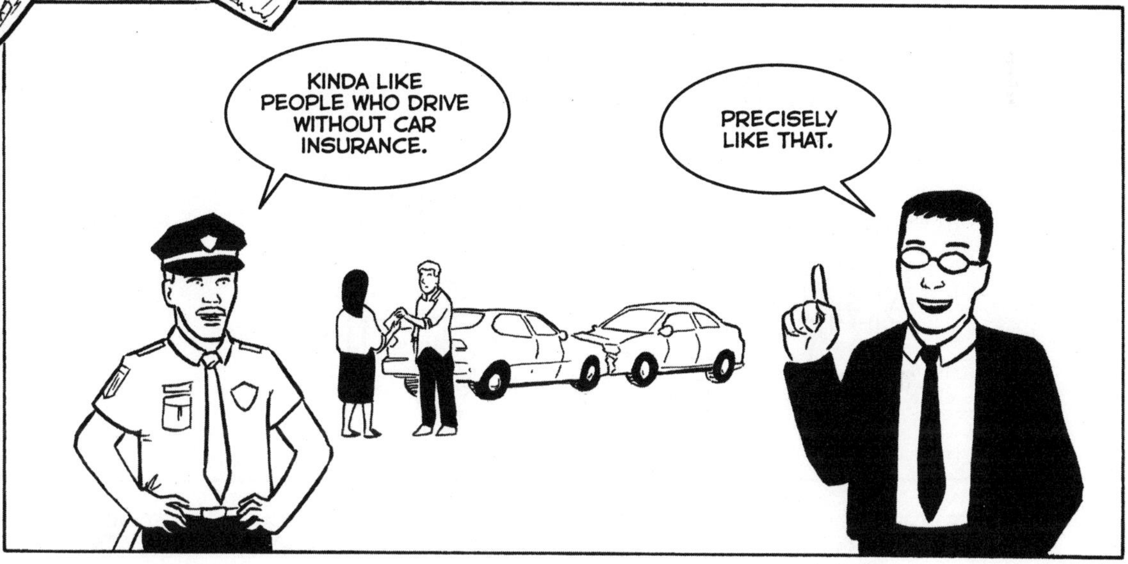

HEALTH CARE

KINDA LIKE PEOPLE WHO DRIVE WITHOUT CAR INSURANCE.

PRECISELY LIKE THAT.

IF YOU ARE GOING TO MANDATE THAT PEOPLE GET INSURANCE, YOU HAVE TO SPECIFY A MINIMUM LEVEL OF COVERAGE TO QUALIFY.

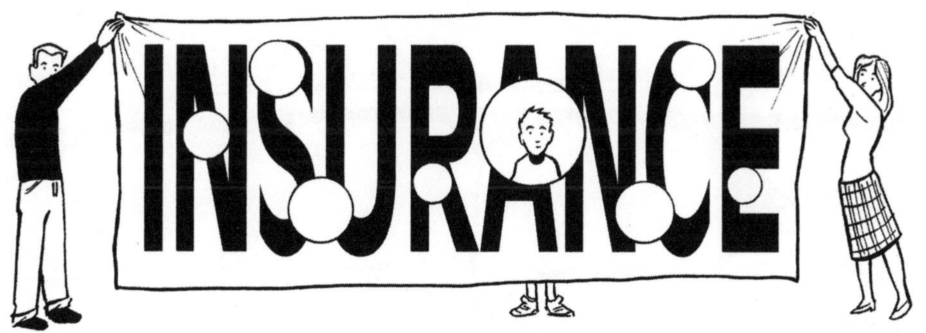

MILLIONS OF AMERICANS THINK THEY ARE FULLY INSURED BUT ACTUALLY HAVE INSURANCE WITH ENORMOUS GAPS.

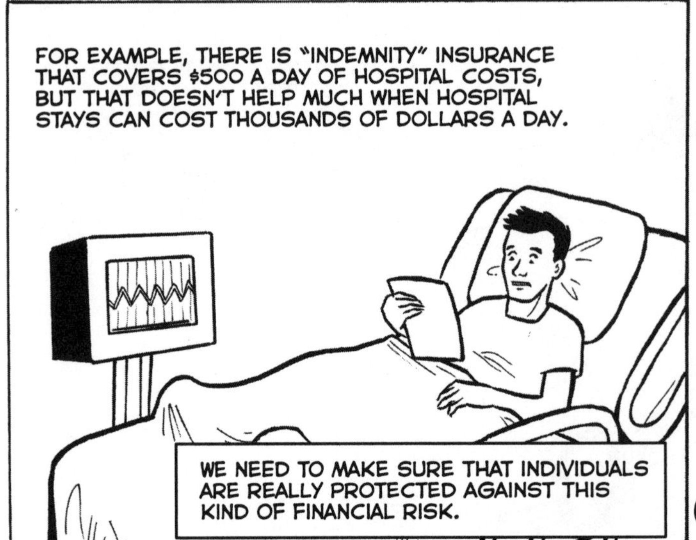
FOR EXAMPLE, THERE IS "INDEMNITY" INSURANCE THAT COVERS $500 A DAY OF HOSPITAL COSTS, BUT THAT DOESN'T HELP MUCH WHEN HOSPITAL STAYS CAN COST THOUSANDS OF DOLLARS A DAY.
WE NEED TO MAKE SURE THAT INDIVIDUALS ARE REALLY PROTECTED AGAINST THIS KIND OF FINANCIAL RISK.

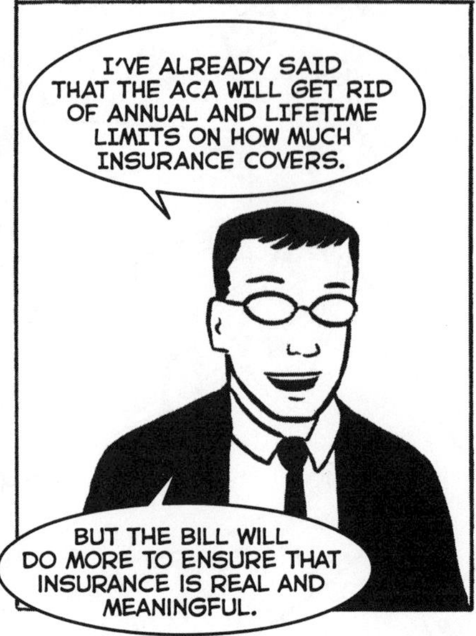
I'VE ALREADY SAID THAT THE ACA WILL GET RID OF ANNUAL AND LIFETIME LIMITS ON HOW MUCH INSURANCE COVERS.
BUT THE BILL WILL DO MORE TO ENSURE THAT INSURANCE IS REAL AND MEANINGFUL.

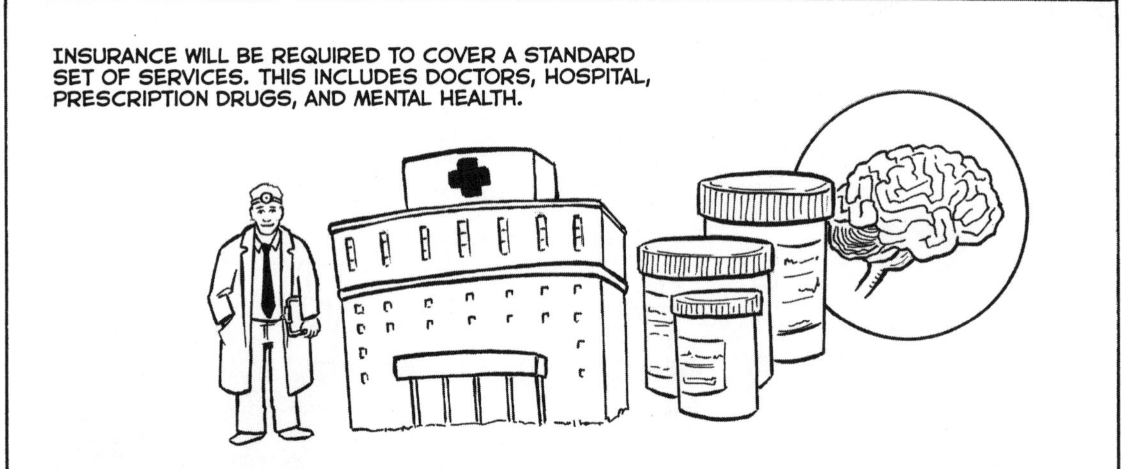
INSURANCE WILL BE REQUIRED TO COVER A STANDARD SET OF SERVICES. THIS INCLUDES DOCTORS, HOSPITAL, PRESCRIPTION DRUGS, AND MENTAL HEALTH.

MOREOVER, THE TOTAL OUT-OF-POCKET EXPENSES FACING INDIVIDUALS CAN'T EXCEED $6,000 A YEAR. THIS ENSURES THAT FOLKS AREN'T GOING TO BE BANKRUPTED BY MEDICAL COSTS.

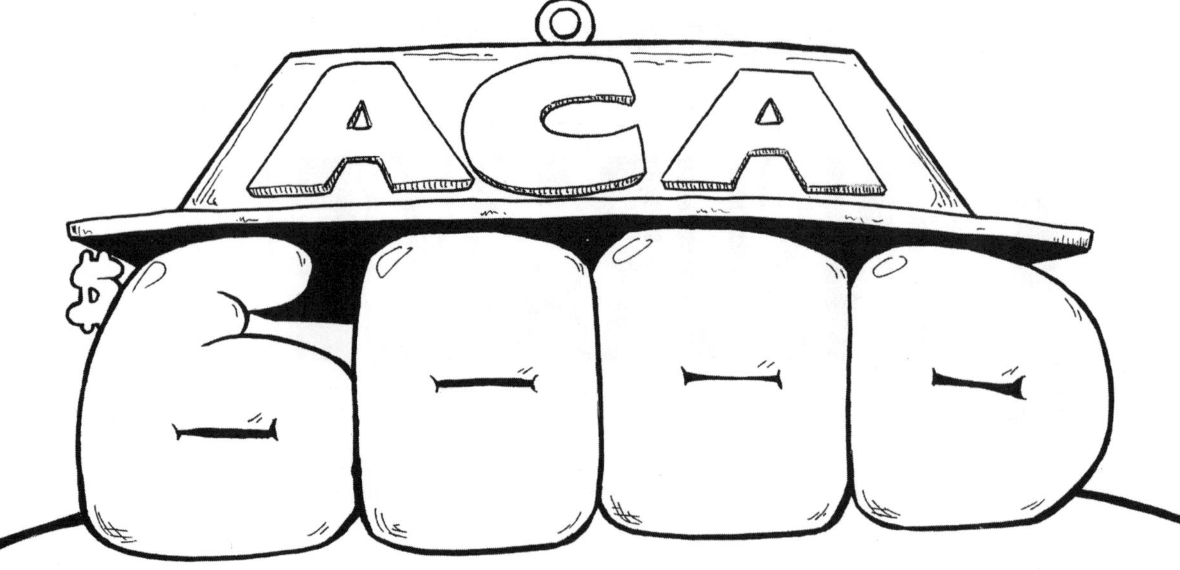

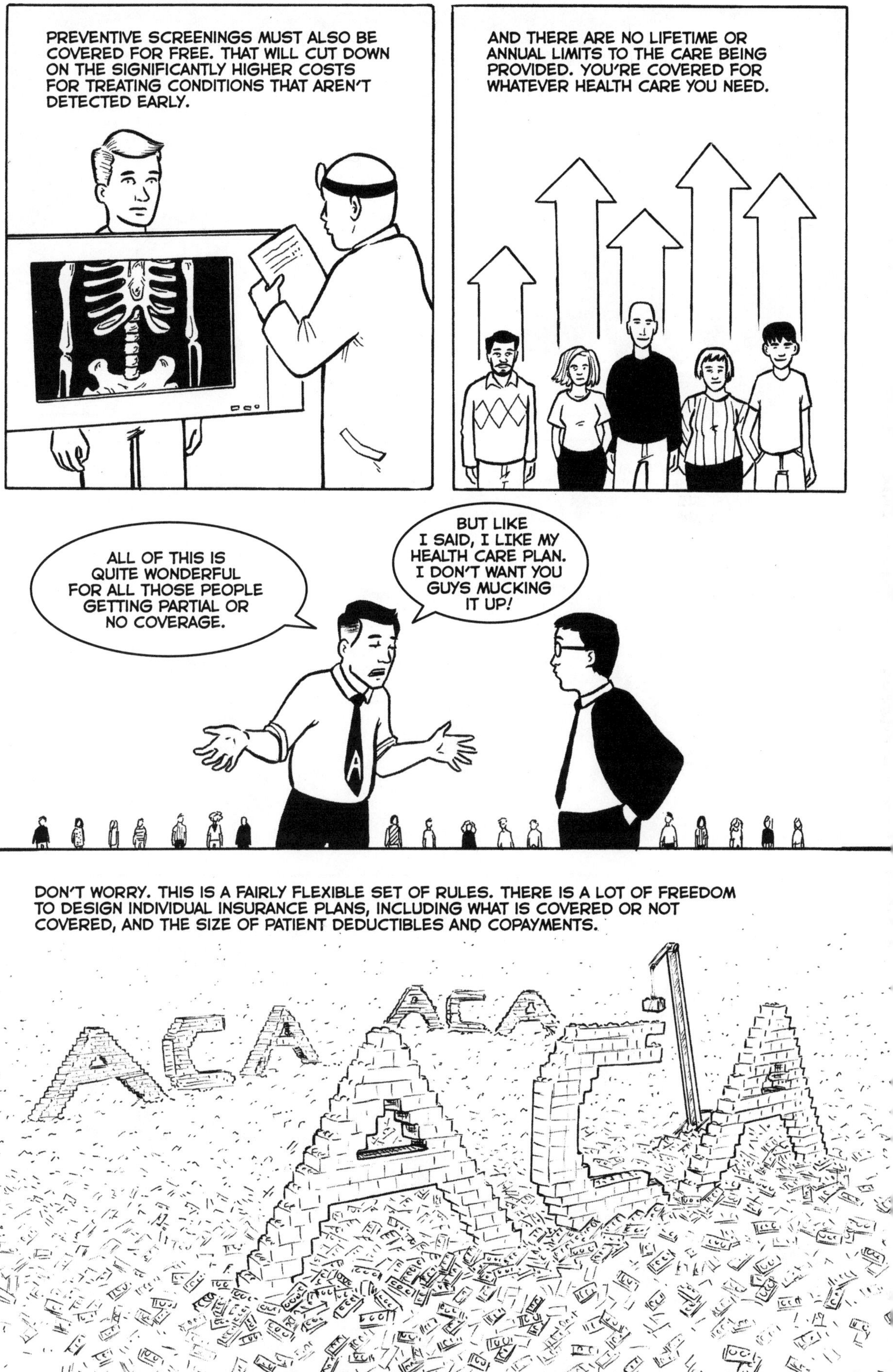

PREVENTIVE SCREENINGS MUST ALSO BE COVERED FOR FREE. THAT WILL CUT DOWN ON THE SIGNIFICANTLY HIGHER COSTS FOR TREATING CONDITIONS THAT AREN'T DETECTED EARLY.

AND THERE ARE NO LIFETIME OR ANNUAL LIMITS TO THE CARE BEING PROVIDED. YOU'RE COVERED FOR WHATEVER HEALTH CARE YOU NEED.

ALL OF THIS IS QUITE WONDERFUL FOR ALL THOSE PEOPLE GETTING PARTIAL OR NO COVERAGE.

BUT LIKE I SAID, I LIKE MY HEALTH CARE PLAN. I DON'T WANT YOU GUYS MUCKING IT UP!

DON'T WORRY. THIS IS A FAIRLY FLEXIBLE SET OF RULES. THERE IS A LOT OF FREEDOM TO DESIGN INDIVIDUAL INSURANCE PLANS, INCLUDING WHAT IS COVERED OR NOT COVERED, AND THE SIZE OF PATIENT DEDUCTIBLES AND COPAYMENTS.

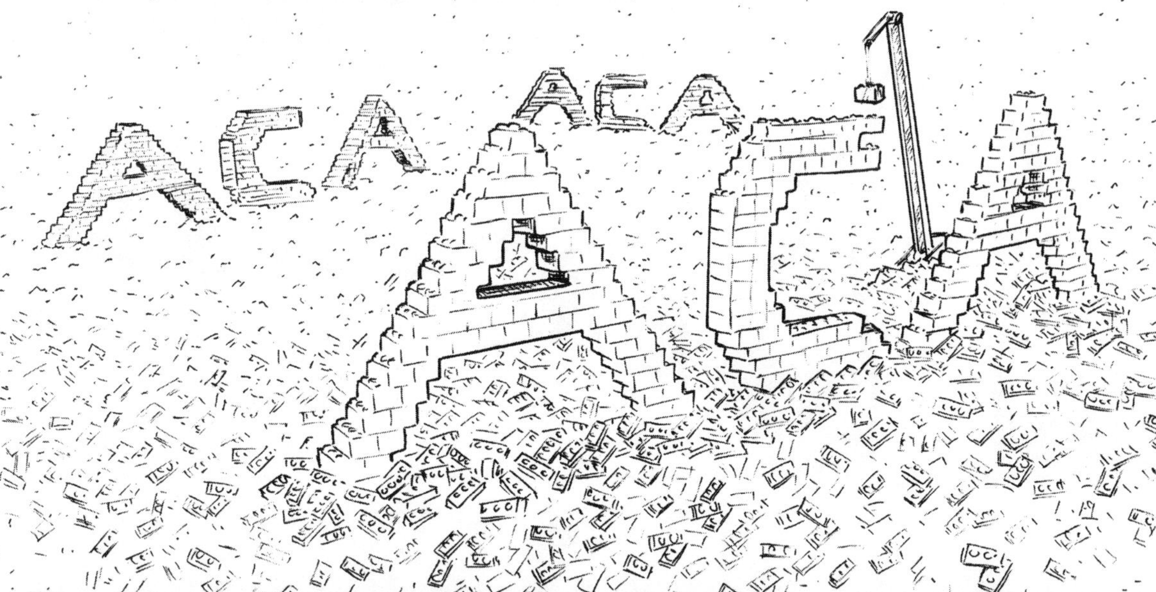

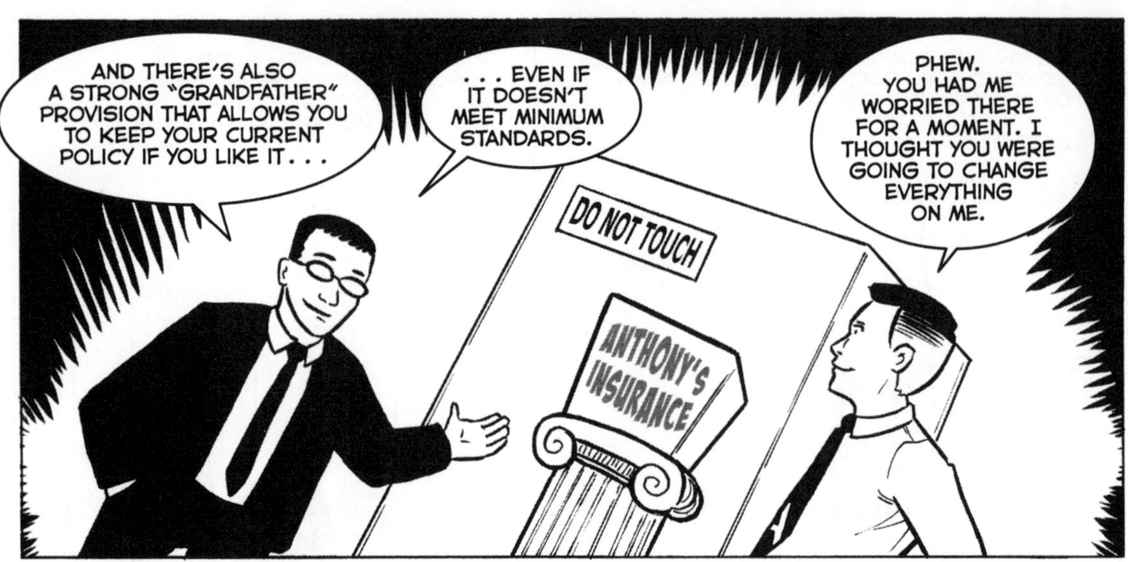
AND THERE'S ALSO A STRONG "GRANDFATHER" PROVISION THAT ALLOWS YOU TO KEEP YOUR CURRENT POLICY IF YOU LIKE IT . . .
. . . EVEN IF IT DOESN'T MEET MINIMUM STANDARDS.
PHEW. YOU HAD ME WORRIED THERE FOR A MOMENT. I THOUGHT YOU WERE GOING TO CHANGE EVERYTHING ON ME.
DO NOT TOUCH
ANTHONY'S INSURANCE

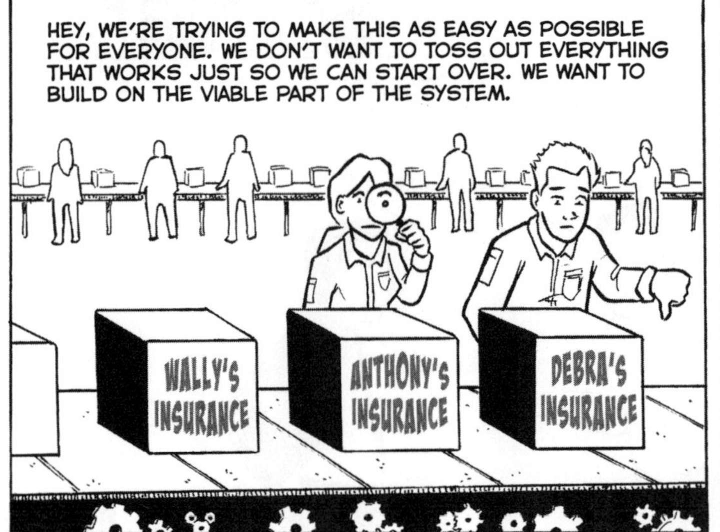
HEY, WE'RE TRYING TO MAKE THIS AS EASY AS POSSIBLE FOR EVERYONE. WE DON'T WANT TO TOSS OUT EVERYTHING THAT WORKS JUST SO WE CAN START OVER. WE WANT TO BUILD ON THE VIABLE PART OF THE SYSTEM.
WALLY'S INSURANCE
ANTHONY'S INSURANCE
DEBRA'S INSURANCE

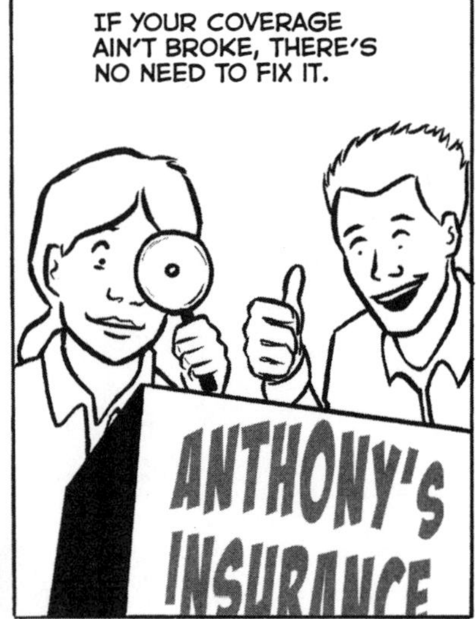
IF YOUR COVERAGE AIN'T BROKE, THERE'S NO NEED TO FIX IT.
ANTHONY'S

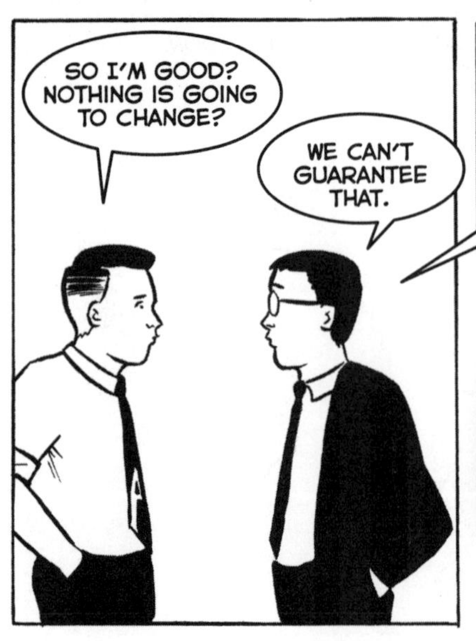
SO I'M GOOD? NOTHING IS GOING TO CHANGE?
WE CAN'T GUARANTEE THAT.

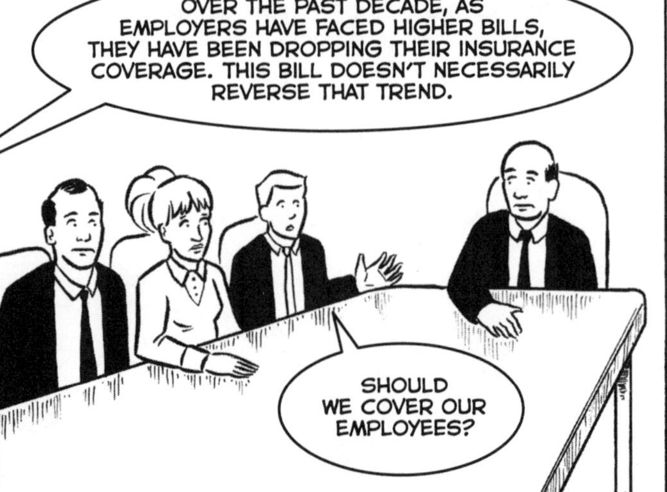
OVER THE PAST DECADE, AS EMPLOYERS HAVE FACED HIGHER BILLS, THEY HAVE BEEN DROPPING THEIR INSURANCE COVERAGE. THIS BILL DOESN'T NECESSARILY REVERSE THAT TREND.
SHOULD WE COVER OUR EMPLOYEES?

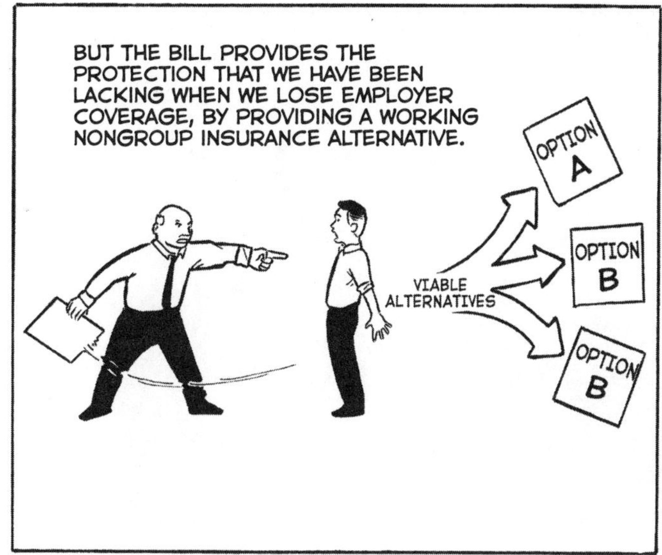
BUT THE BILL PROVIDES THE PROTECTION THAT WE HAVE BEEN LACKING WHEN WE LOSE EMPLOYER COVERAGE, BY PROVIDING A WORKING NONGROUP INSURANCE ALTERNATIVE.
VIABLE ALTERNATIVES
OPTION A
OPTION B
OPTION B

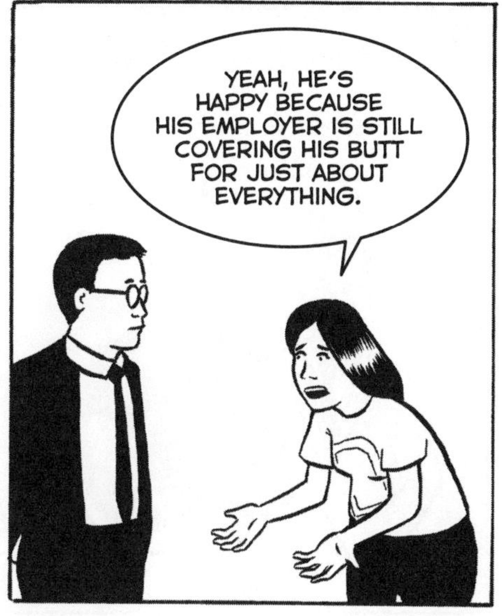
YEAH, HE'S HAPPY BECAUSE HIS EMPLOYER IS STILL COVERING HIS BUTT FOR JUST ABOUT EVERYTHING.

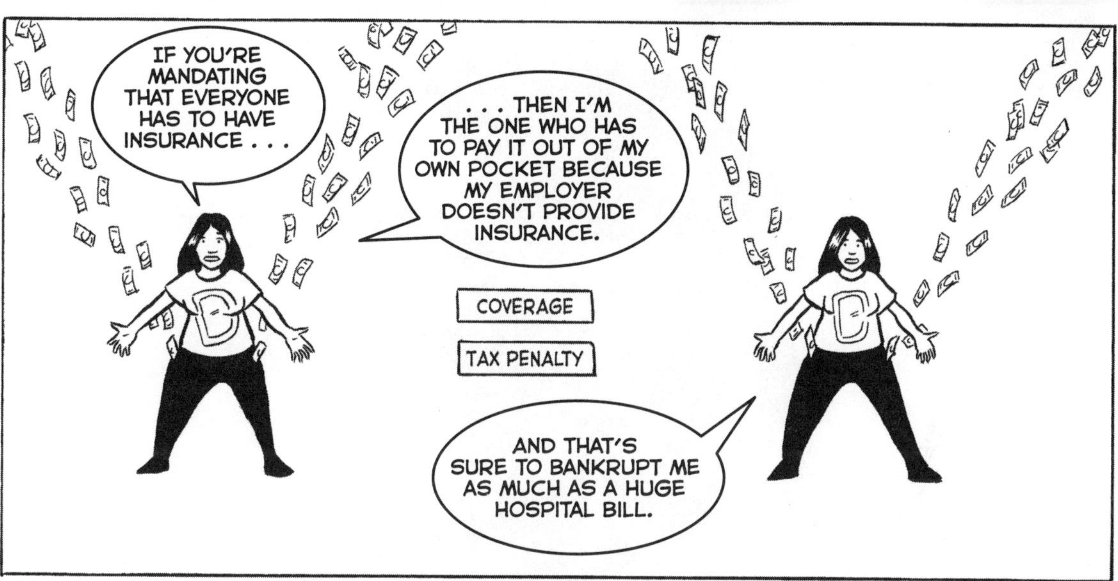
IF YOU'RE MANDATING THAT EVERYONE HAS TO HAVE INSURANCE . . .
. . . THEN I'M THE ONE WHO HAS TO PAY IT OUT OF MY OWN POCKET BECAUSE MY EMPLOYER DOESN'T PROVIDE INSURANCE.
COVERAGE
TAX PENALTY
AND THAT'S SURE TO BANKRUPT ME AS MUCH AS A HUGE HOSPITAL BILL.

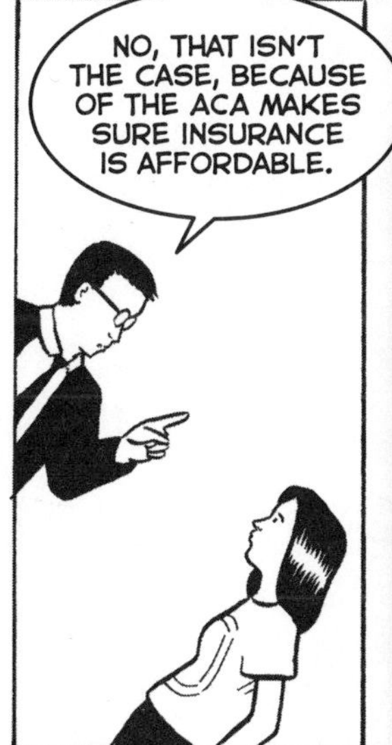
NO, THAT ISN'T THE CASE, BECAUSE OF THE ACA MAKES SURE INSURANCE IS AFFORDABLE.

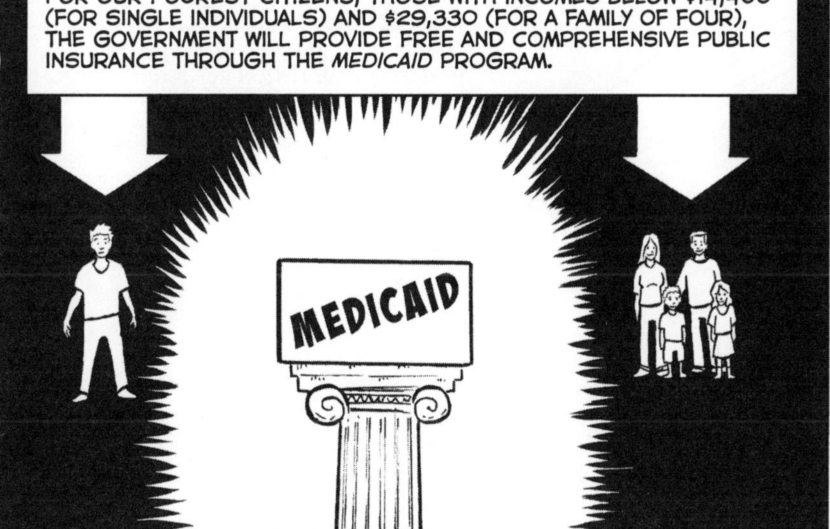
FOR OUR POOREST CITIZENS, THOSE WITH INCOMES BELOW $14,400 (FOR SINGLE INDIVIDUALS) AND $29,330 (FOR A FAMILY OF FOUR), THE GOVERNMENT WILL PROVIDE FREE AND COMPREHENSIVE PUBLIC INSURANCE THROUGH THE *MEDICAID* PROGRAM.
MEDICAID

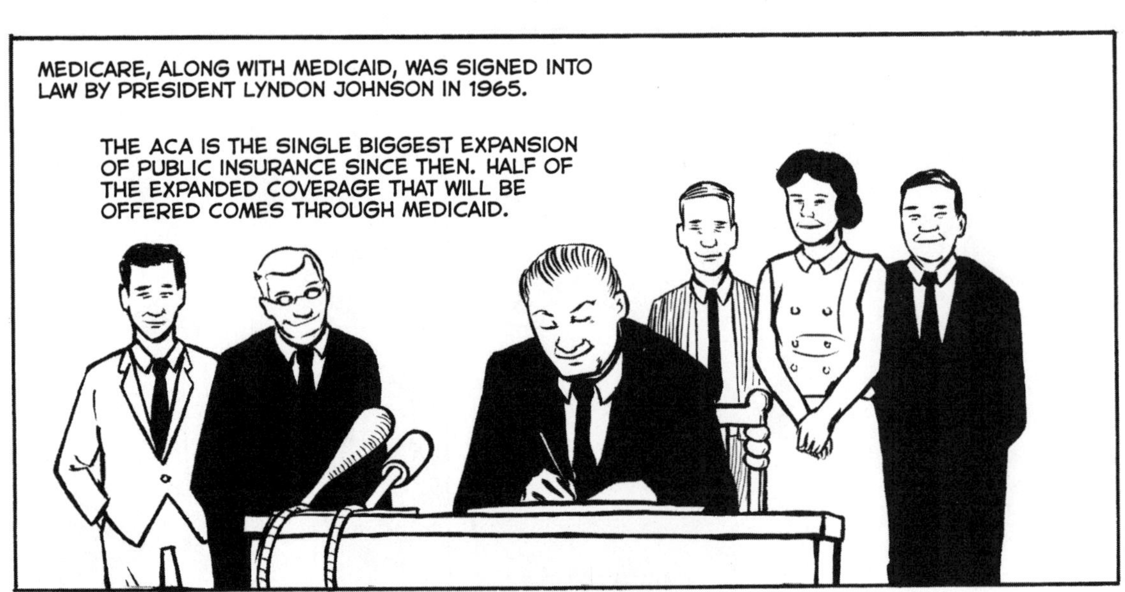
MEDICARE, ALONG WITH MEDICAID, WAS SIGNED INTO LAW BY PRESIDENT LYNDON JOHNSON IN 1965.
THE ACA IS THE SINGLE BIGGEST EXPANSION OF PUBLIC INSURANCE SINCE THEN. HALF OF THE EXPANDED COVERAGE THAT WILL BE OFFERED COMES THROUGH MEDICAID.

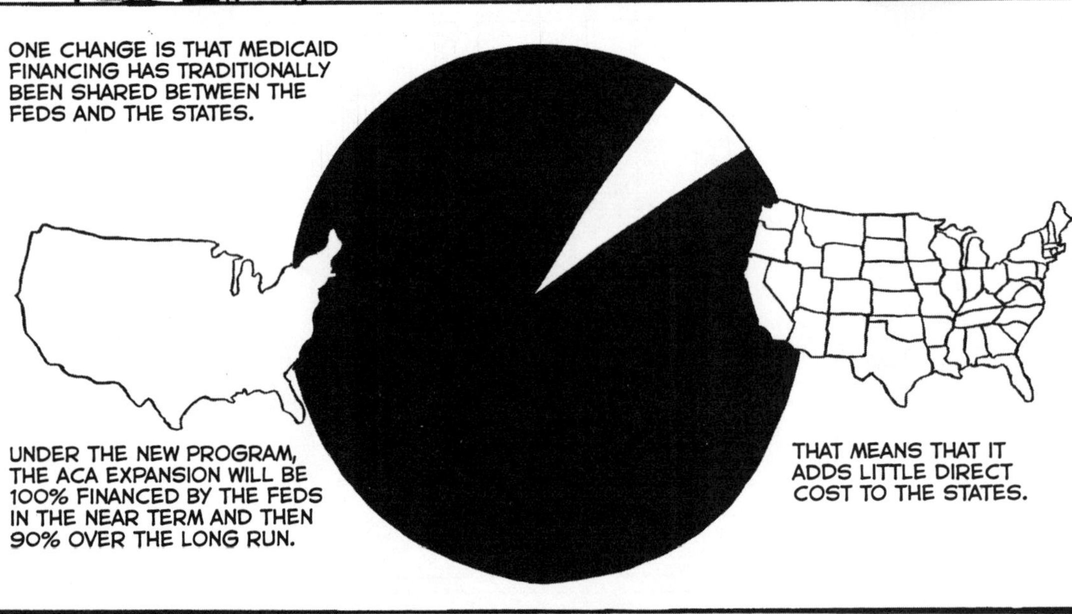
ONE CHANGE IS THAT MEDICAID FINANCING HAS TRADITIONALLY BEEN SHARED BETWEEN THE FEDS AND THE STATES.
UNDER THE NEW PROGRAM, THE ACA EXPANSION WILL BE 100% FINANCED BY THE FEDS IN THE NEAR TERM AND THEN 90% OVER THE LONG RUN.
THAT MEANS THAT IT ADDS LITTLE DIRECT COST TO THE STATES.

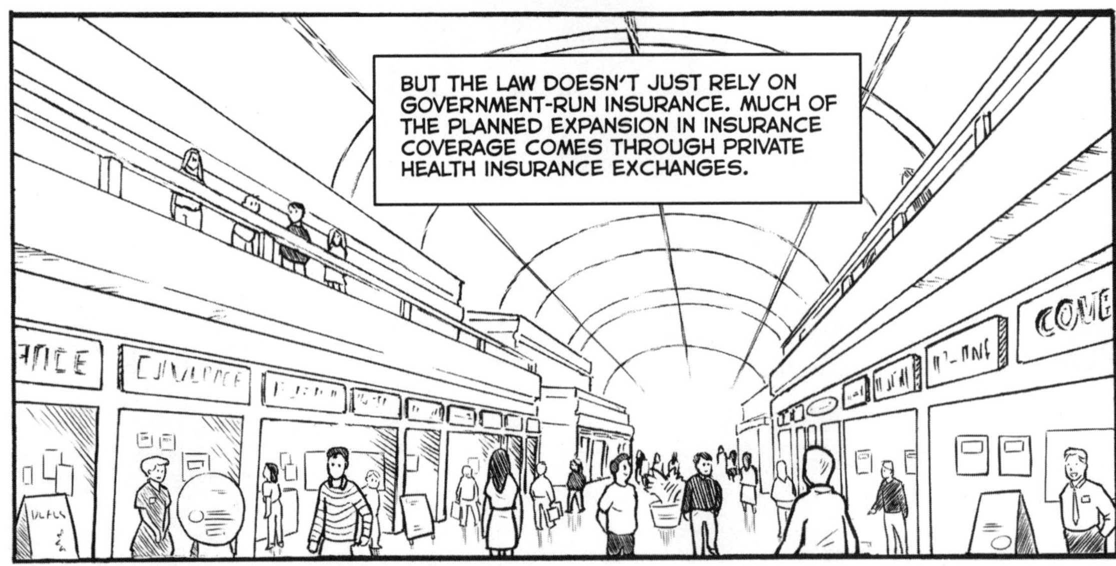
BUT THE LAW DOESN'T JUST RELY ON GOVERNMENT-RUN INSURANCE. MUCH OF THE PLANNED EXPANSION IN INSURANCE COVERAGE COMES THROUGH PRIVATE HEALTH INSURANCE EXCHANGES.

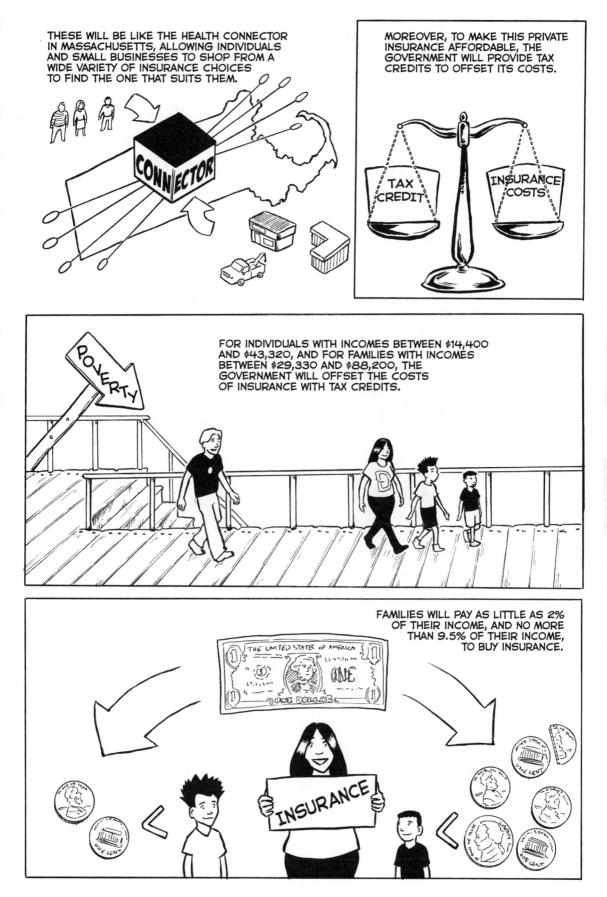

THESE WILL BE LIKE THE HEALTH CONNECTOR IN MASSACHUSETTS, ALLOWING INDIVIDUALS AND SMALL BUSINESSES TO SHOP FROM A WIDE VARIETY OF INSURANCE CHOICES TO FIND THE ONE THAT SUITS THEM.
CONNECTOR

MOREOVER, TO MAKE THIS PRIVATE INSURANCE AFFORDABLE, THE GOVERNMENT WILL PROVIDE TAX CREDITS TO OFFSET ITS COSTS.
TAX CREDIT
INSURANCE COSTS

FOR INDIVIDUALS WITH INCOMES BETWEEN $14,400 AND $43,320, AND FOR FAMILIES WITH INCOMES BETWEEN $29,330 AND $88,200, THE GOVERNMENT WILL OFFSET THE COSTS OF INSURANCE WITH TAX CREDITS.
POVERTY

FAMILIES WILL PAY AS LITTLE AS 2% OF THEIR INCOME, AND NO MORE THAN 9.5% OF THEIR INCOME, TO BUY INSURANCE.
THE UNITED STATES OF AMERICA
ONE DOLLAR
INSURANCE
ONE CENT

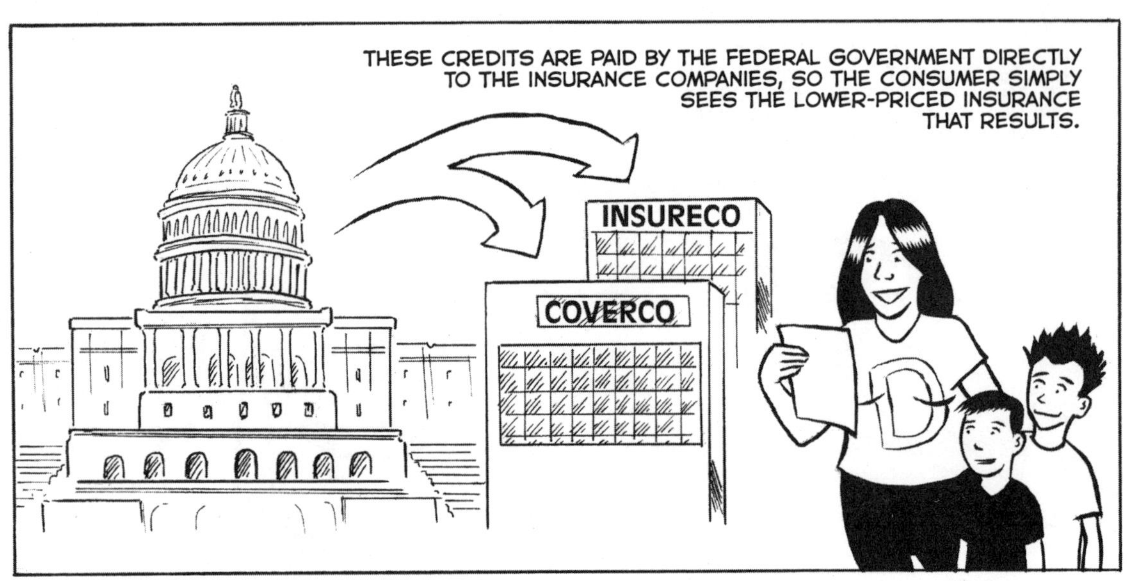
THESE CREDITS ARE PAID BY THE FEDERAL GOVERNMENT DIRECTLY TO THE INSURANCE COMPANIES, SO THE CONSUMER SIMPLY SEES THE LOWER-PRICED INSURANCE THAT RESULTS.
INSURECO
COVERCO

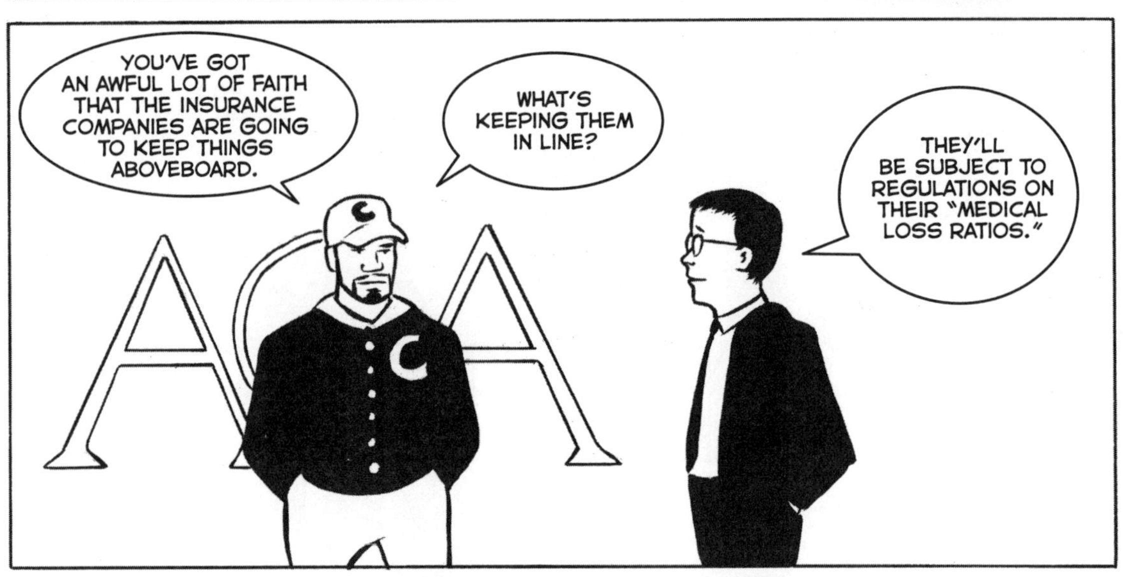
YOU'VE GOT AN AWFUL LOT OF FAITH THAT THE INSURANCE COMPANIES ARE GOING TO KEEP THINGS ABOVEBOARD.
WHAT'S KEEPING THEM IN LINE?
THEY'LL BE SUBJECT TO REGULATIONS ON THEIR "MEDICAL LOSS RATIOS."

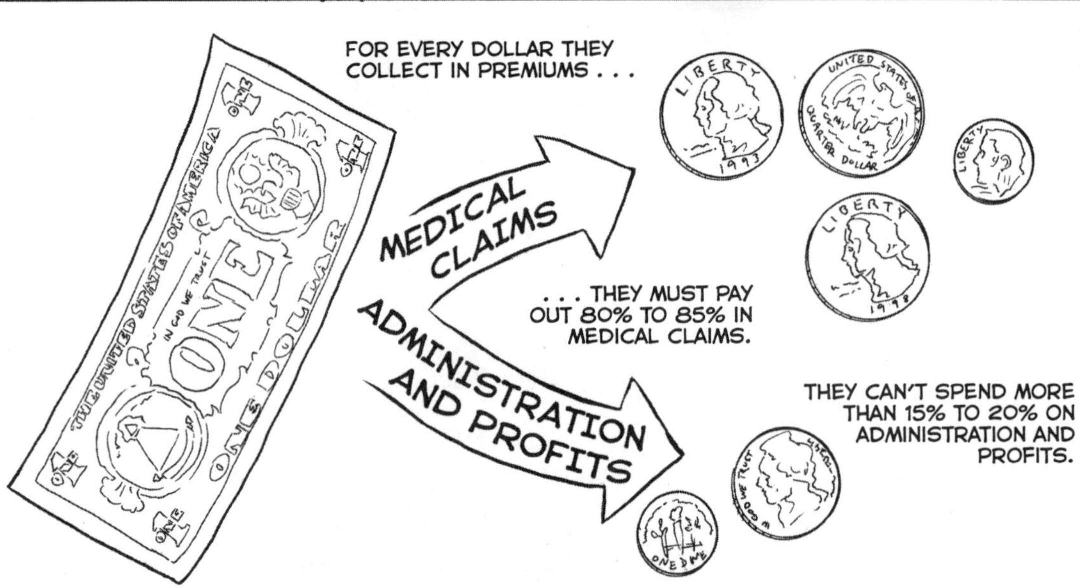
FOR EVERY DOLLAR THEY COLLECT IN PREMIUMS . . .
MEDICAL CLAIMS
. . . THEY MUST PAY OUT 80% TO 85% IN MEDICAL CLAIMS.
ADMINISTRATION AND PROFITS
THEY CAN'T SPEND MORE THAN 15% TO 20% ON ADMINISTRATION AND PROFITS.

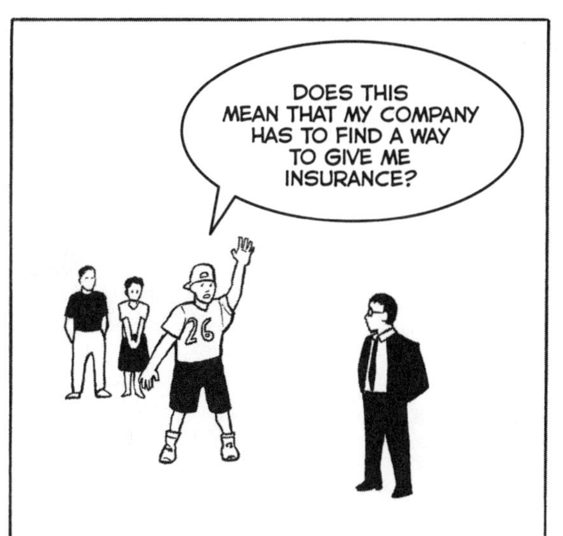
DOES THIS MEAN THAT MY COMPANY HAS TO FIND A WAY TO GIVE ME INSURANCE?

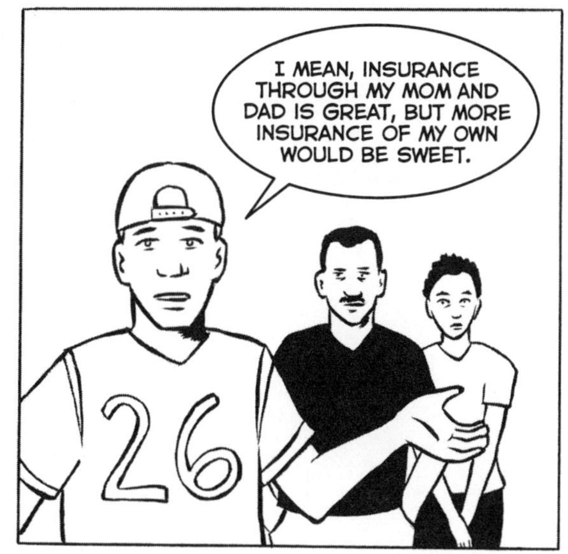
I MEAN, INSURANCE THROUGH MY MOM AND DAD IS GREAT, BUT MORE INSURANCE OF MY OWN WOULD BE SWEET.

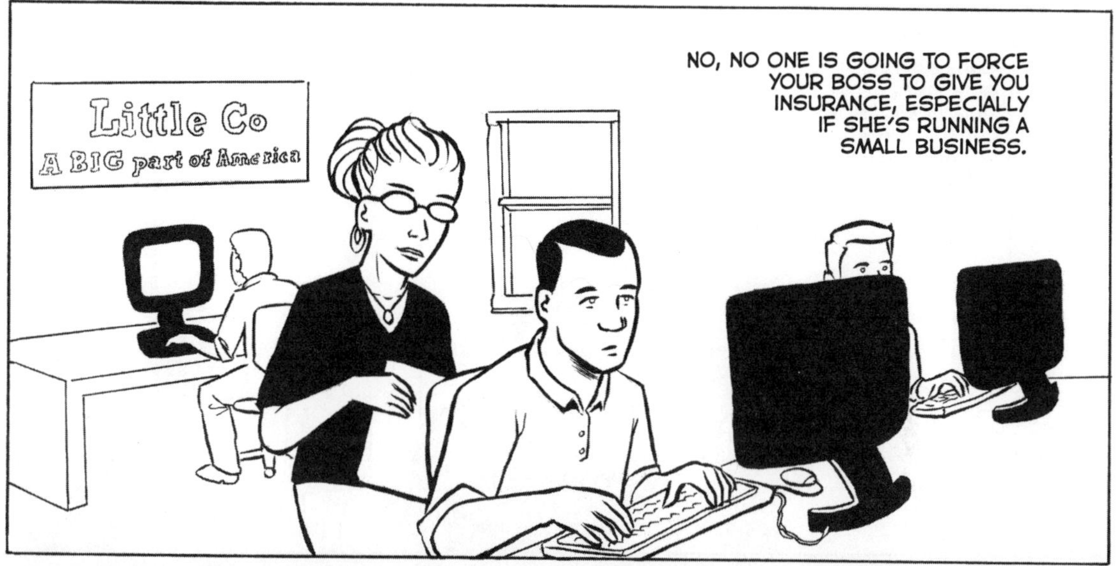
NO, NO ONE IS GOING TO FORCE YOUR BOSS TO GIVE YOU INSURANCE, ESPECIALLY IF SHE'S RUNNING A SMALL BUSINESS.
Little Co
A BIG part of America

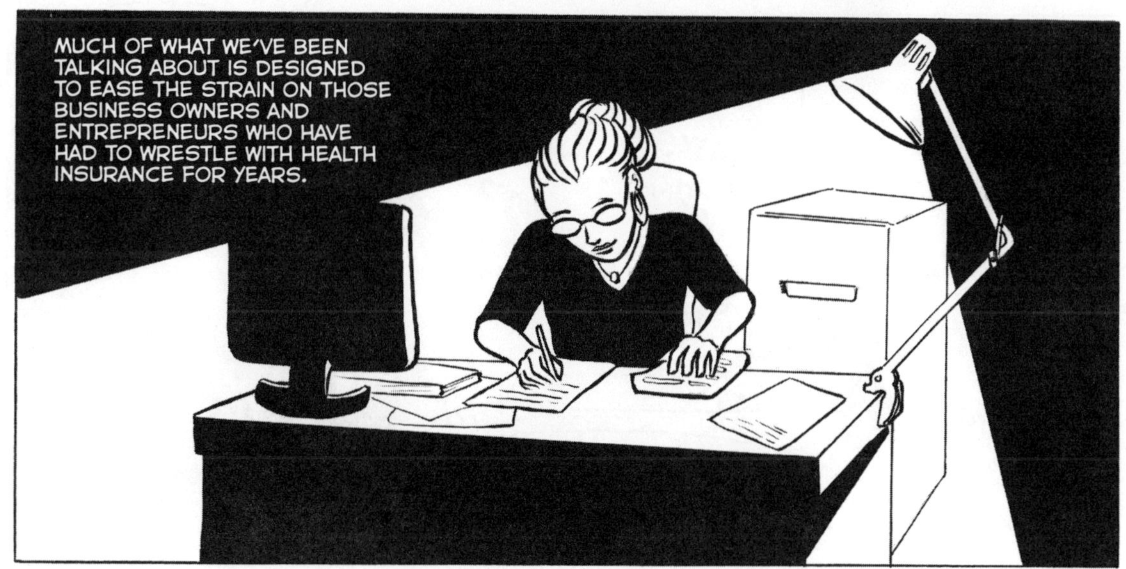
MUCH OF WHAT WE'VE BEEN TALKING ABOUT IS DESIGNED TO EASE THE STRAIN ON THOSE BUSINESS OWNERS AND ENTREPRENEURS WHO HAVE HAD TO WRESTLE WITH HEALTH INSURANCE FOR YEARS.

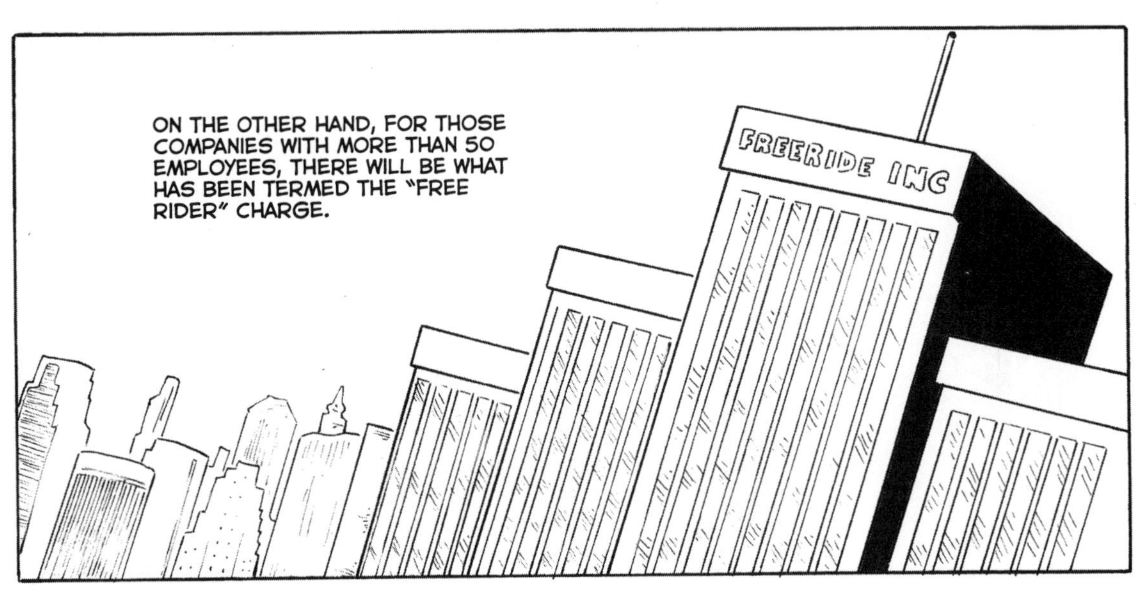
ON THE OTHER HAND, FOR THOSE COMPANIES WITH MORE THAN 50 EMPLOYEES, THERE WILL BE WHAT HAS BEEN TERMED THE "FREE RIDER" CHARGE.
FREERIDE INC

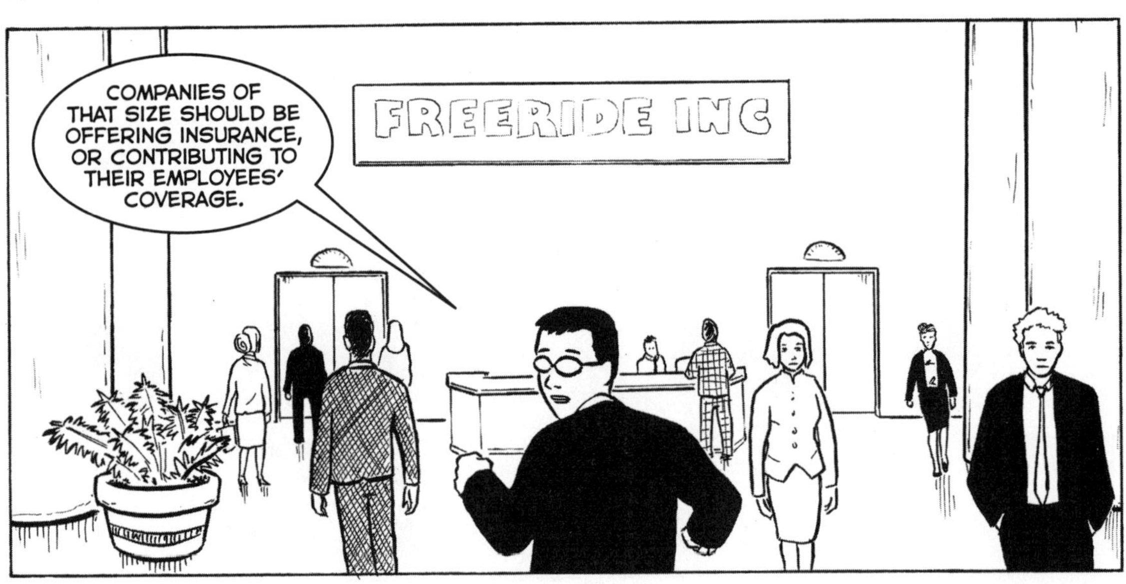
COMPANIES OF THAT SIZE SHOULD BE OFFERING INSURANCE, OR CONTRIBUTING TO THEIR EMPLOYEES' COVERAGE.
FREERIDE INC

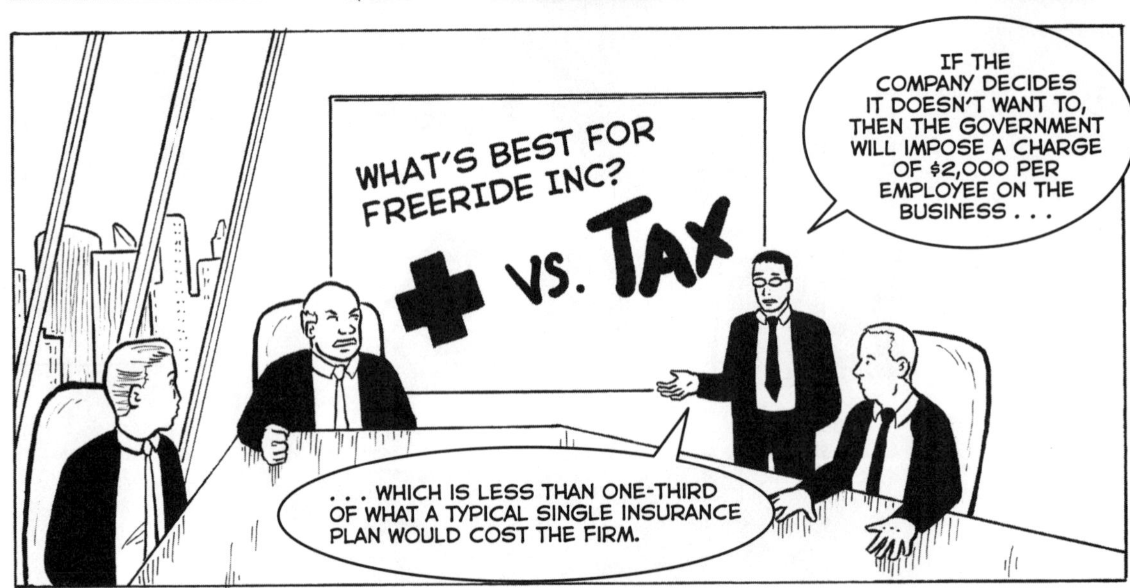
WHAT'S BEST FOR FREERIDE INC?
VS. TAX
IF THE COMPANY DECIDES IT DOESN'T WANT TO, THEN THE GOVERNMENT WILL IMPOSE A CHARGE OF $2,000 PER EMPLOYEE ON THE BUSINESS . . .
. . . WHICH IS LESS THAN ONE-THIRD OF WHAT A TYPICAL SINGLE INSURANCE PLAN WOULD COST THE FIRM.

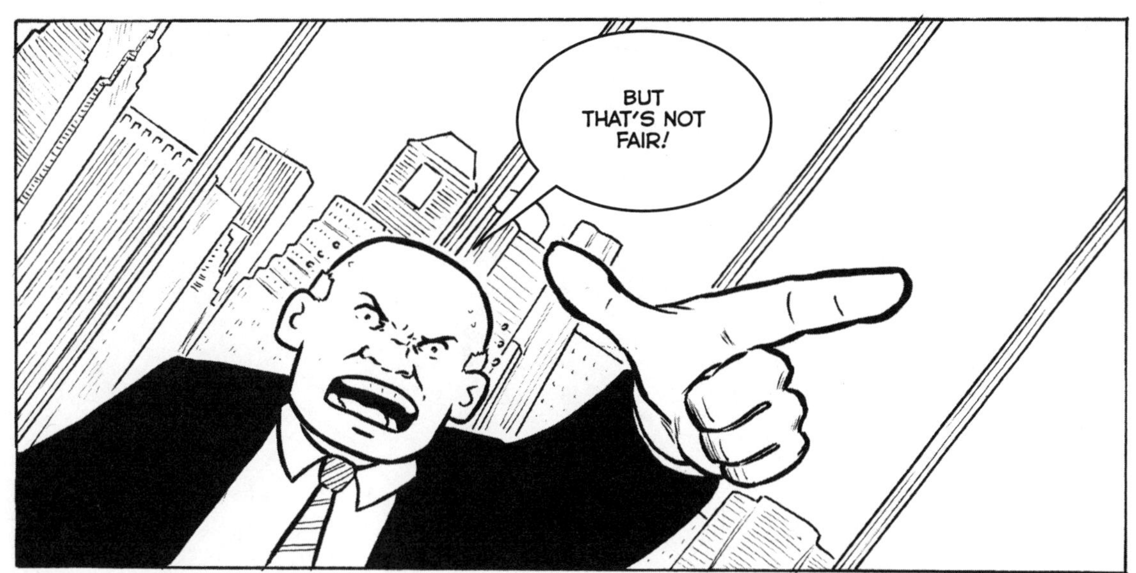
BUT THAT'S NOT FAIR!

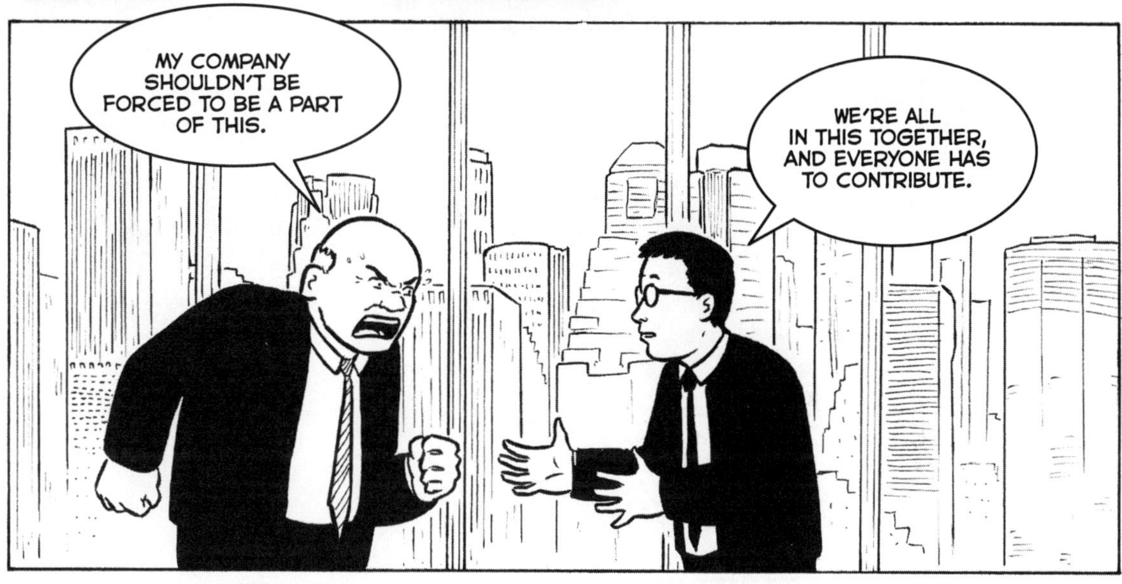
MY COMPANY SHOULDN'T BE FORCED TO BE A PART OF THIS.
WE'RE ALL IN THIS TOGETHER, AND EVERYONE HAS TO CONTRIBUTE.

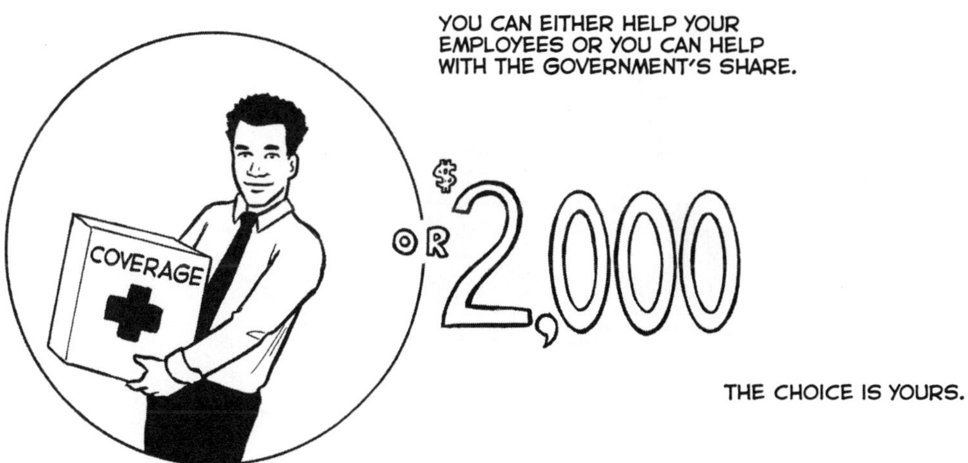
YOU CAN EITHER HELP YOUR EMPLOYEES OR YOU CAN HELP WITH THE GOVERNMENT'S SHARE.
COVERAGE
OR
$2,000
THE CHOICE IS YOURS.

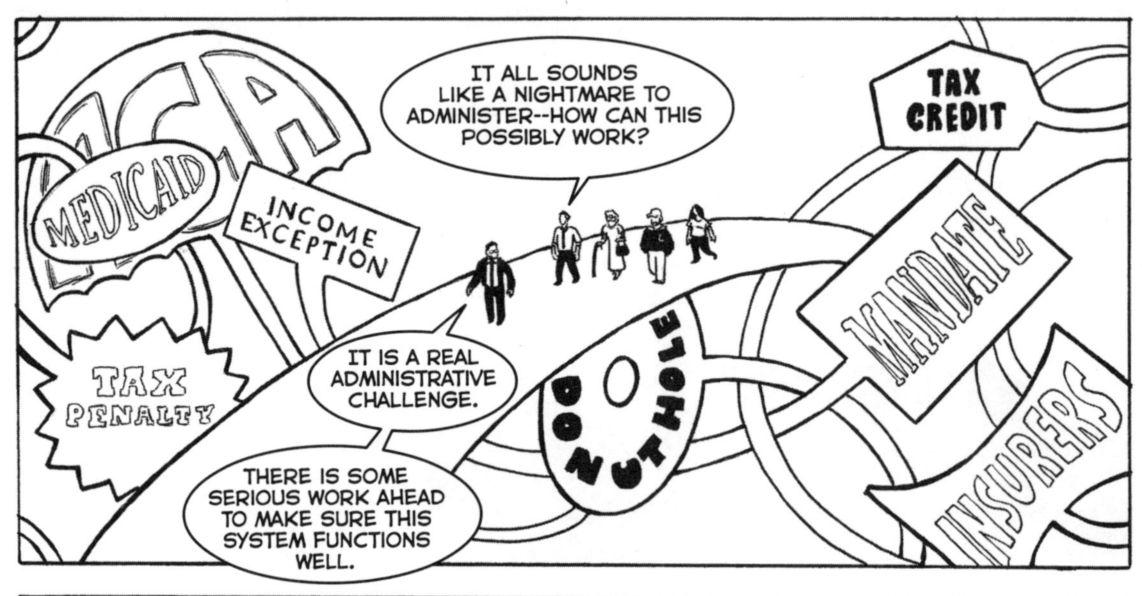
ACA
MEDICAID
INCOME EXCEPTION
IT ALL SOUNDS LIKE A NIGHTMARE TO ADMINISTER--HOW CAN THIS POSSIBLY WORK?
TAX CREDIT
MANDATE
TAX PENALTY
IT IS A REAL ADMINISTRATIVE CHALLENGE.
DONUT HOLE
THERE IS SOME SERIOUS WORK AHEAD TO MAKE SURE THIS SYSTEM FUNCTIONS WELL.
INSURERS

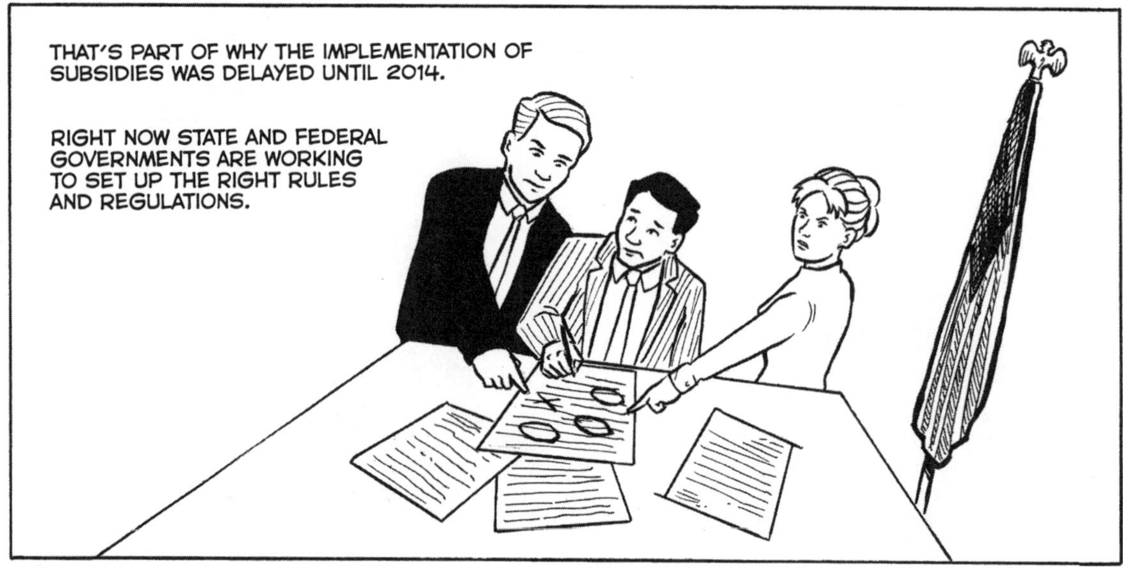
THAT'S PART OF WHY THE IMPLEMENTATION OF SUBSIDIES WAS DELAYED UNTIL 2014.
RIGHT NOW STATE AND FEDERAL GOVERNMENTS ARE WORKING TO SET UP THE RIGHT RULES AND REGULATIONS.

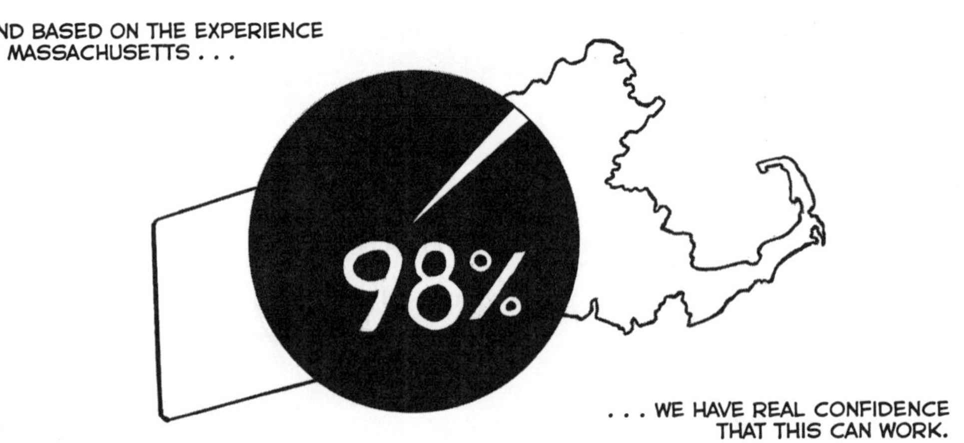
AND BASED ON THE EXPERIENCE IN MASSACHUSETTS . . .
98%
. . . WE HAVE REAL CONFIDENCE THAT THIS CAN WORK.

CHAPTER 8 SELLING FEAR INSTEAD OF FACTS

SO WHAT IS THE UPSHOT OF ALL THIS?
HOW WILL THE NATION BENEFIT?

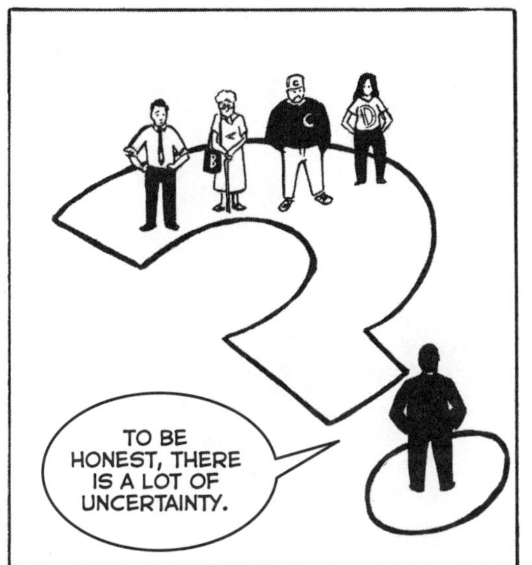

TO BE HONEST, THERE IS A LOT OF UNCERTAINTY.

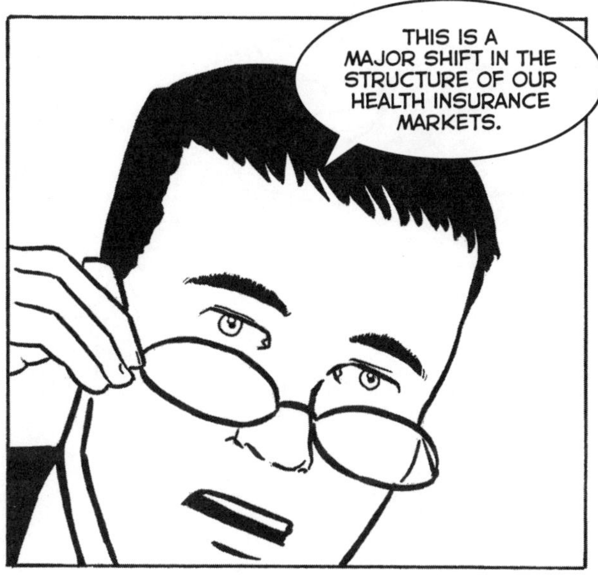

THIS IS A MAJOR SHIFT IN THE STRUCTURE OF OUR HEALTH INSURANCE MARKETS.

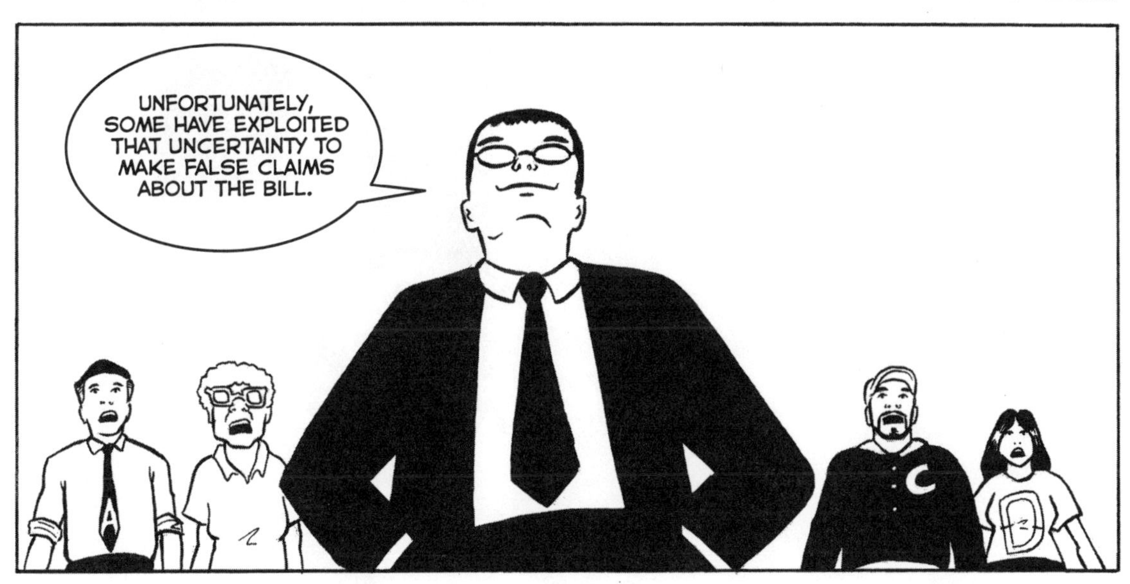

UNFORTUNATELY, SOME HAVE EXPLOITED THAT UNCERTAINTY TO MAKE FALSE CLAIMS ABOUT THE BILL.

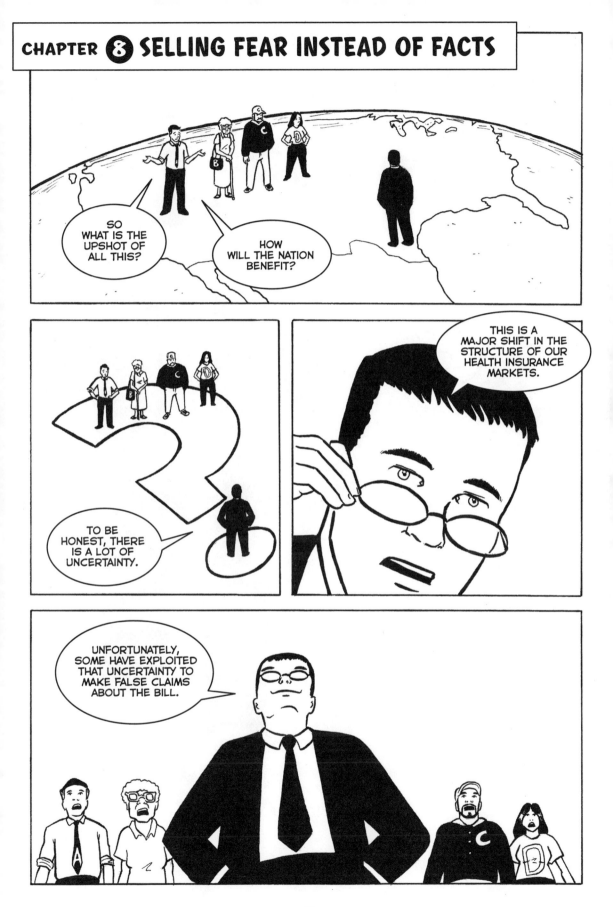

WE WON'T COVER THE UNINSURED!

IT WILL BE THE END OF THE EMPLOYER-PROVIDED INSURANCE!

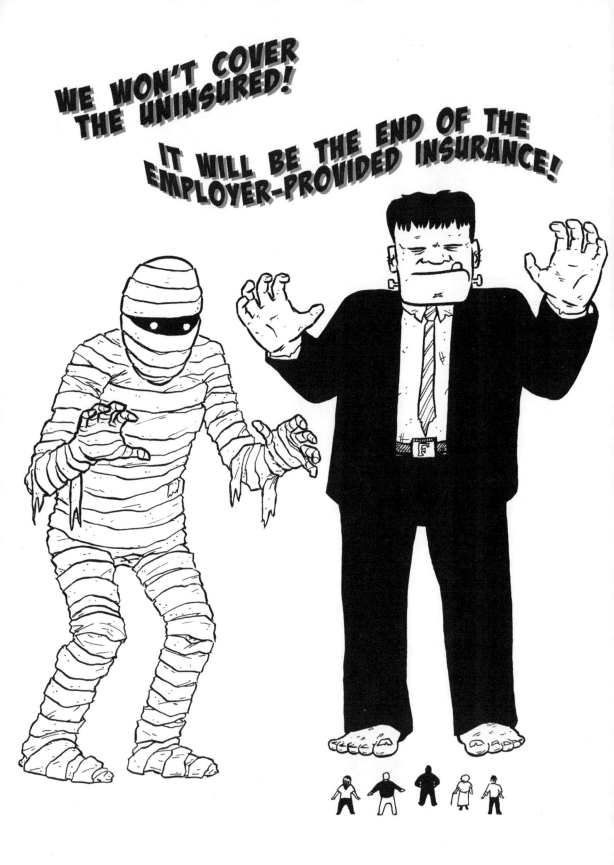

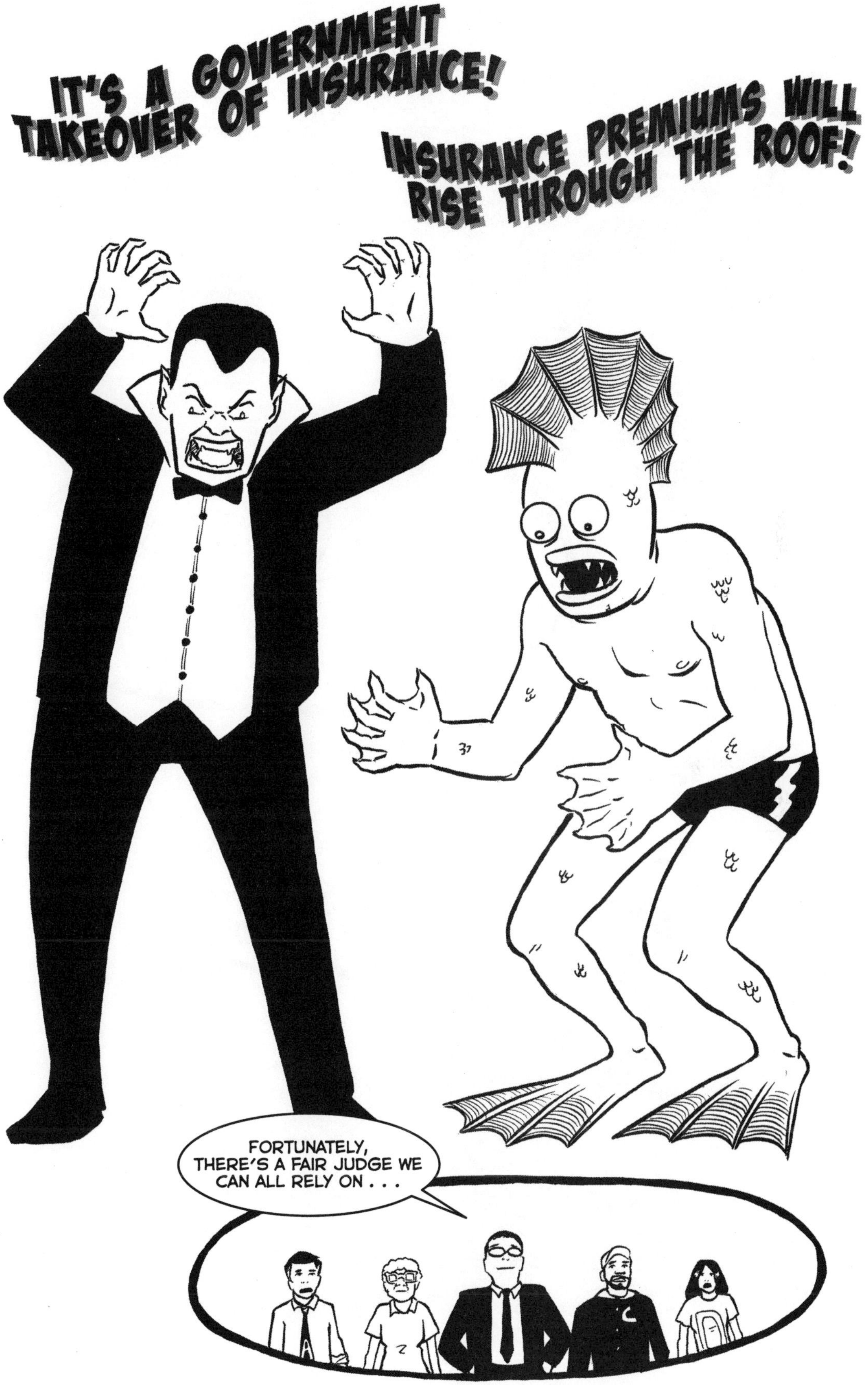

IT'S A GOVERNMENT TAKEOVER OF INSURANCE!

INSURANCE PREMIUMS WILL RISE THROUGH THE ROOF!

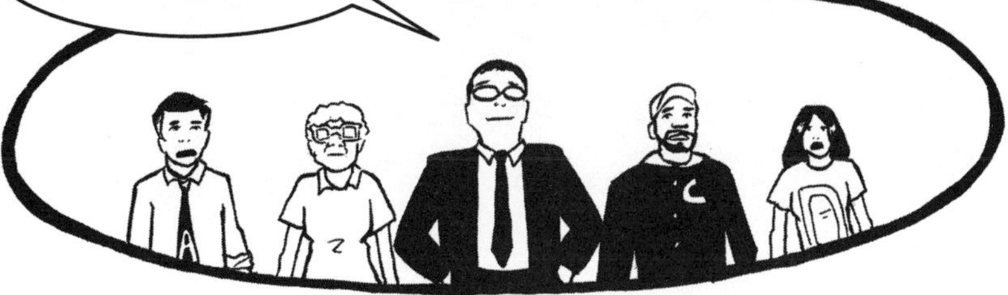
FORTUNATELY, THERE'S A FAIR JUDGE WE CAN ALL RELY ON . . .

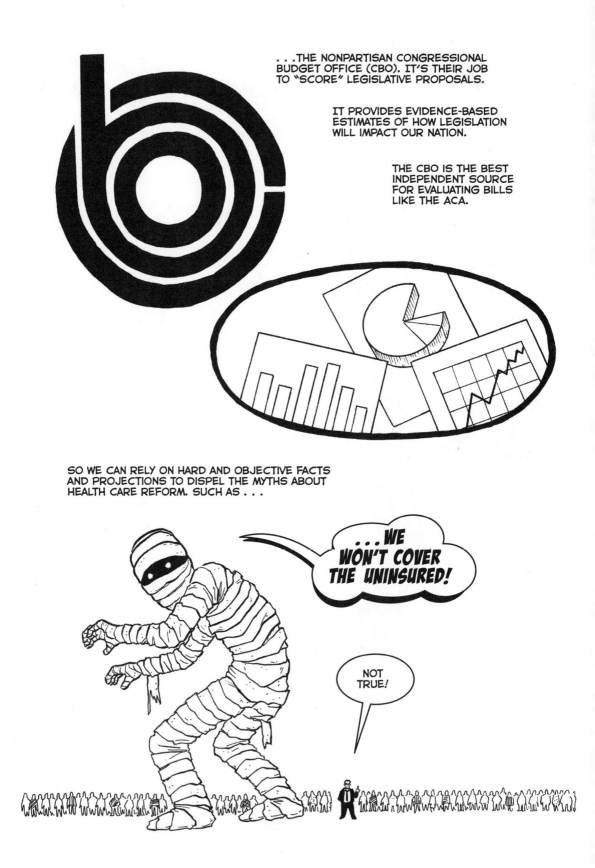

. . .THE NONPARTISAN CONGRESSIONAL BUDGET OFFICE (CBO). IT'S THEIR JOB TO "SCORE" LEGISLATIVE PROPOSALS.

IT PROVIDES EVIDENCE-BASED ESTIMATES OF HOW LEGISLATION WILL IMPACT OUR NATION.

THE CBO IS THE BEST INDEPENDENT SOURCE FOR EVALUATING BILLS LIKE THE ACA.

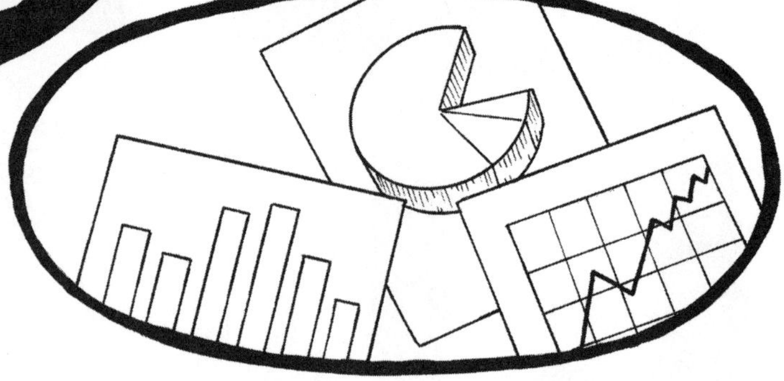

SO WE CAN RELY ON HARD AND OBJECTIVE FACTS AND PROJECTIONS TO DISPEL THE MYTHS ABOUT HEALTH CARE REFORM. SUCH AS . . .

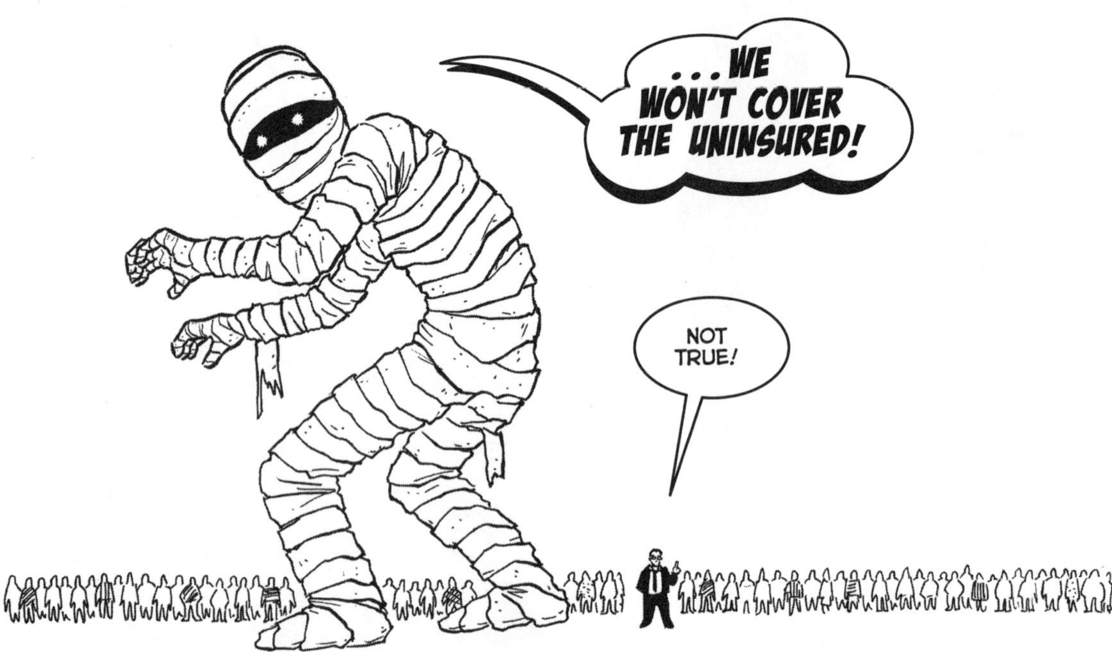

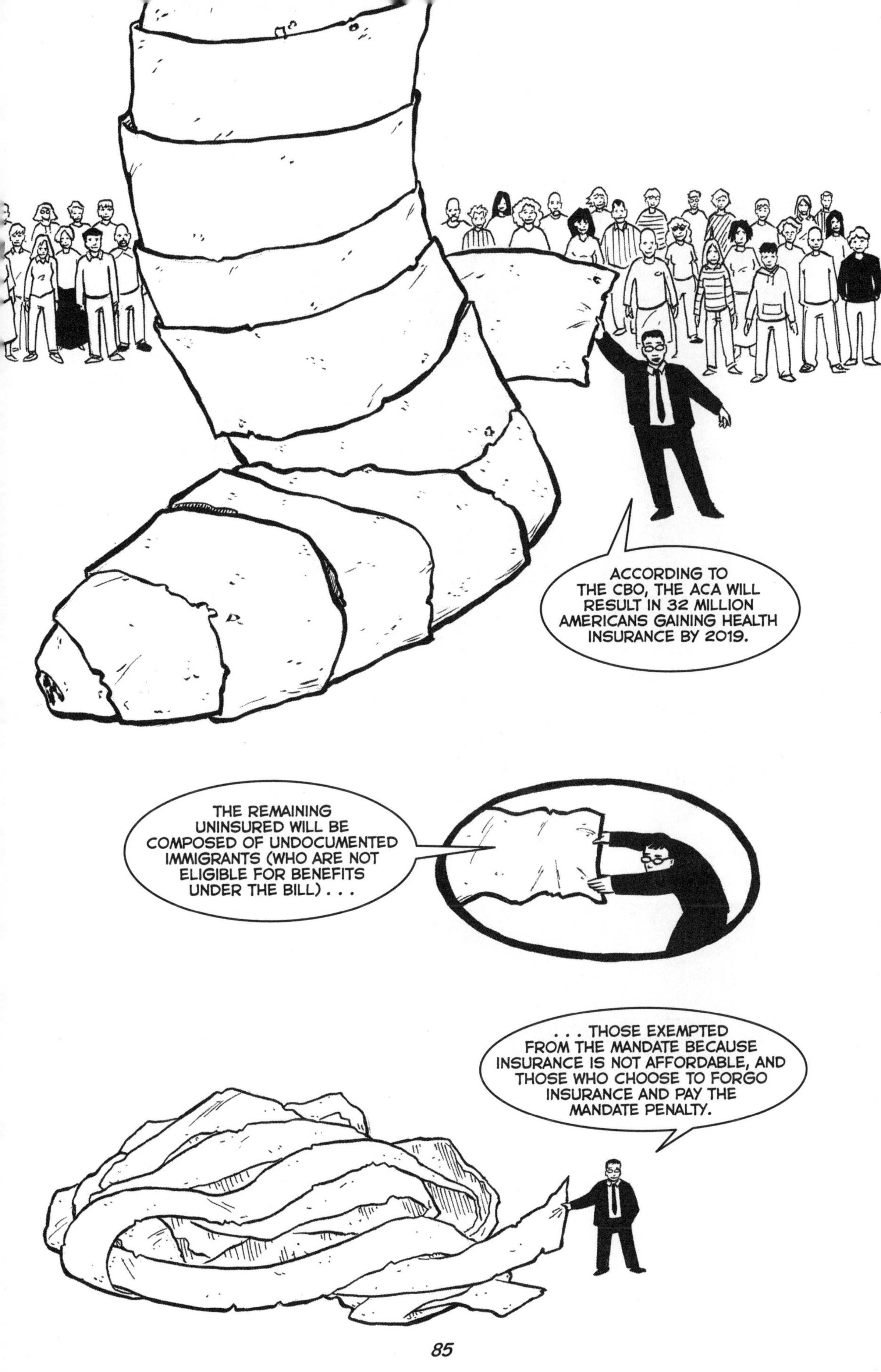
ACCORDING TO THE CBO, THE ACA WILL RESULT IN 32 MILLION AMERICANS GAINING HEALTH INSURANCE BY 2019.
THE REMAINING UNINSURED WILL BE COMPOSED OF UNDOCUMENTED IMMIGRANTS (WHO ARE NOT ELIGIBLE FOR BENEFITS UNDER THE BILL) . . .
. . . THOSE EXEMPTED FROM THE MANDATE BECAUSE INSURANCE IS NOT AFFORDABLE, AND THOSE WHO CHOOSE TO FORGO INSURANCE AND PAY THE MANDATE PENALTY.

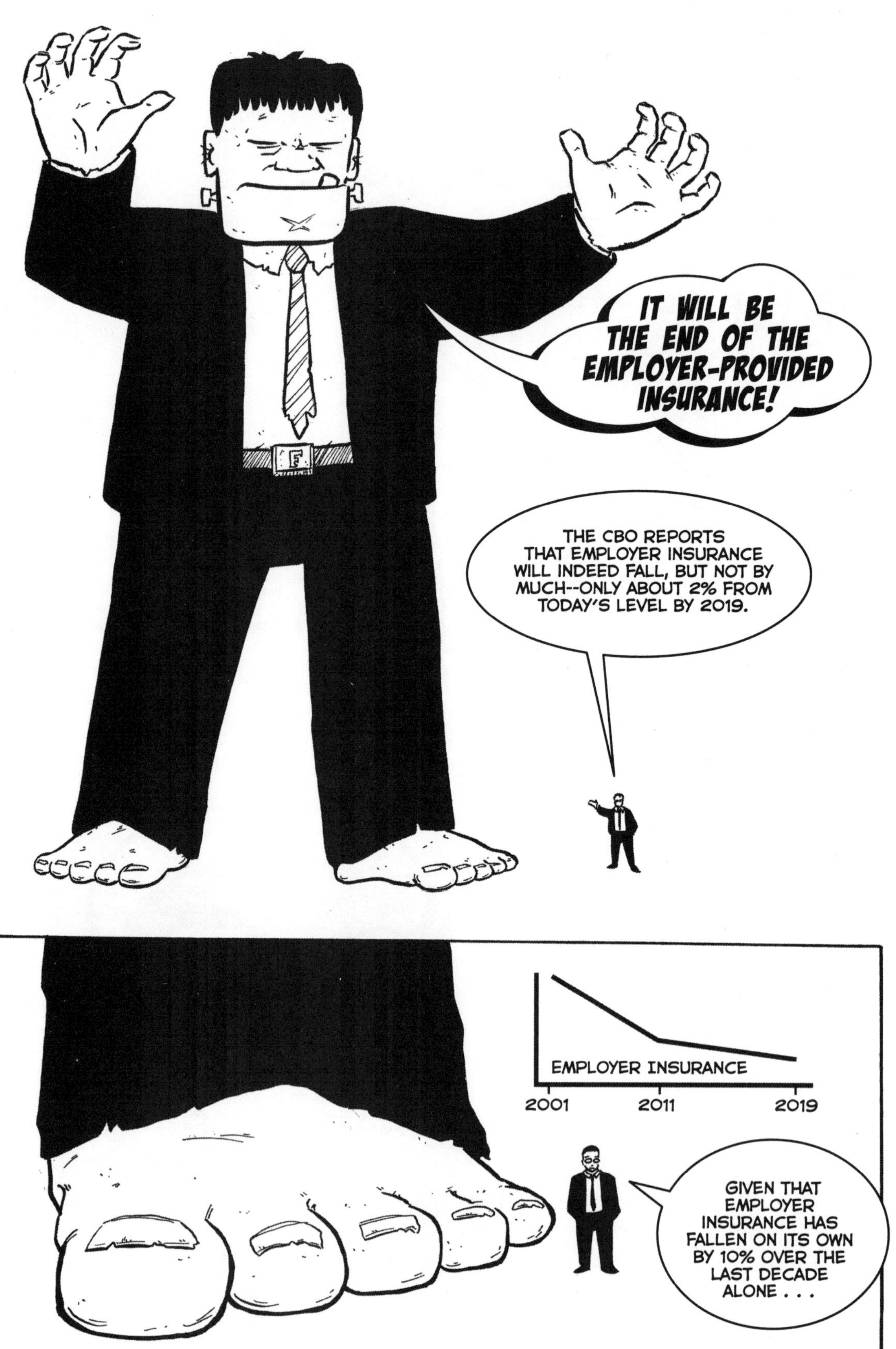
IT WILL BE THE END OF THE EMPLOYER-PROVIDED INSURANCE!
THE CBO REPORTS THAT EMPLOYER INSURANCE WILL INDEED FALL, BUT NOT BY MUCH--ONLY ABOUT 2% FROM TODAY'S LEVEL BY 2019.
F
EMPLOYER INSURANCE
2001
2011
2019
GIVEN THAT EMPLOYER INSURANCE HAS FALLEN ON ITS OWN BY 10% OVER THE LAST DECADE ALONE . . .

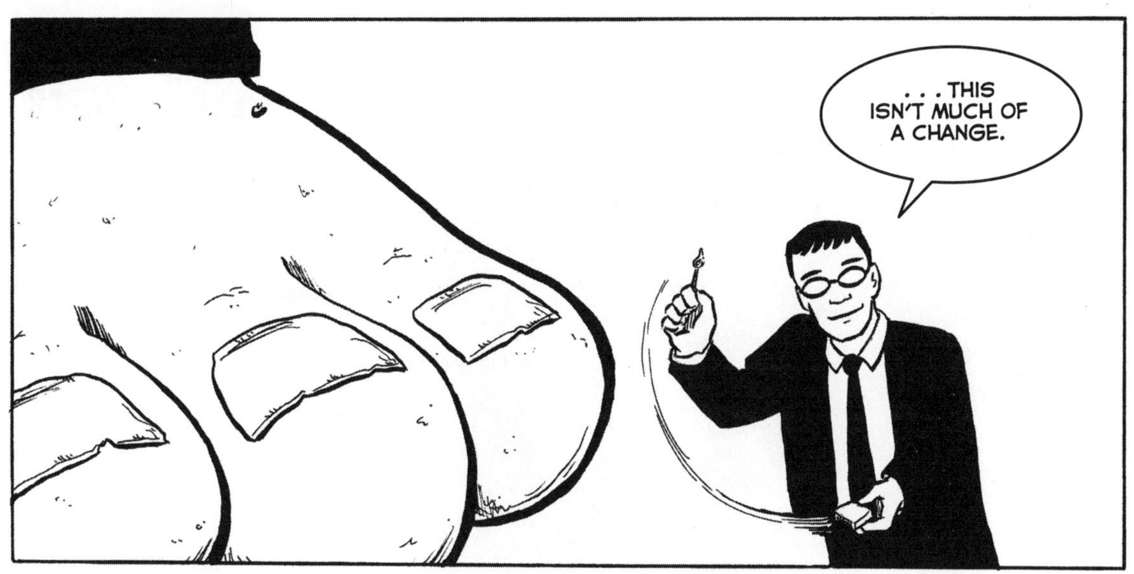
. . . THIS ISN'T MUCH OF A CHANGE.

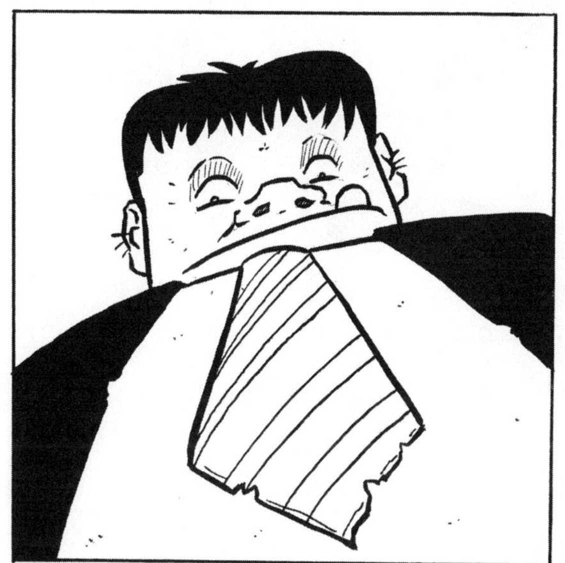

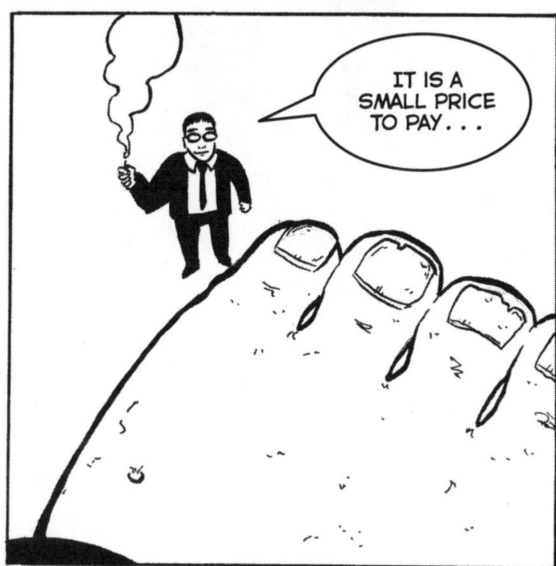
IT IS A SMALL PRICE TO PAY . . .

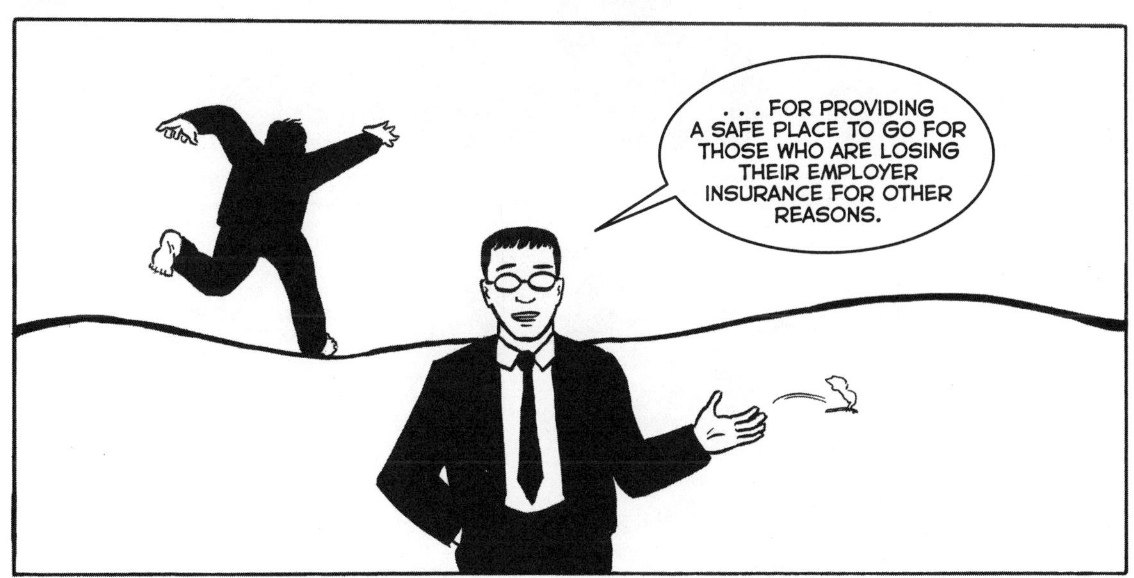
. . . FOR PROVIDING A SAFE PLACE TO GO FOR THOSE WHO ARE LOSING THEIR EMPLOYER INSURANCE FOR OTHER REASONS.

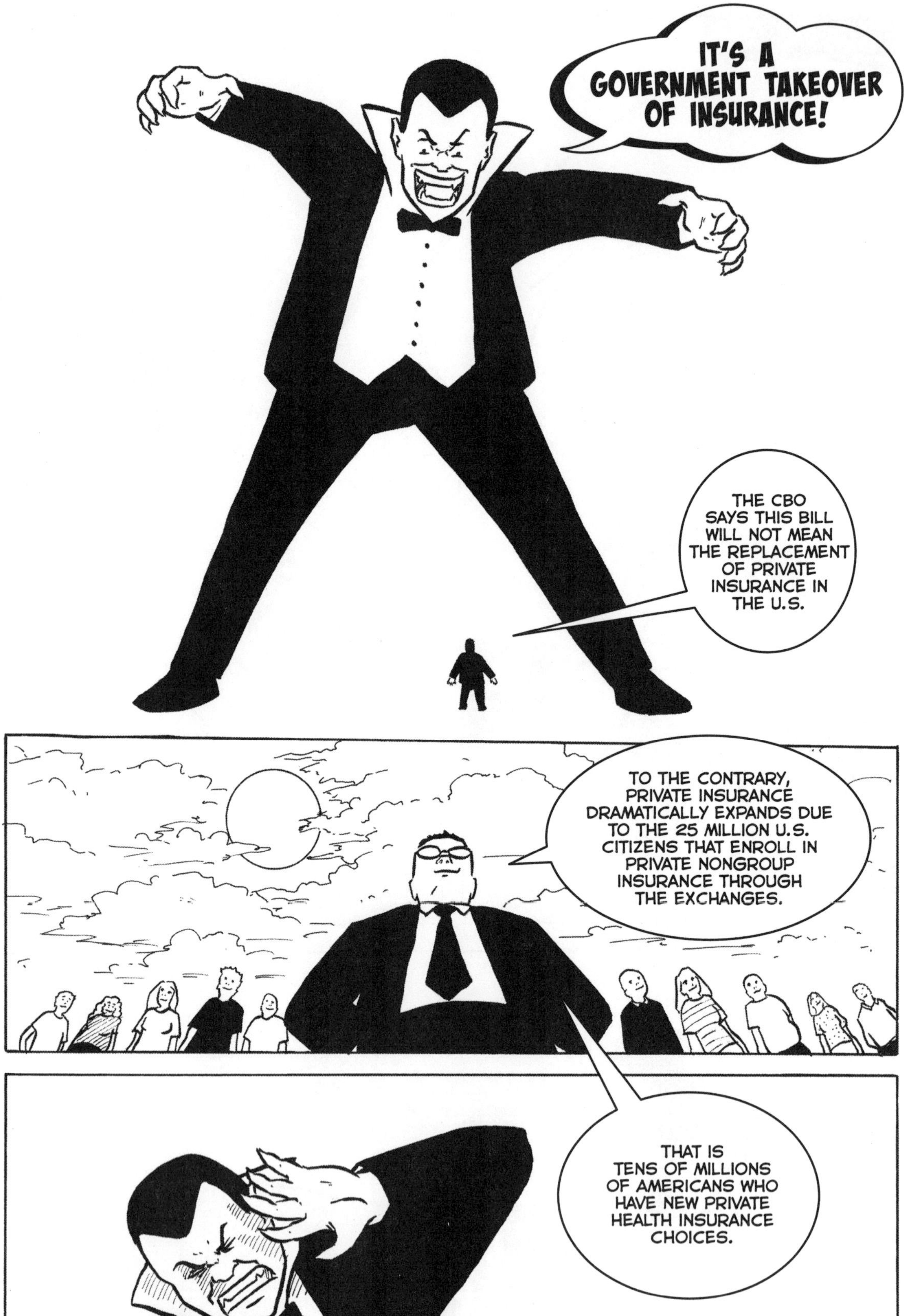

IT'S A GOVERNMENT TAKEOVER OF INSURANCE!

THE CBO SAYS THIS BILL WILL NOT MEAN THE REPLACEMENT OF PRIVATE INSURANCE IN THE U.S.

TO THE CONTRARY, PRIVATE INSURANCE DRAMATICALLY EXPANDS DUE TO THE 25 MILLION U.S. CITIZENS THAT ENROLL IN PRIVATE NONGROUP INSURANCE THROUGH THE EXCHANGES.

THAT IS TENS OF MILLIONS OF AMERICANS WHO HAVE NEW PRIVATE HEALTH INSURANCE CHOICES.

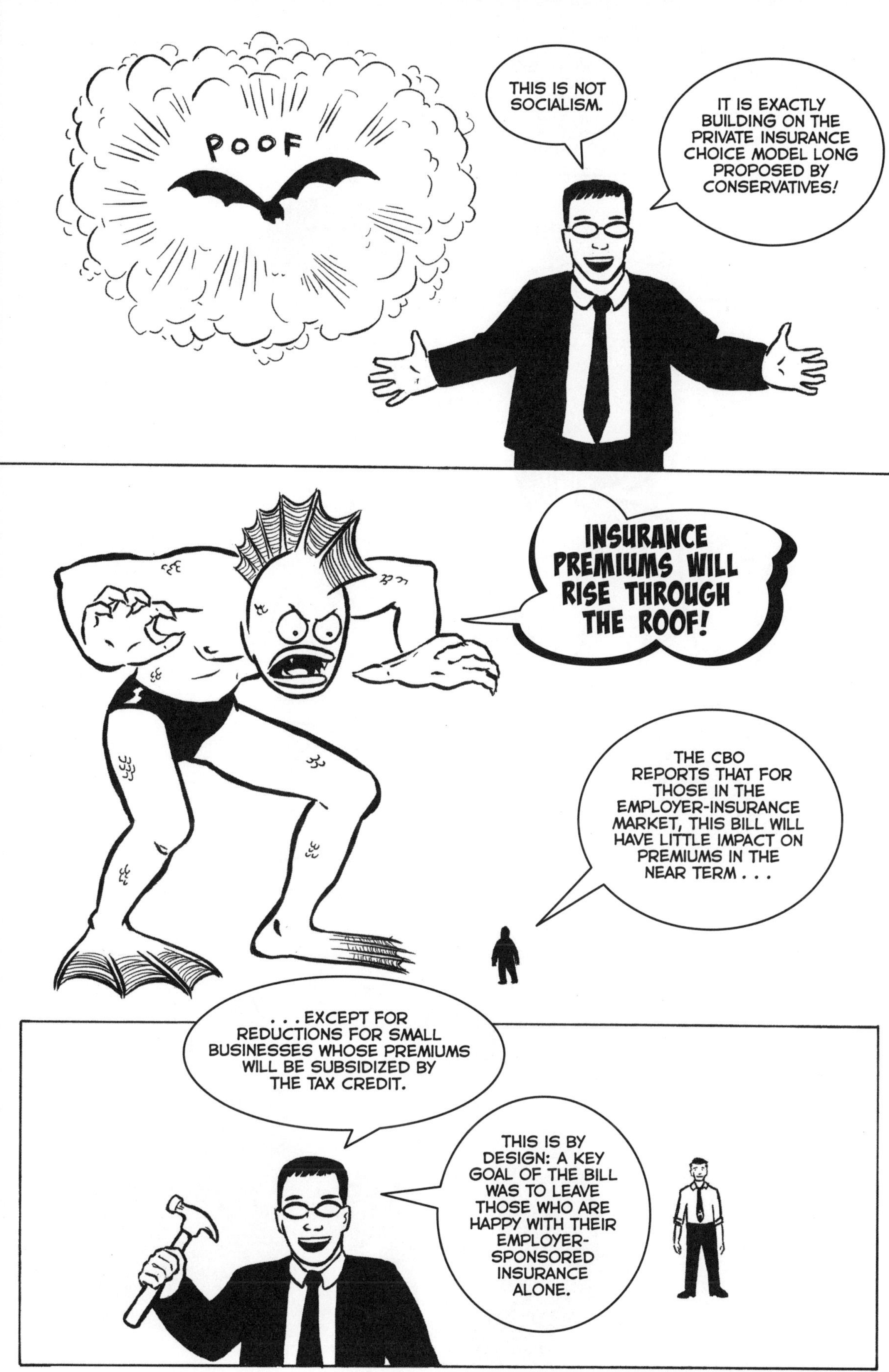
POOF
THIS IS NOT SOCIALISM.
IT IS EXACTLY BUILDING ON THE PRIVATE INSURANCE CHOICE MODEL LONG PROPOSED BY CONSERVATIVES!
INSURANCE PREMIUMS WILL RISE THROUGH THE ROOF!
THE CBO REPORTS THAT FOR THOSE IN THE EMPLOYER-INSURANCE MARKET, THIS BILL WILL HAVE LITTLE IMPACT ON PREMIUMS IN THE NEAR TERM . . .
. . . EXCEPT FOR REDUCTIONS FOR SMALL BUSINESSES WHOSE PREMIUMS WILL BE SUBSIDIZED BY THE TAX CREDIT.
THIS IS BY DESIGN: A KEY GOAL OF THE BILL WAS TO LEAVE THOSE WHO ARE HAPPY WITH THEIR EMPLOYER-SPONSORED INSURANCE ALONE.

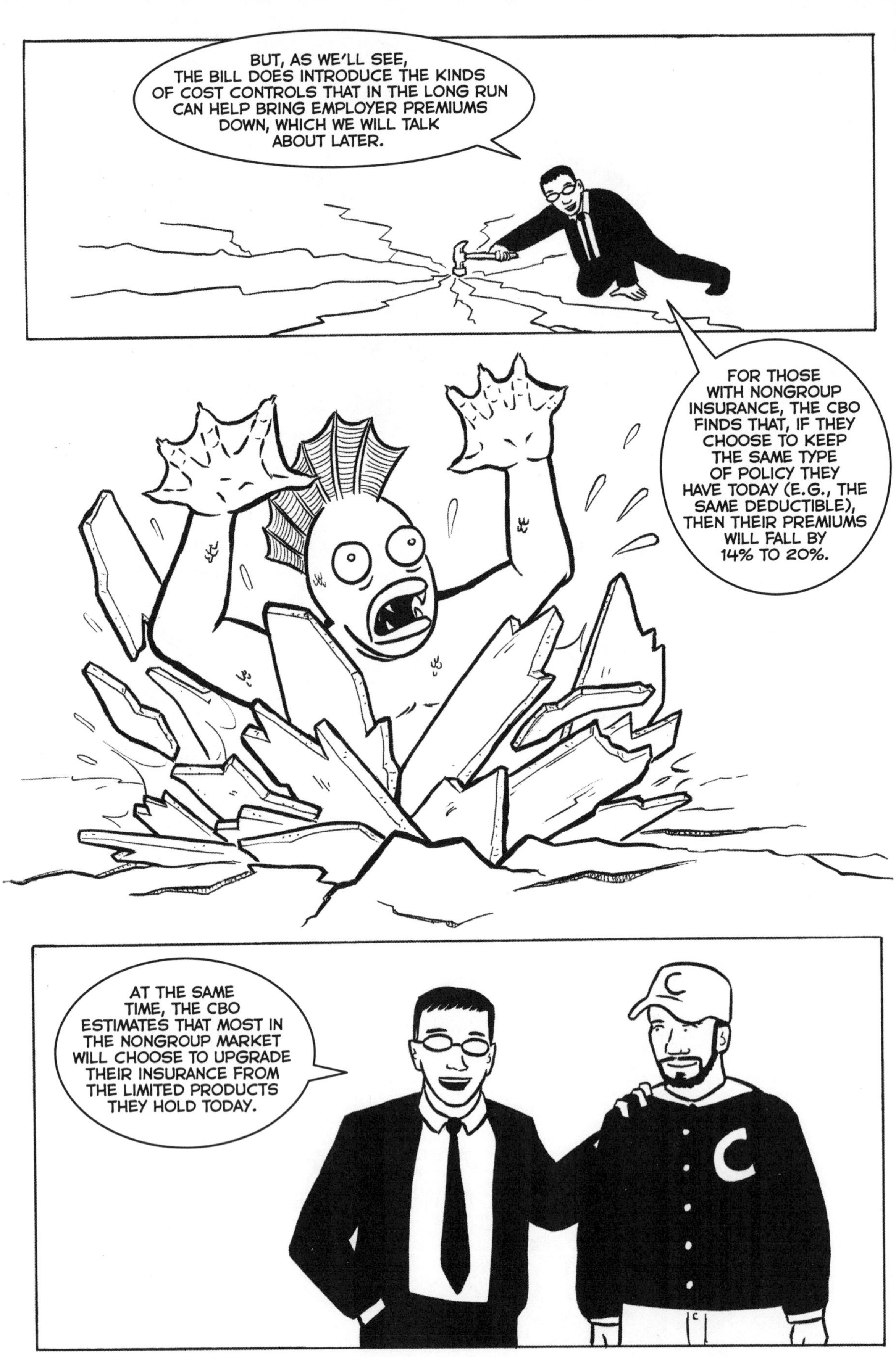
BUT, AS WE'LL SEE, THE BILL DOES INTRODUCE THE KINDS OF COST CONTROLS THAT IN THE LONG RUN CAN HELP BRING EMPLOYER PREMIUMS DOWN, WHICH WE WILL TALK ABOUT LATER.
FOR THOSE WITH NONGROUP INSURANCE, THE CBO FINDS THAT, IF THEY CHOOSE TO KEEP THE SAME TYPE OF POLICY THEY HAVE TODAY (E.G., THE SAME DEDUCTIBLE), THEN THEIR PREMIUMS WILL FALL BY 14% TO 20%.
AT THE SAME TIME, THE CBO ESTIMATES THAT MOST IN THE NONGROUP MARKET WILL CHOOSE TO UPGRADE THEIR INSURANCE FROM THE LIMITED PRODUCTS THEY HOLD TODAY.

CHAPTER 9 PICKING UP THE CHECK

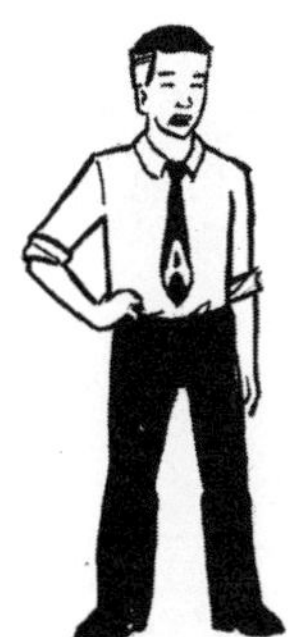
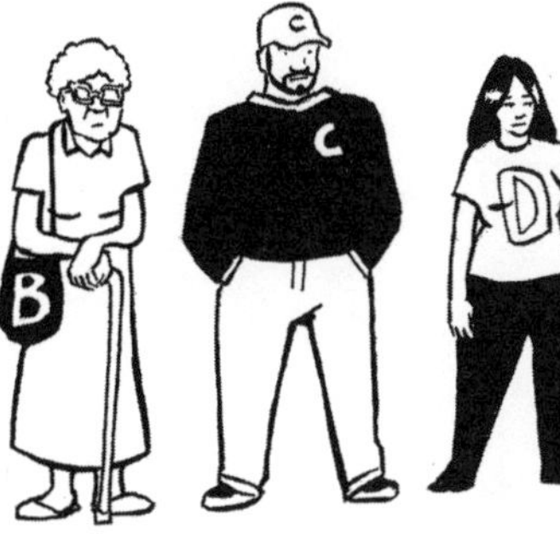
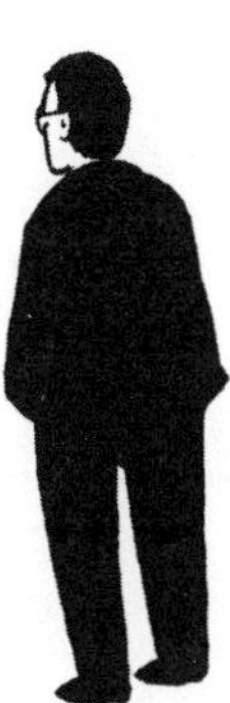

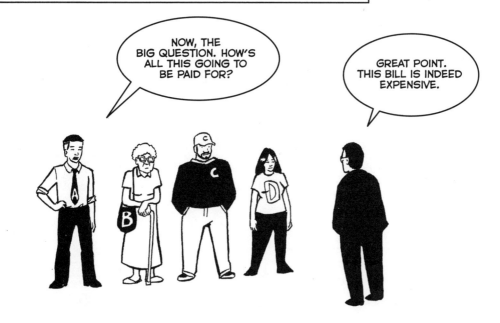

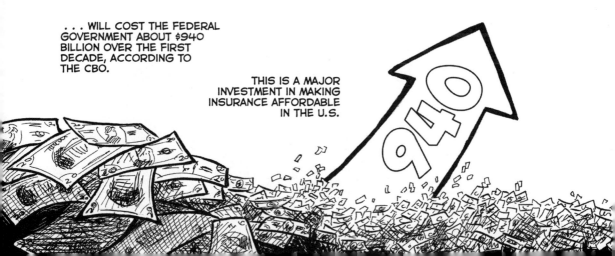

THE EXPANSION IN MEDICAID TO OUR POOREST CITIZENS, AND THE NEW SYSTEMS OF TAX CREDITS THAT MAKES INSURANCE AFFORDABLE FOR OTHER LOW-INCOME FAMILIES AND SMALL BUSINESSES . . .

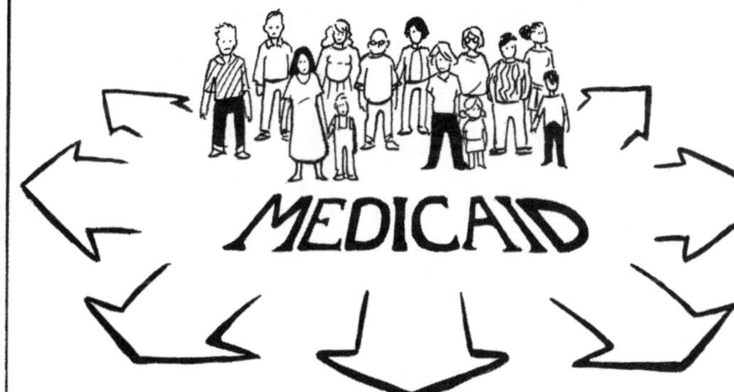

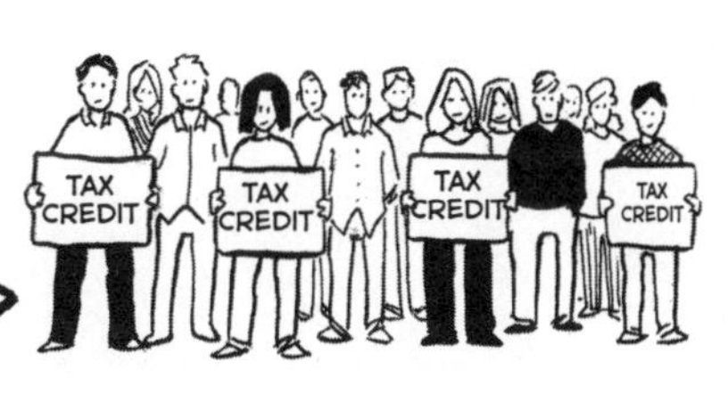

. . . WILL COST THE FEDERAL GOVERNMENT ABOUT $940 BILLION OVER THE FIRST DECADE, ACCORDING TO THE CBO.

THIS IS A MAJOR INVESTMENT IN MAKING INSURANCE AFFORDABLE IN THE U.S.

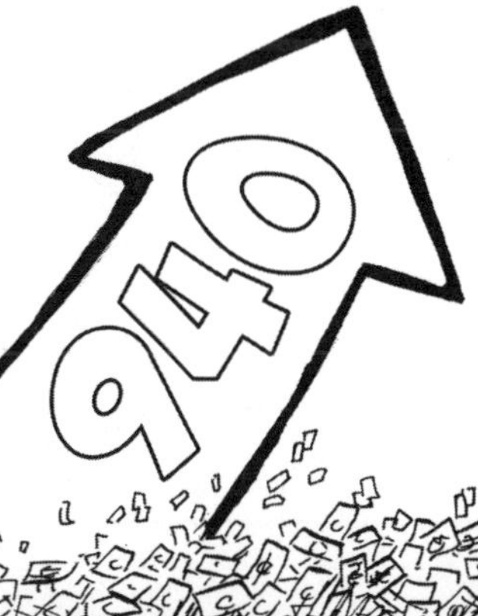

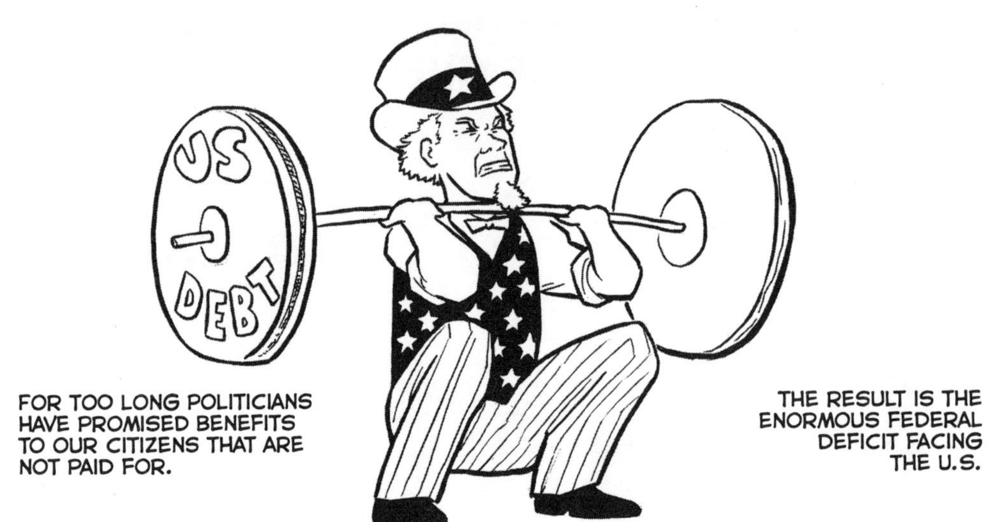
US
DEBT
FOR TOO LONG POLITICIANS HAVE PROMISED BENEFITS TO OUR CITIZENS THAT ARE NOT PAID FOR.
THE RESULT IS THE ENORMOUS FEDERAL DEFICIT FACING THE U.S.

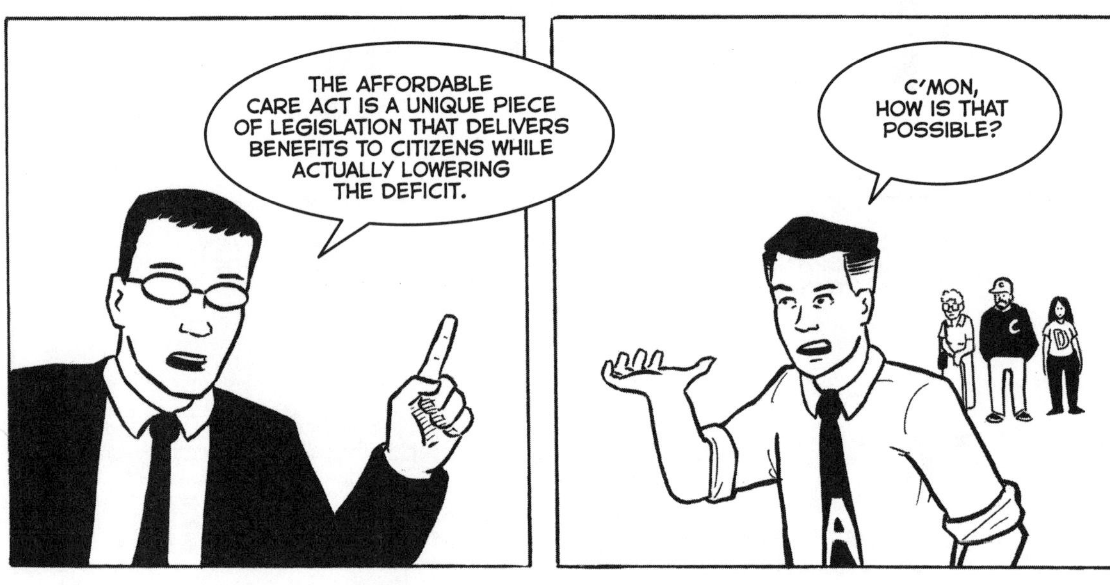
THE AFFORDABLE CARE ACT IS A UNIQUE PIECE OF LEGISLATION THAT DELIVERS BENEFITS TO CITIZENS WHILE ACTUALLY LOWERING THE DEFICIT.
C'MON, HOW IS THAT POSSIBLE?

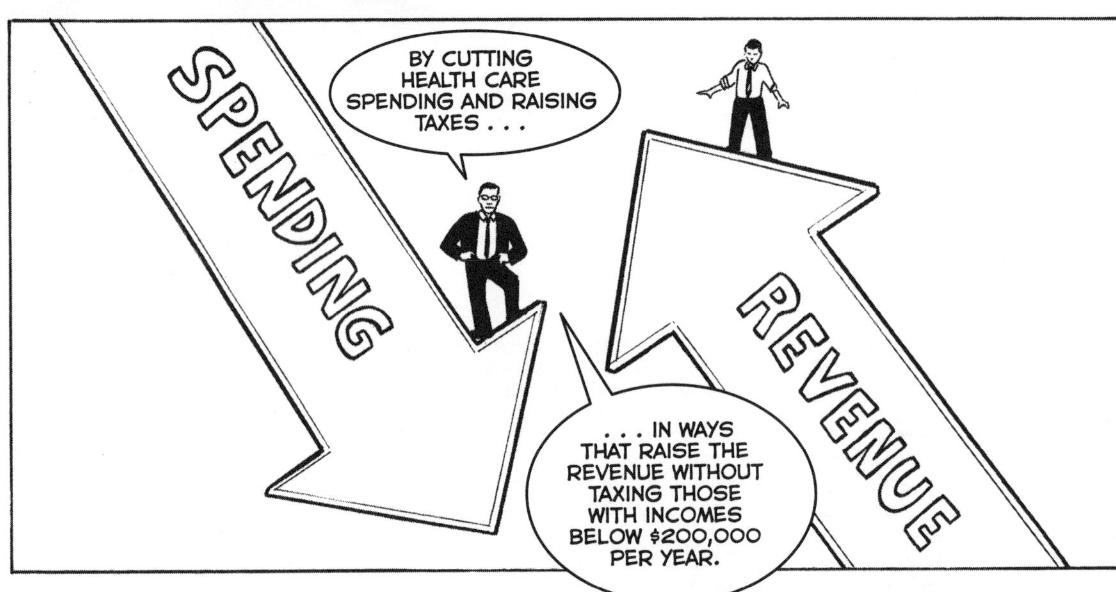
SPENDING
BY CUTTING HEALTH CARE SPENDING AND RAISING TAXES . . .
REVENUE
. . . IN WAYS THAT RAISE THE REVENUE WITHOUT TAXING THOSE WITH INCOMES BELOW $200,000 PER YEAR.

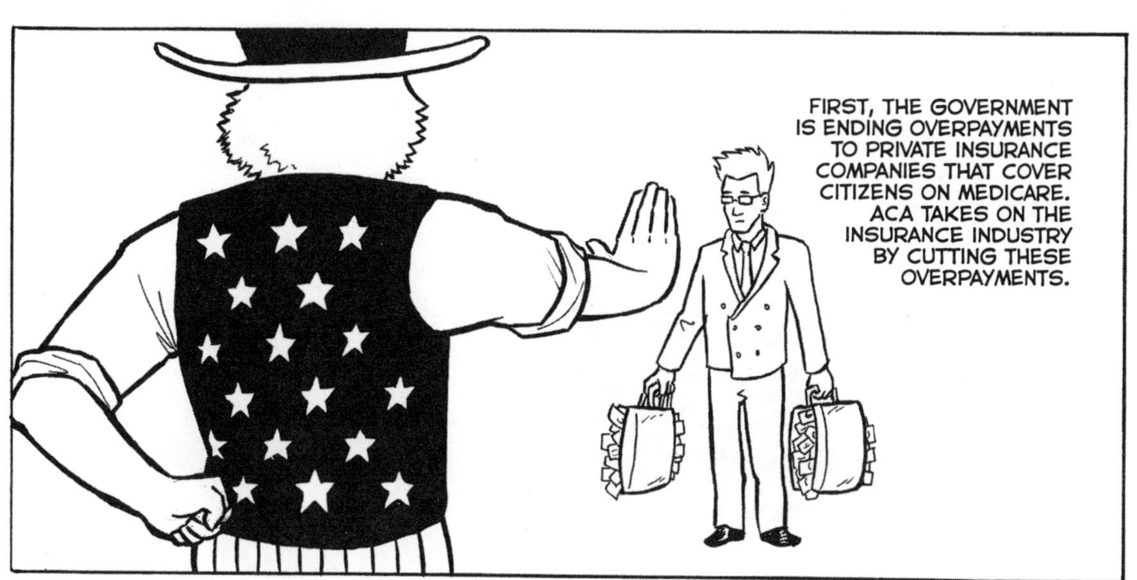

FIRST, THE GOVERNMENT IS ENDING OVERPAYMENTS TO PRIVATE INSURANCE COMPANIES THAT COVER CITIZENS ON MEDICARE. ACA TAKES ON THE INSURANCE INDUSTRY BY CUTTING THESE OVERPAYMENTS.

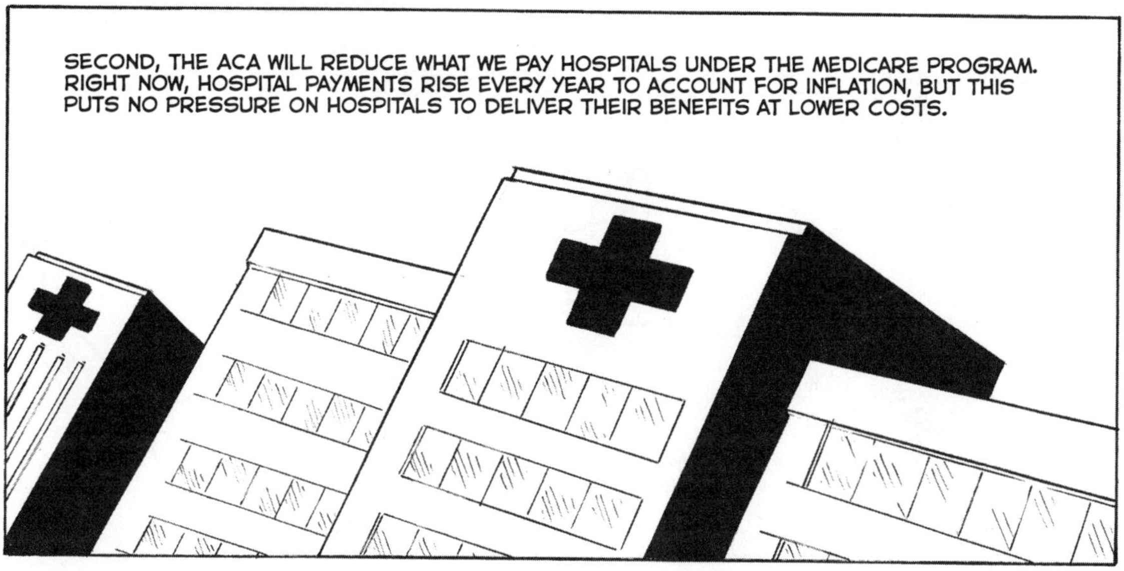

SECOND, THE ACA WILL REDUCE WHAT WE PAY HOSPITALS UNDER THE MEDICARE PROGRAM. RIGHT NOW, HOSPITAL PAYMENTS RISE EVERY YEAR TO ACCOUNT FOR INFLATION, BUT THIS PUTS NO PRESSURE ON HOSPITALS TO DELIVER THEIR BENEFITS AT LOWER COSTS.

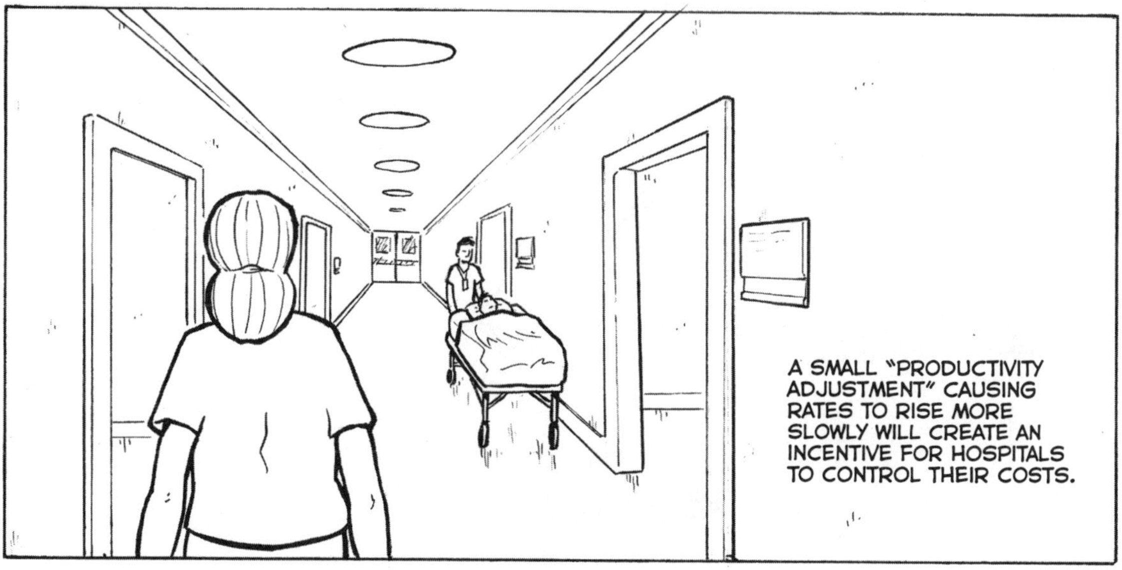

A SMALL "PRODUCTIVITY ADJUSTMENT" CAUSING RATES TO RISE MORE SLOWLY WILL CREATE AN INCENTIVE FOR HOSPITALS TO CONTROL THEIR COSTS.

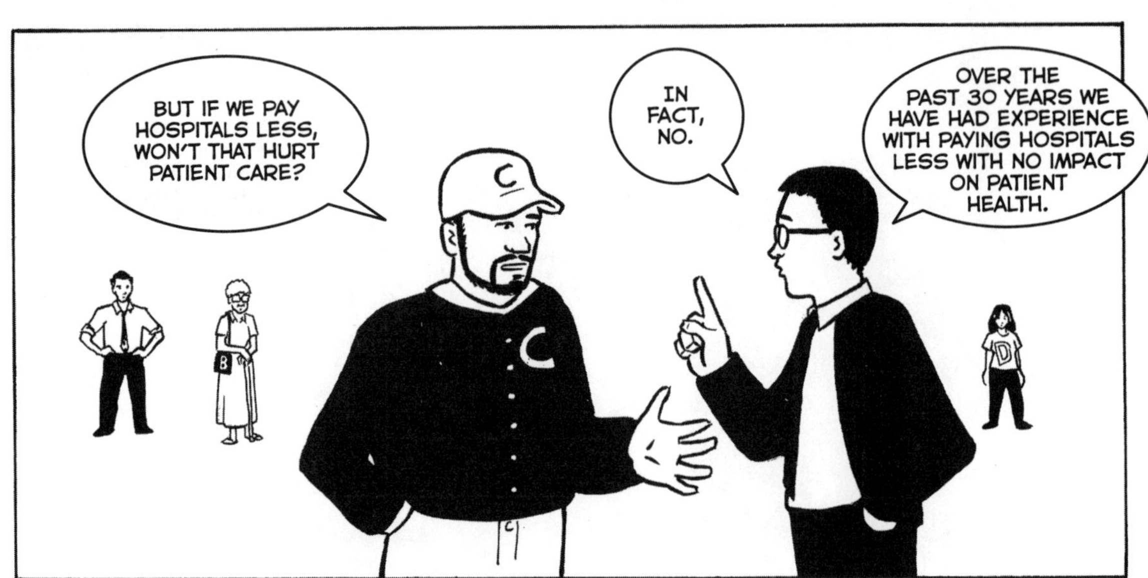
BUT IF WE PAY HOSPITALS LESS, WON'T THAT HURT PATIENT CARE?
IN FACT, NO.
OVER THE PAST 30 YEARS WE HAVE HAD EXPERIENCE WITH PAYING HOSPITALS LESS WITH NO IMPACT ON PATIENT HEALTH.

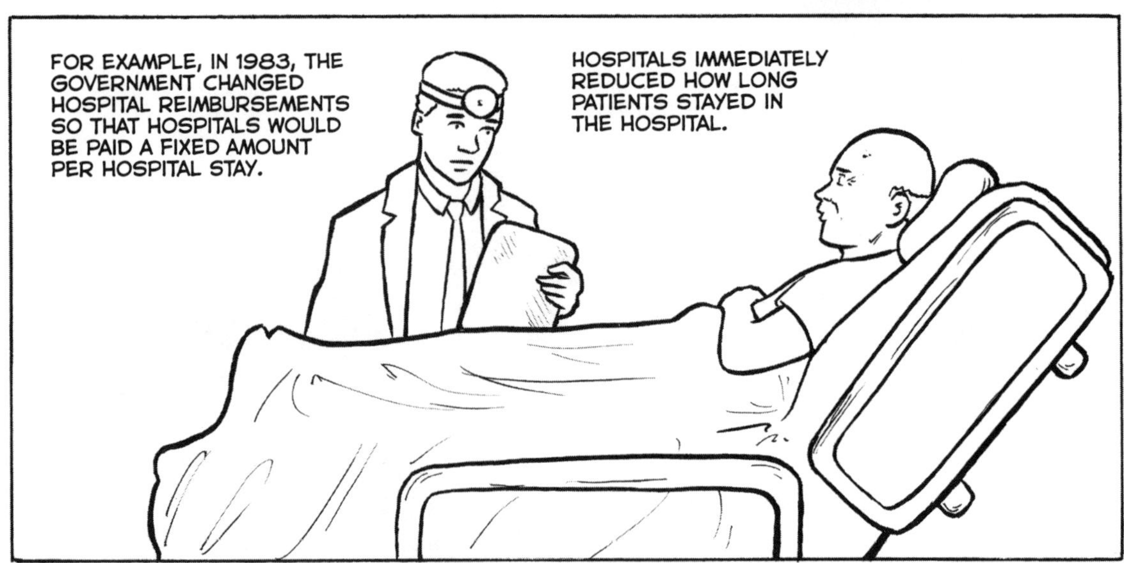
FOR EXAMPLE, IN 1983, THE GOVERNMENT CHANGED HOSPITAL REIMBURSEMENTS SO THAT HOSPITALS WOULD BE PAID A FIXED AMOUNT PER HOSPITAL STAY.
HOSPITALS IMMEDIATELY REDUCED HOW LONG PATIENTS STAYED IN THE HOSPITAL.

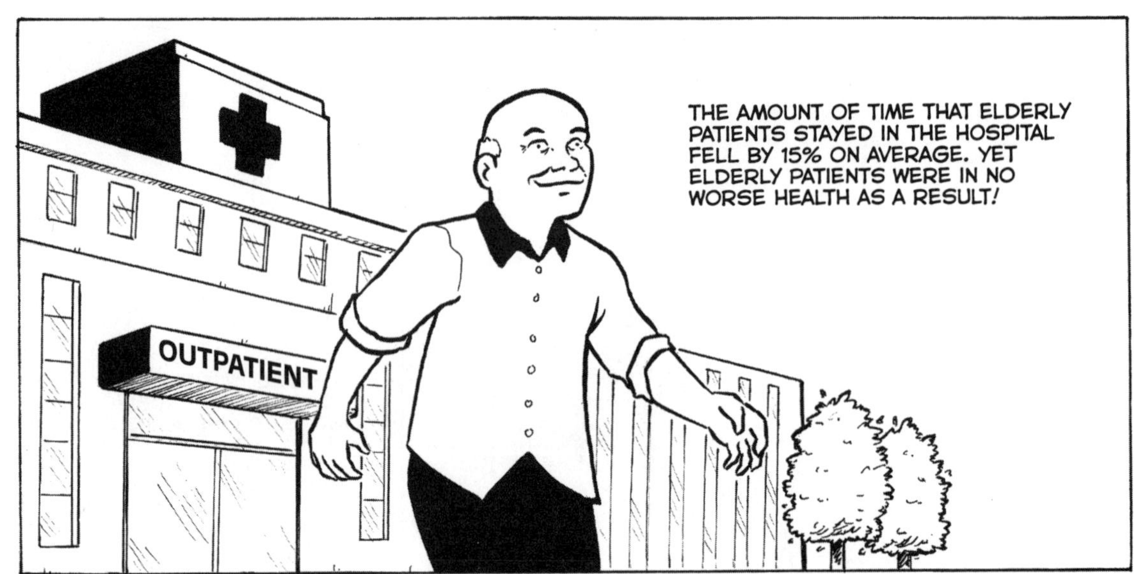
OUTPATIENT
THE AMOUNT OF TIME THAT ELDERLY PATIENTS STAYED IN THE HOSPITAL FELL BY 15% ON AVERAGE. YET ELDERLY PATIENTS WERE IN NO WORSE HEALTH AS A RESULT!

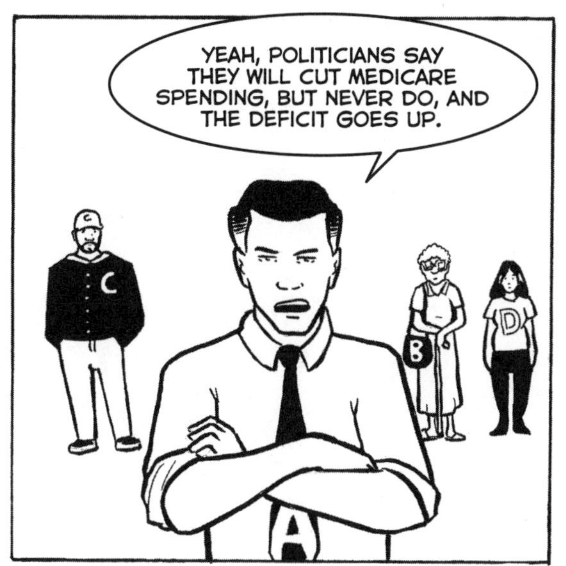
YEAH, POLITICIANS SAY THEY WILL CUT MEDICARE SPENDING, BUT NEVER DO, AND THE DEFICIT GOES UP.
C
B
D
A

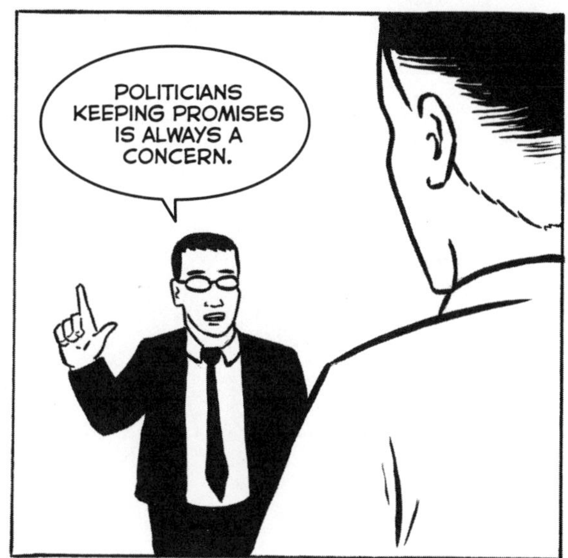
POLITICIANS KEEPING PROMISES IS ALWAYS A CONCERN.

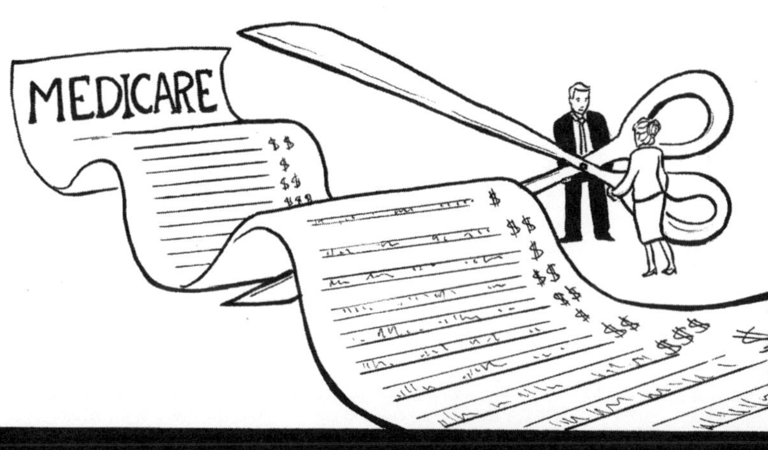
BUT THE HISTORY OF THE MEDICARE PROGRAM IS VERY ENCOURAGING. OVER THE PAST 20 YEARS, VIRTUALLY ALL PROPOSED MEDICARE CUTS HAVE BEEN ENACTED. THERE IS NO REASON TO THINK THAT CONGRESS CAN'T KEEP ITS PROMISES ON THIS ONE.
MEDICARE

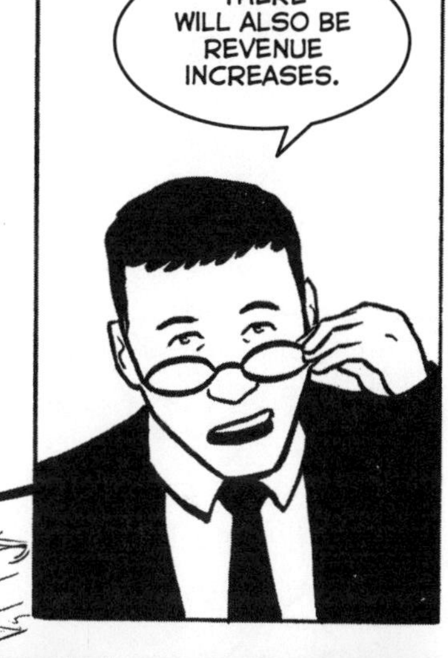
THERE WILL ALSO BE REVENUE INCREASES.

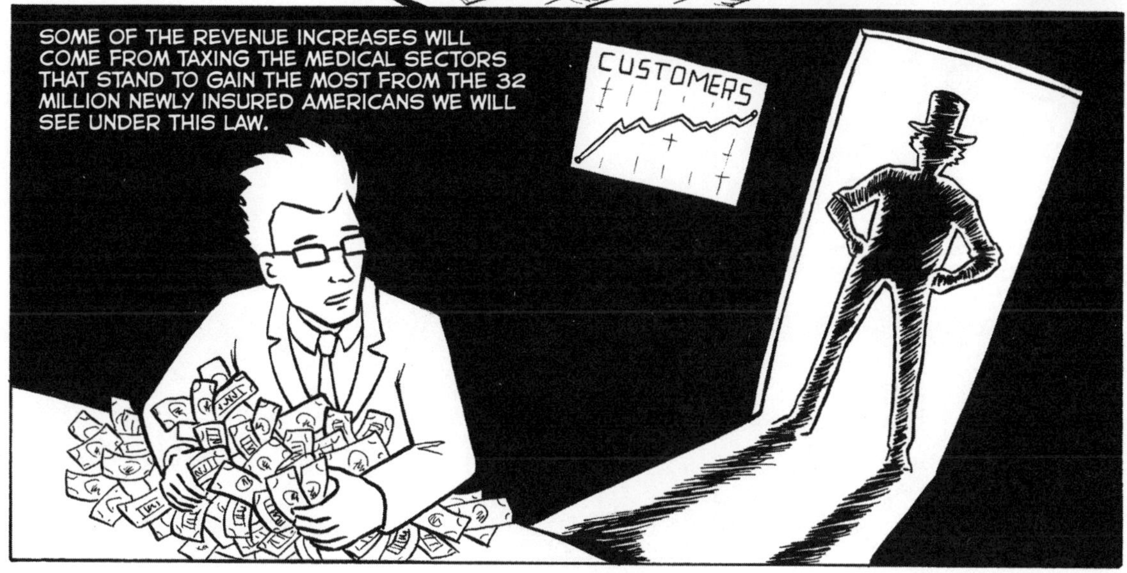
SOME OF THE REVENUE INCREASES WILL COME FROM TAXING THE MEDICAL SECTORS THAT STAND TO GAIN THE MOST FROM THE 32 MILLION NEWLY INSURED AMERICANS WE WILL SEE UNDER THIS LAW.
CUSTOMERS

THIS INCLUDES THE PHARMACEUTICAL COMPANIES, MEDICAL DEVICE COMPANIES, AND THE INSURANCE INDUSTRY.

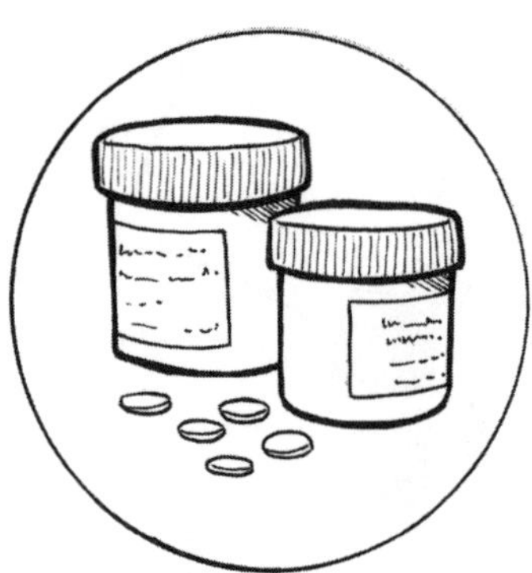

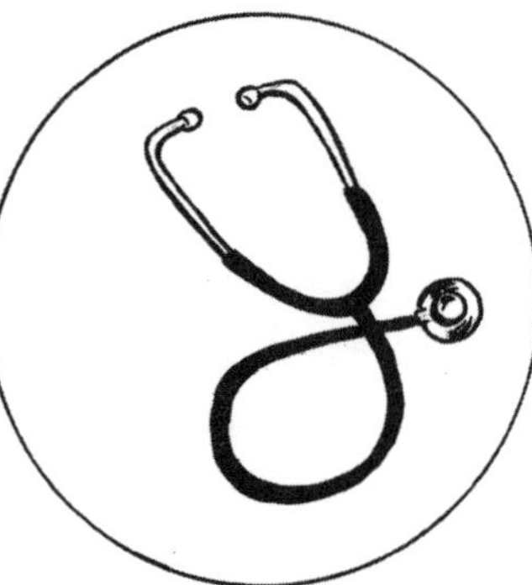

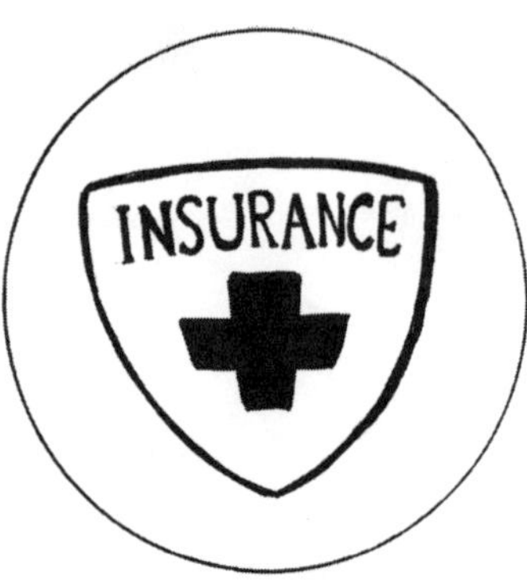

MOST OF THE REMAINING REVENUE WILL COME FROM INCREASED TAXES ON THE RICHEST AMERICANS.

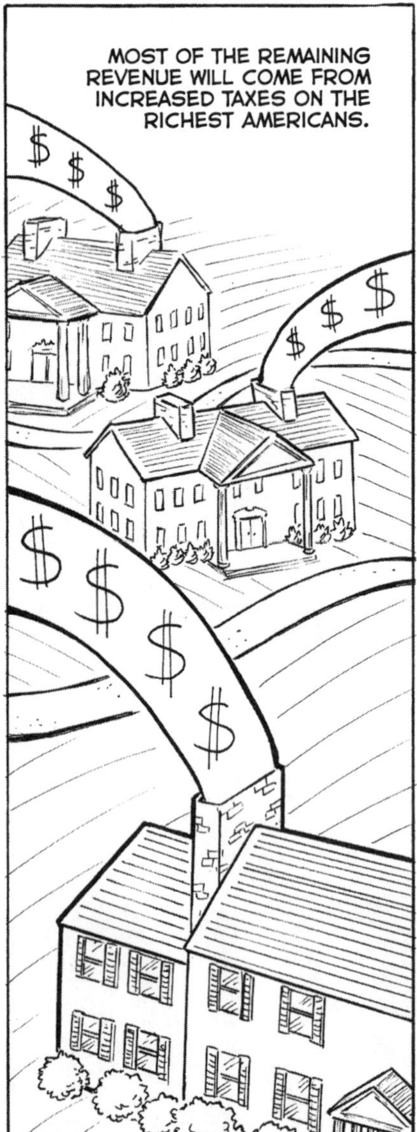

THE PAYROLL TAX THAT FINANCES THE MEDICARE PROGRAM WILL RISE BY ALMOST 1% ON THOSE INDIVIDUALS WITH INCOMES ABOVE $200,000 PER YEAR AND THOSE FAMILIES WITH INCOMES ABOVE $250,000 PER YEAR.

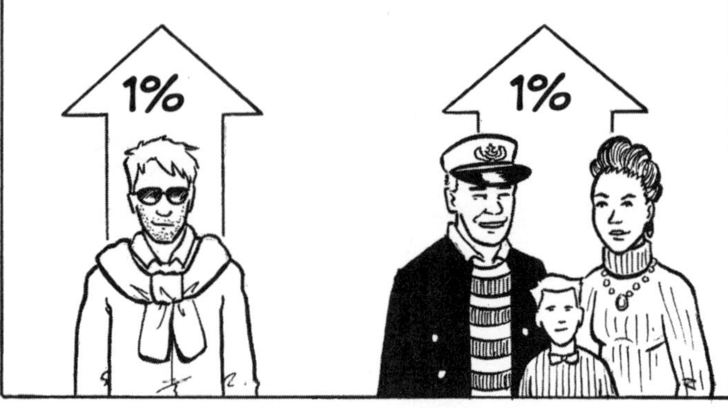

AND FOR THE FIRST TIME, THIS TAX WILL APPLY NOT ONLY TO WAGES, BUT ALSO TO MONEY MADE FROM INVESTMENTS.

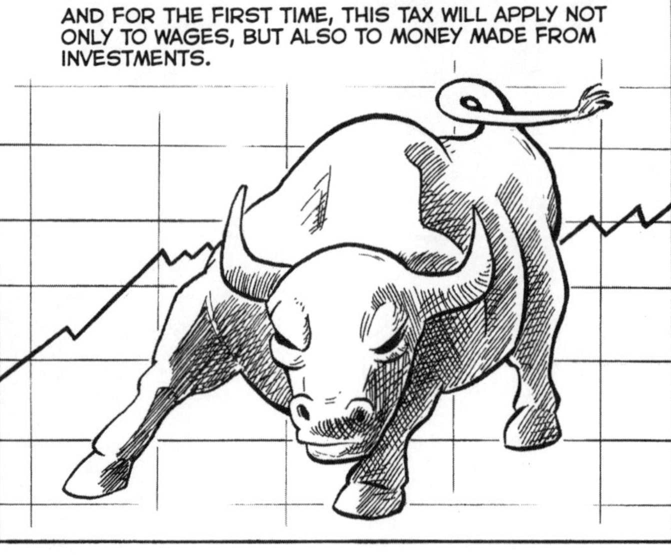

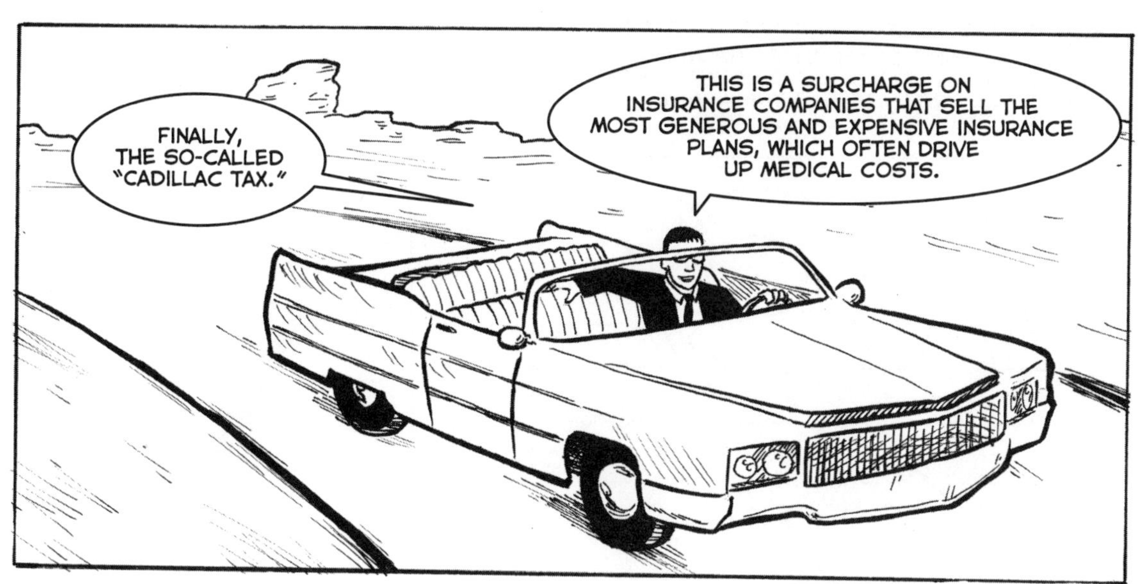
FINALLY, THE SO-CALLED "CADILLAC TAX."
THIS IS A SURCHARGE ON INSURANCE COMPANIES THAT SELL THE MOST GENEROUS AND EXPENSIVE INSURANCE PLANS, WHICH OFTEN DRIVE UP MEDICAL COSTS.

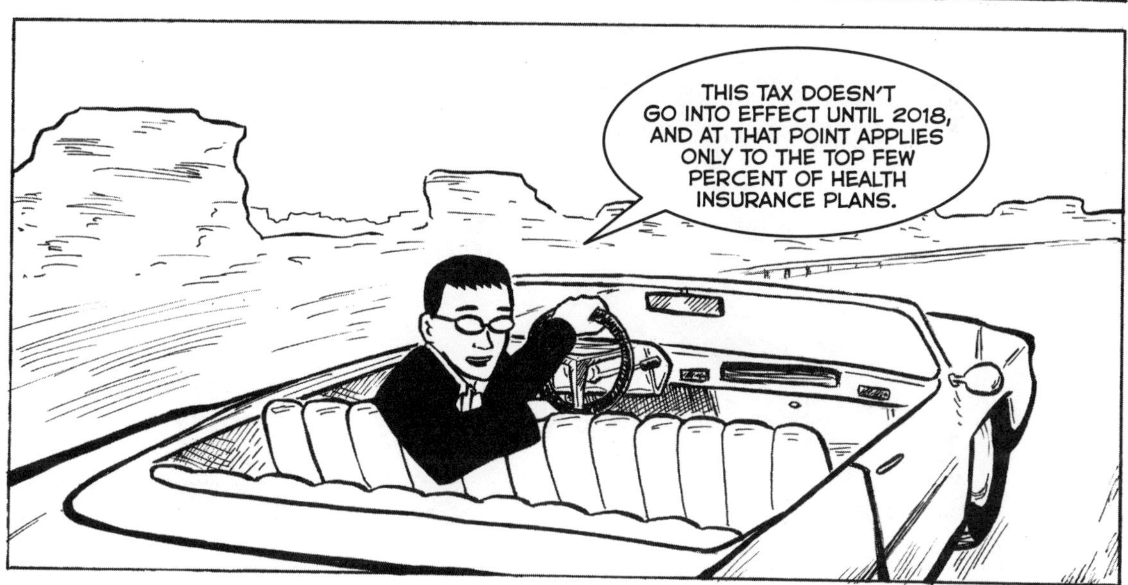
THIS TAX DOESN'T GO INTO EFFECT UNTIL 2018, AND AT THAT POINT APPLIES ONLY TO THE TOP FEW PERCENT OF HEALTH INSURANCE PLANS.

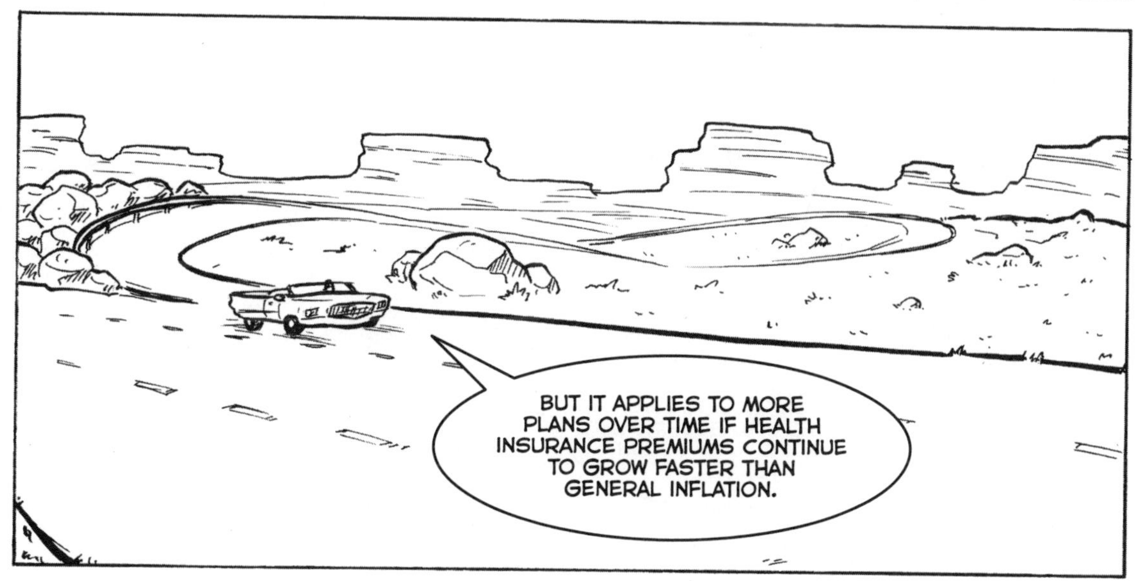
BUT IT APPLIES TO MORE PLANS OVER TIME IF HEALTH INSURANCE PREMIUMS CONTINUE TO GROW FASTER THAN GENERAL INFLATION.

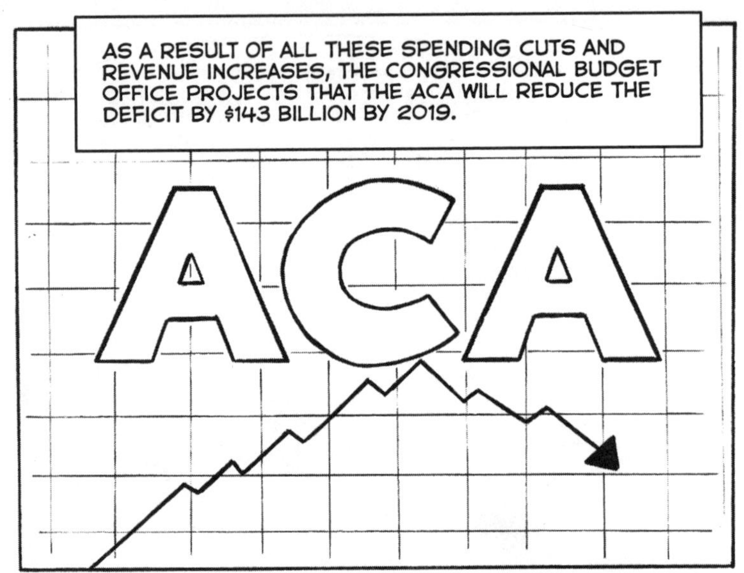

AS A RESULT OF ALL THESE SPENDING CUTS AND REVENUE INCREASES, THE CONGRESSIONAL BUDGET OFFICE PROJECTS THAT THE ACA WILL REDUCE THE DEFICIT BY $143 BILLION BY 2019.

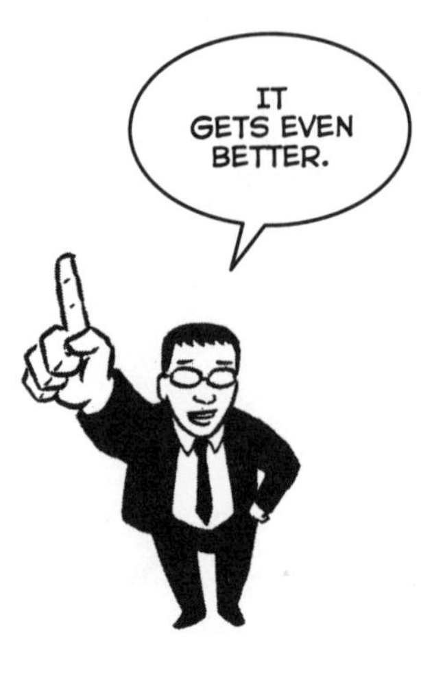

IT GETS EVEN BETTER.

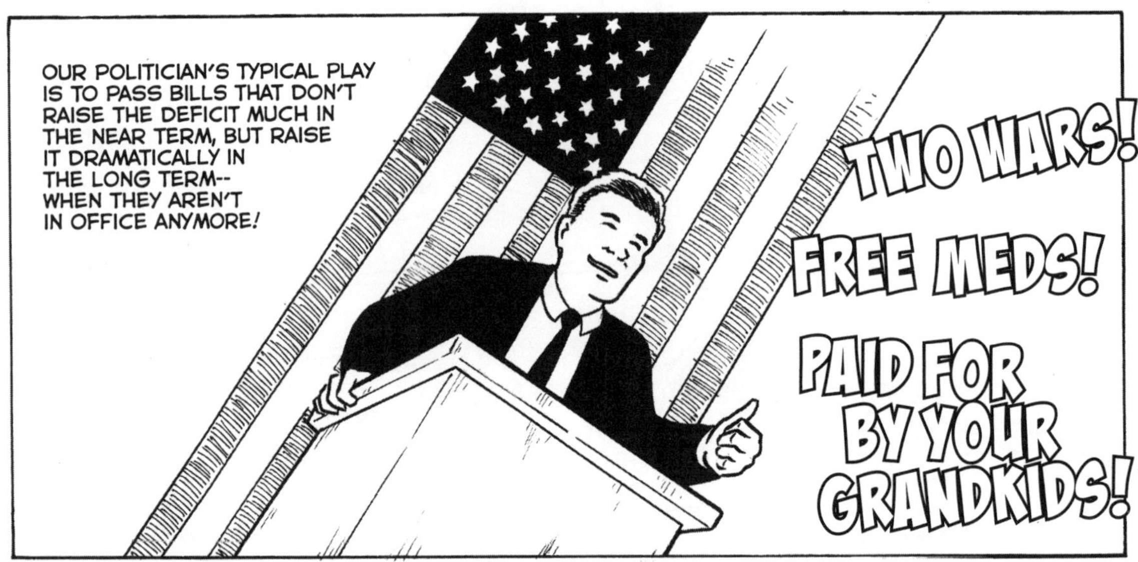

OUR POLITICIAN'S TYPICAL PLAY IS TO PASS BILLS THAT DON'T RAISE THE DEFICIT MUCH IN THE NEAR TERM, BUT RAISE IT DRAMATICALLY IN THE LONG TERM-- WHEN THEY AREN'T IN OFFICE ANYMORE!
TWO WARS!
FREE MEDS!
PAID FOR BY YOUR GRANDKIDS!

BUT THE ACA IS THE OPPOSITE: THE DEFICIT-REDUCING EFFECTS OF THIS LEGISLATION GROW OVER TIME, SO THAT OVER ITS SECOND DECADE THE ACA CUTS MORE THAN $1 TRILLION FROM THE DEFICIT!

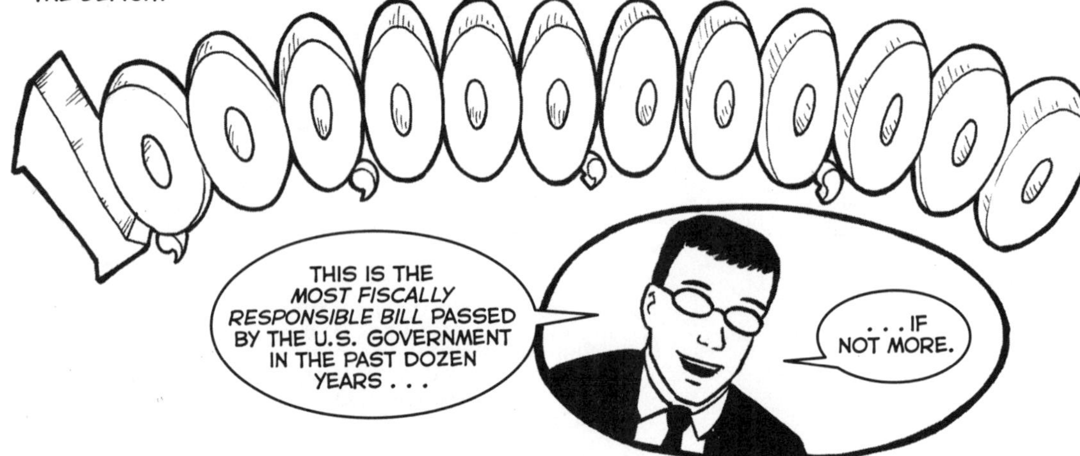

1,000,000,000,000
THIS IS THE *MOST FISCALLY RESPONSIBLE BILL* PASSED BY THE U.S. GOVERNMENT IN THE PAST DOZEN YEARS . . .
. . . IF NOT MORE.

CHAPTER 10 TAKING ON COST CONTROL

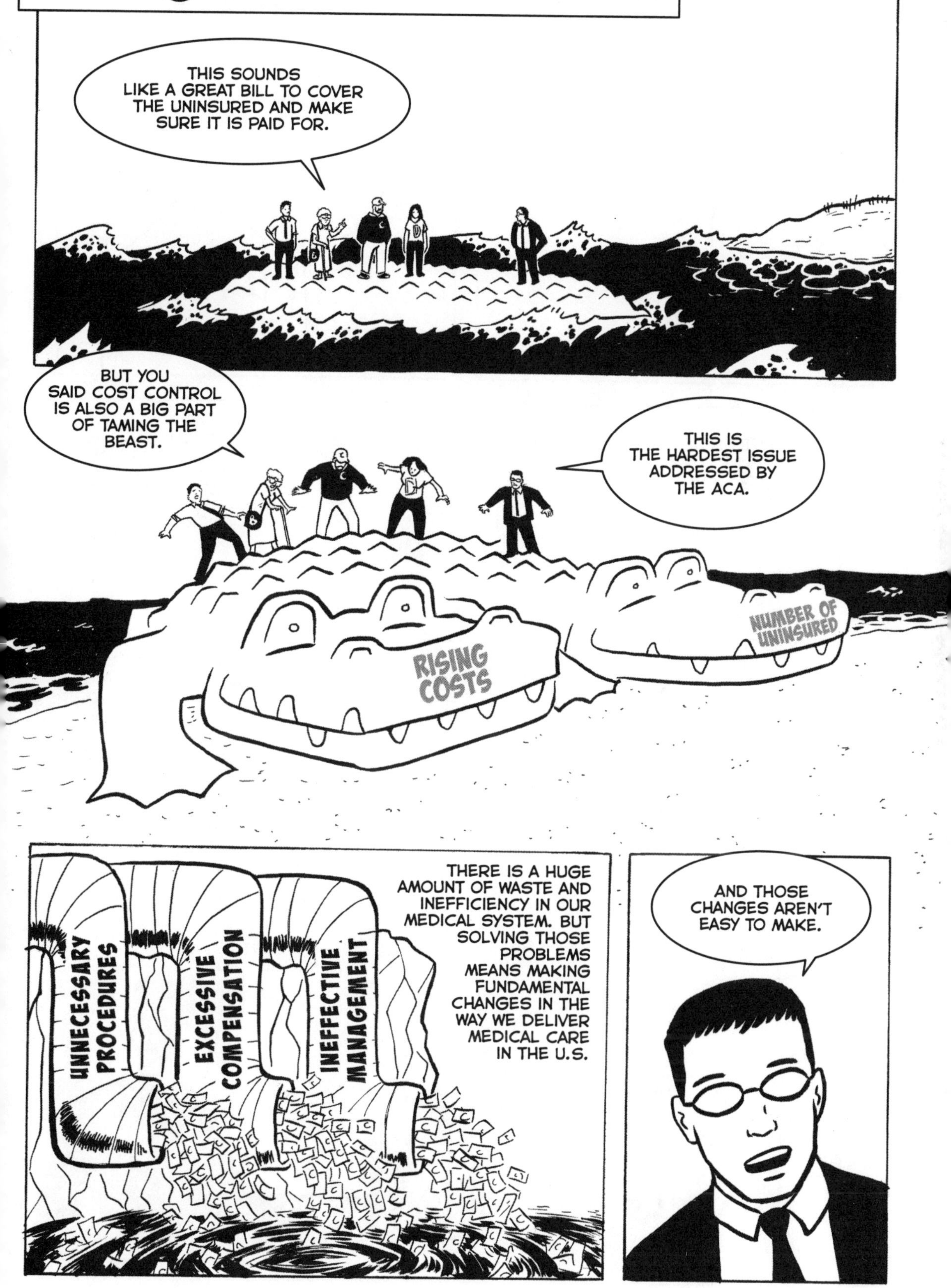

THIS SOUNDS LIKE A GREAT BILL TO COVER THE UNINSURED AND MAKE SURE IT IS PAID FOR.

BUT YOU SAID COST CONTROL IS ALSO A BIG PART OF TAMING THE BEAST.

THIS IS THE HARDEST ISSUE ADDRESSED BY THE ACA.

RISING COSTS

NUMBER OF UNINSURED

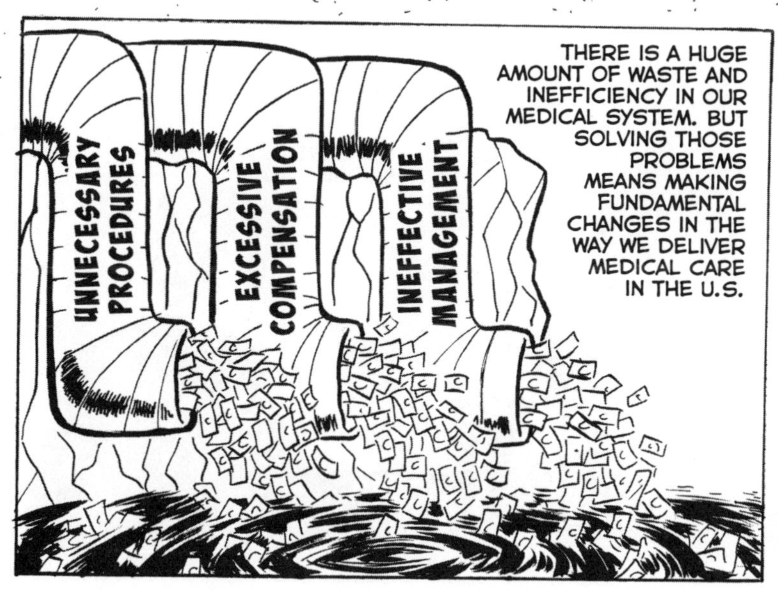

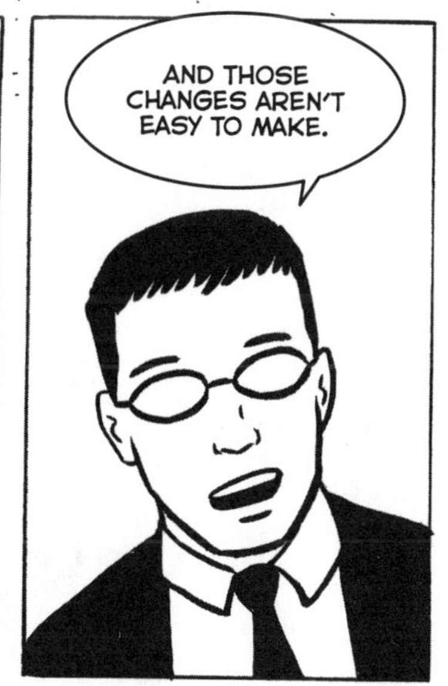

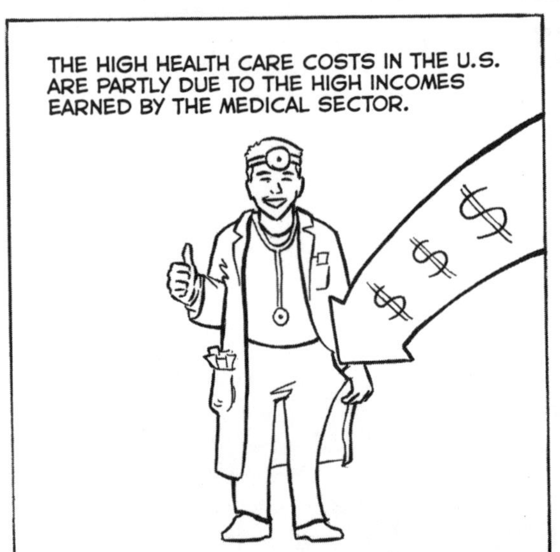
THE HIGH HEALTH CARE COSTS IN THE U.S. ARE PARTLY DUE TO THE HIGH INCOMES EARNED BY THE MEDICAL SECTOR.
$
$
$

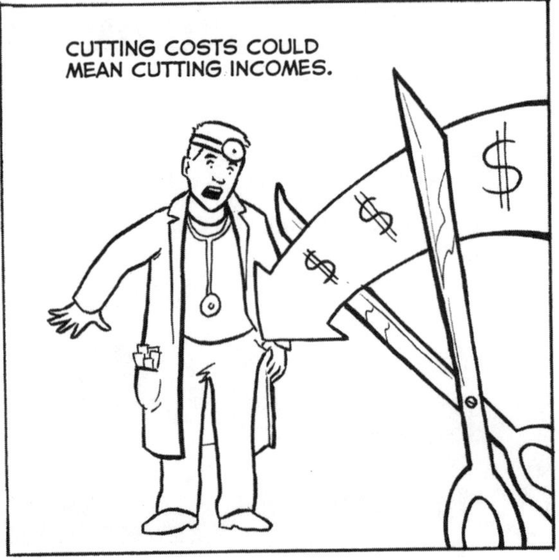
CUTTING COSTS COULD MEAN CUTTING INCOMES.
$
$
$

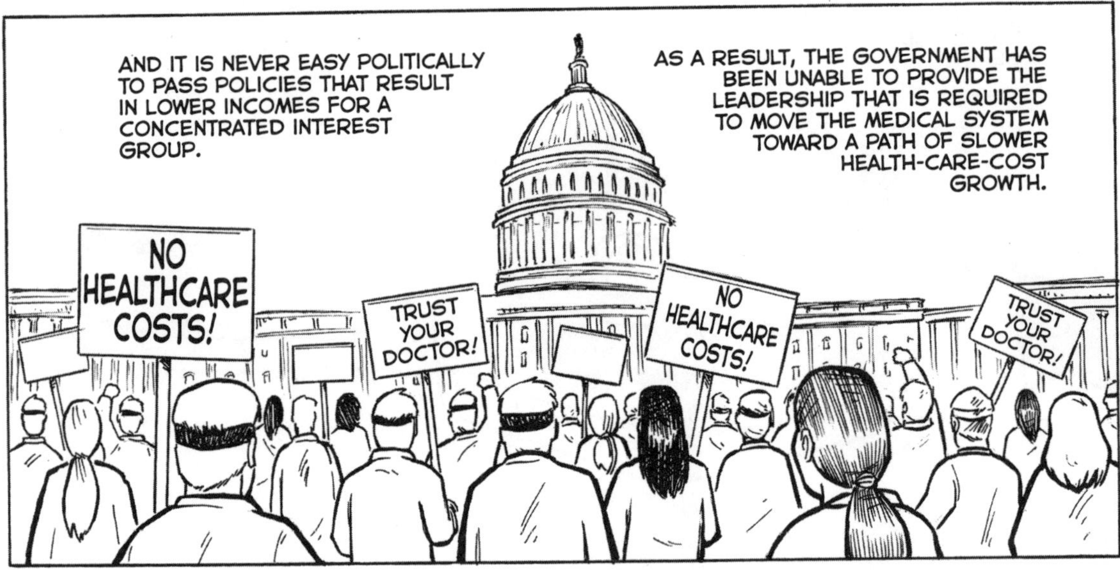
AND IT IS NEVER EASY POLITICALLY TO PASS POLICIES THAT RESULT IN LOWER INCOMES FOR A CONCENTRATED INTEREST GROUP.
AS A RESULT, THE GOVERNMENT HAS BEEN UNABLE TO PROVIDE THE LEADERSHIP THAT IS REQUIRED TO MOVE THE MEDICAL SYSTEM TOWARD A PATH OF SLOWER HEALTH-CARE-COST GROWTH.
NO HEALTHCARE COSTS!
TRUST YOUR DOCTOR!
NO HEALTHCARE COSTS!
TRUST YOUR DOCTOR!

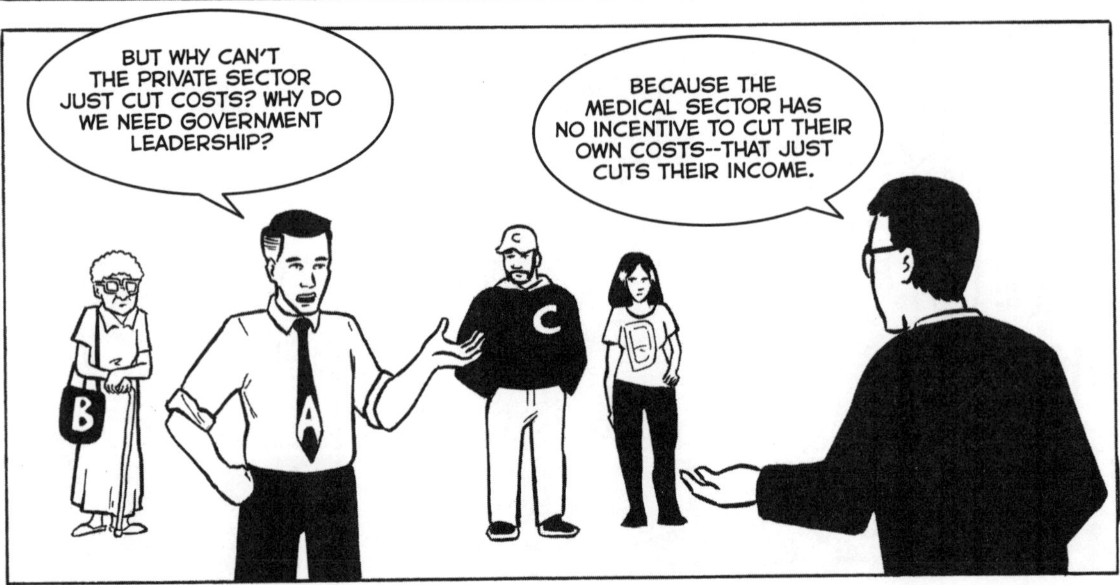
BUT WHY CAN'T THE PRIVATE SECTOR JUST CUT COSTS? WHY DO WE NEED GOVERNMENT LEADERSHIP?
BECAUSE THE MEDICAL SECTOR HAS NO INCENTIVE TO CUT THEIR OWN COSTS--THAT JUST CUTS THEIR INCOME.
B
A
C
C
D

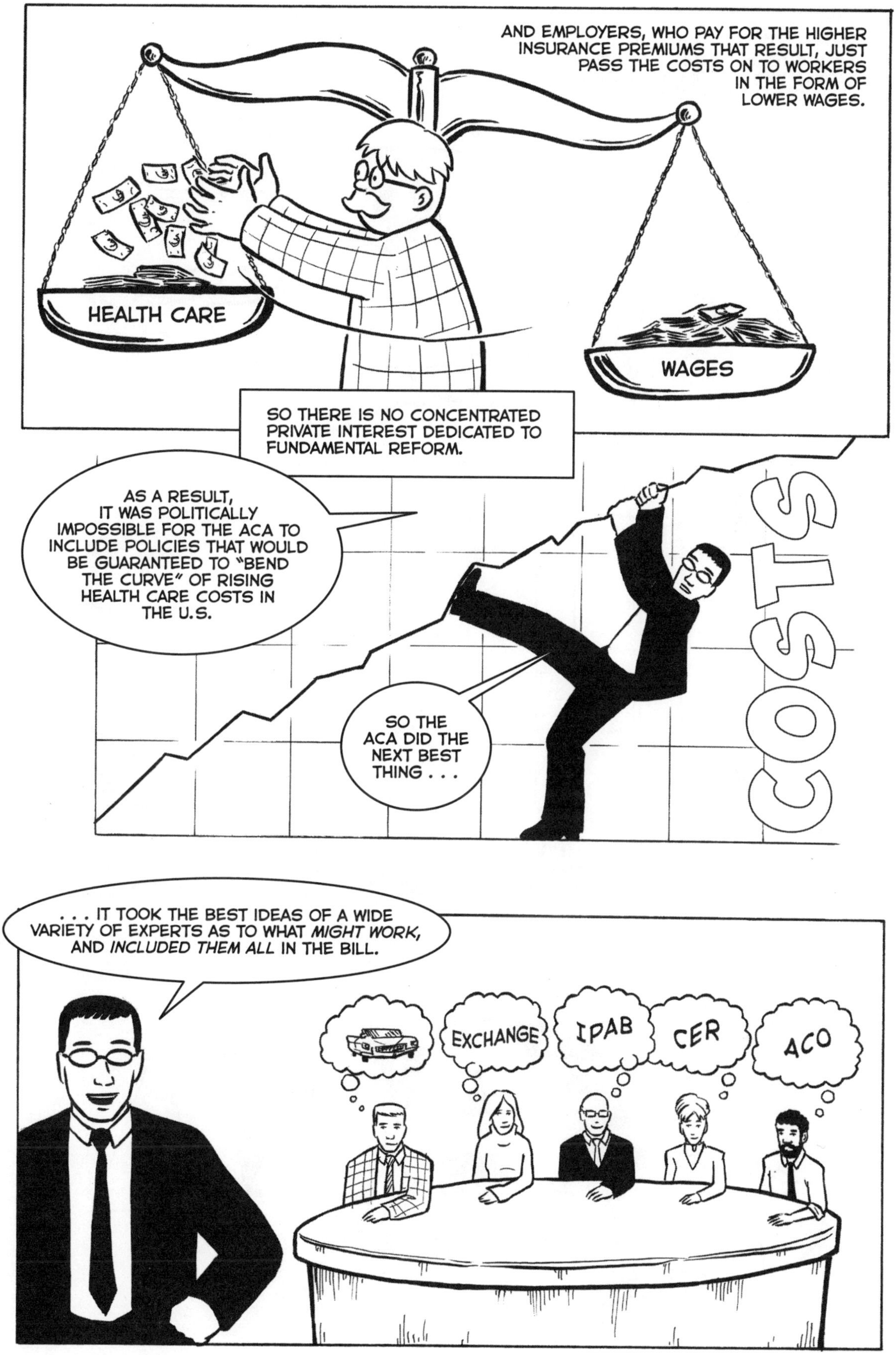

AND EMPLOYERS, WHO PAY FOR THE HIGHER INSURANCE PREMIUMS THAT RESULT, JUST PASS THE COSTS ON TO WORKERS IN THE FORM OF LOWER WAGES.

HEALTH CARE

WAGES

SO THERE IS NO CONCENTRATED PRIVATE INTEREST DEDICATED TO FUNDAMENTAL REFORM.

AS A RESULT, IT WAS POLITICALLY IMPOSSIBLE FOR THE ACA TO INCLUDE POLICIES THAT WOULD BE GUARANTEED TO "BEND THE CURVE" OF RISING HEALTH CARE COSTS IN THE U.S.

COSTS

SO THE ACA DID THE NEXT BEST THING . . .

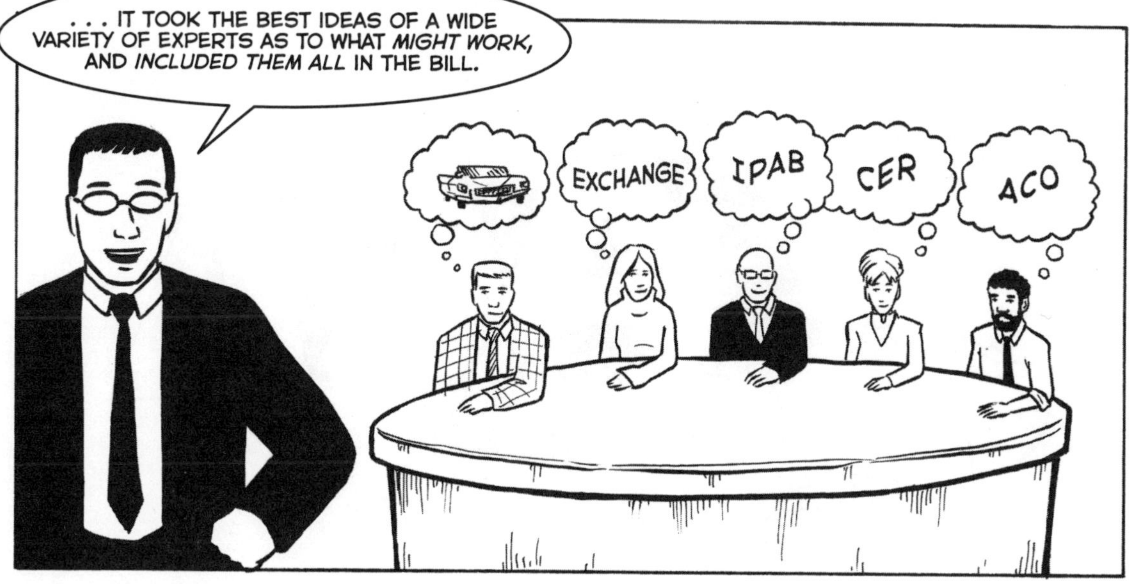

. . . IT TOOK THE BEST IDEAS OF A WIDE VARIETY OF EXPERTS AS TO WHAT *MIGHT WORK,* AND *INCLUDED THEM ALL* IN THE BILL.
EXCHANGE
IPAB
CER
ACO

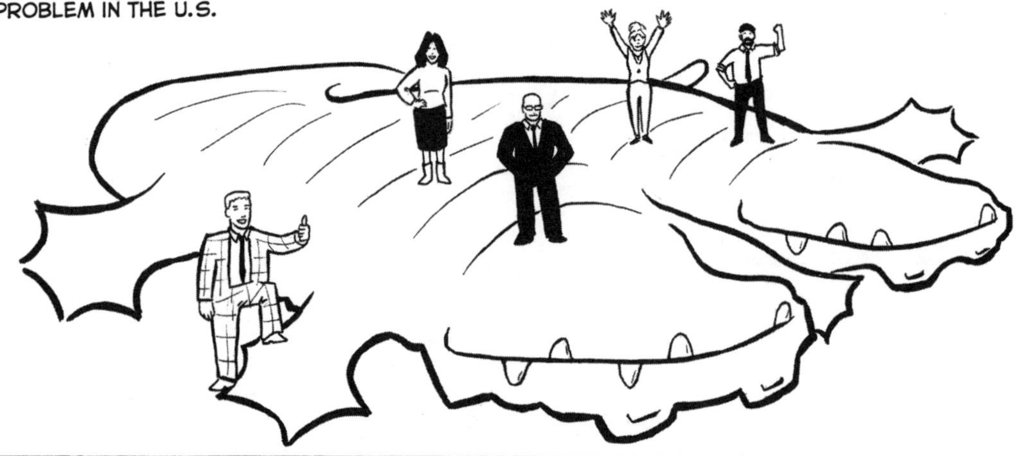
IF THEY ALL WORK OUT, THE ACA WILL END UP SOLVING OUR COST PROBLEM IN THE U.S.

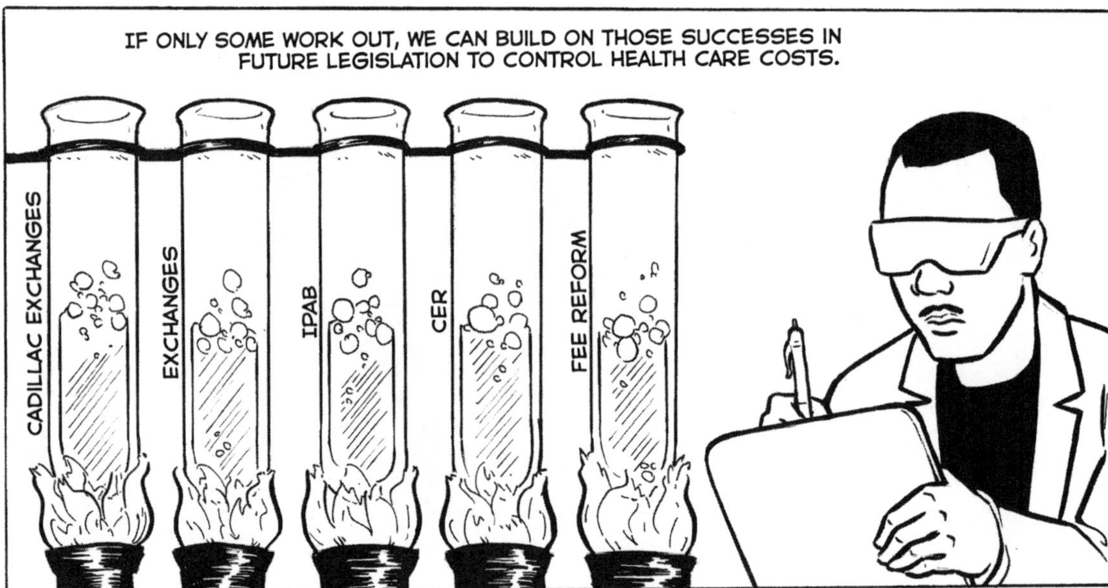
IF ONLY SOME WORK OUT, WE CAN BUILD ON THOSE SUCCESSES IN FUTURE LEGISLATION TO CONTROL HEALTH CARE COSTS.
CADILLAC EXCHANGES
EXCHANGES
IPAB
CER
FEE REFORM

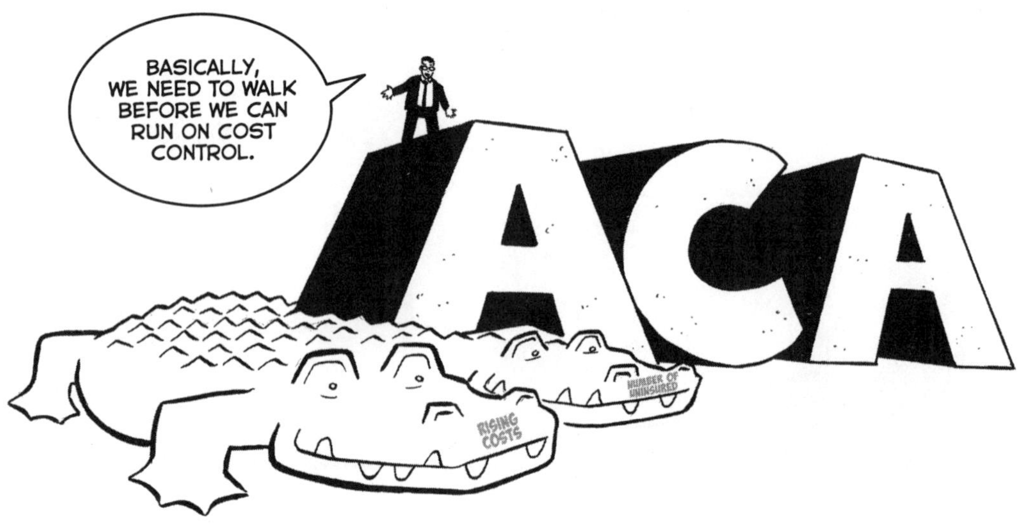
BASICALLY, WE NEED TO WALK BEFORE WE CAN RUN ON COST CONTROL.
ACA
RISING COSTS
NUMBER OF UNINSURED

THROUGH FIVE KEY INNOVATIONS IN COST CONTROL INCLUDED IN THE ACA . . .

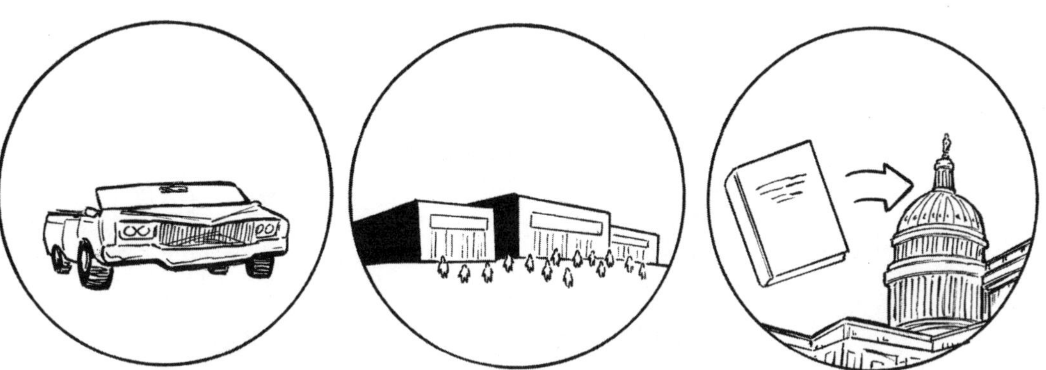

. . . WE WILL LEARN WHAT WORKS AND WHAT DOESN'T . . .

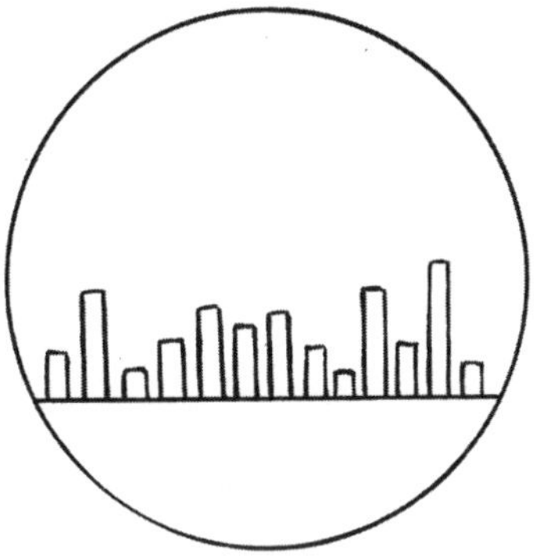

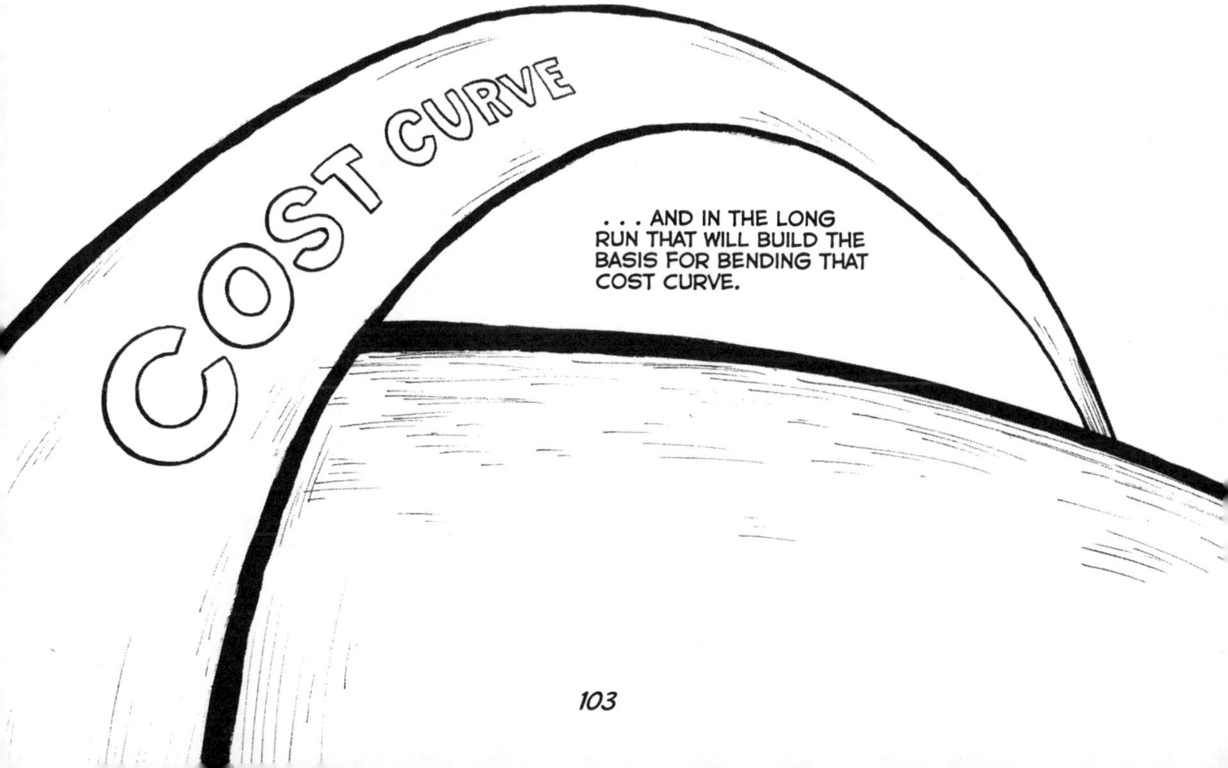

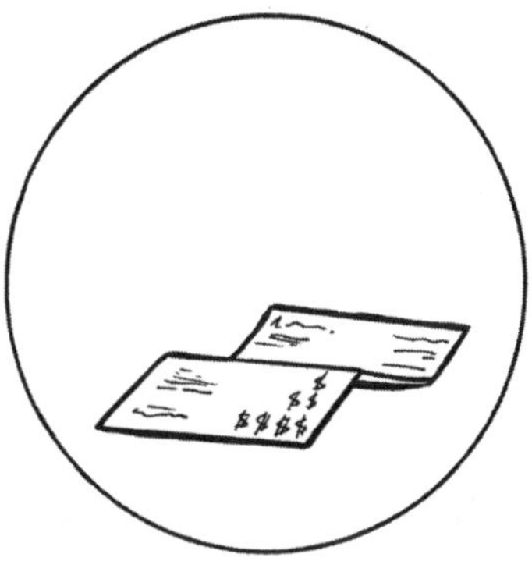

COST CURVE

. . . AND IN THE LONG RUN THAT WILL BUILD THE BASIS FOR BENDING THAT COST CURVE.

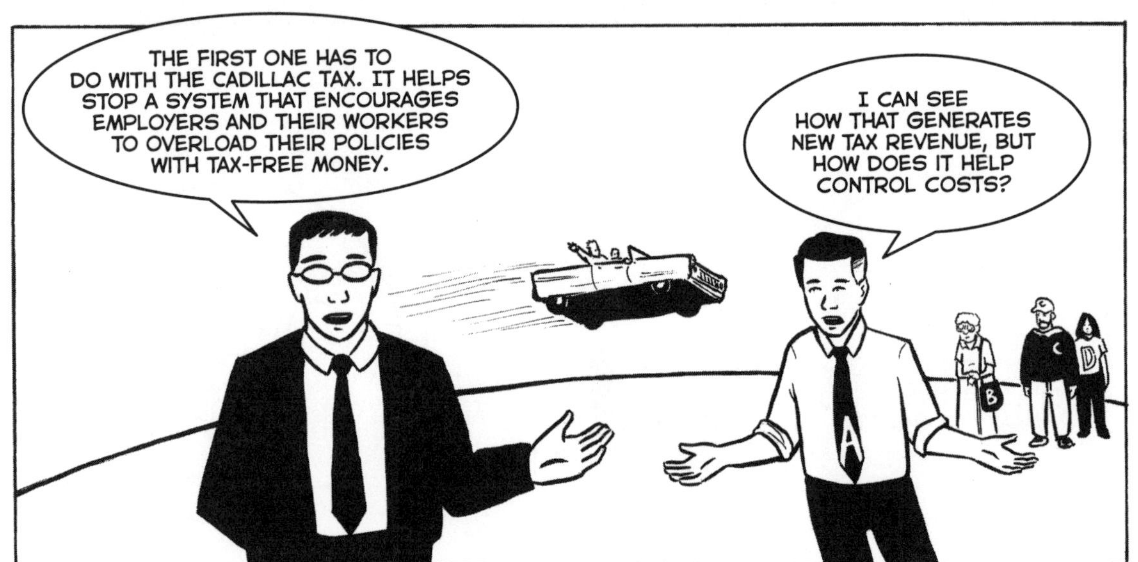
THE FIRST ONE HAS TO DO WITH THE CADILLAC TAX. IT HELPS STOP A SYSTEM THAT ENCOURAGES EMPLOYERS AND THEIR WORKERS TO OVERLOAD THEIR POLICIES WITH TAX-FREE MONEY.
I CAN SEE HOW THAT GENERATES NEW TAX REVENUE, BUT HOW DOES IT HELP CONTROL COSTS?
A
B
C
D

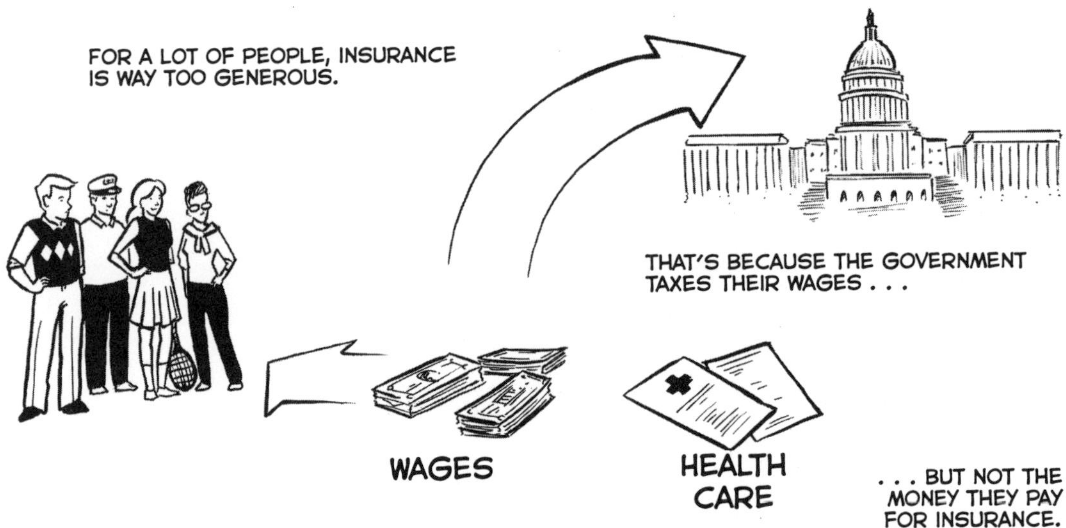
FOR A LOT OF PEOPLE, INSURANCE IS WAY TOO GENEROUS.
THAT'S BECAUSE THE GOVERNMENT TAXES THEIR WAGES . . .
WAGES
HEALTH CARE
. . . BUT NOT THE MONEY THEY PAY FOR INSURANCE.

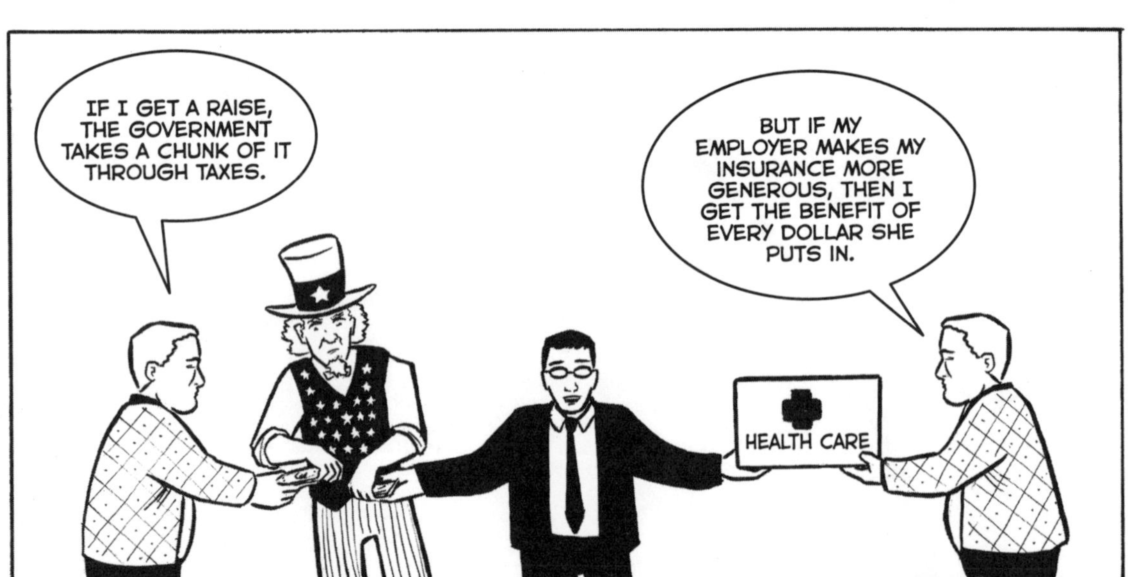
IF I GET A RAISE, THE GOVERNMENT TAKES A CHUNK OF IT THROUGH TAXES.
BUT IF MY EMPLOYER MAKES MY INSURANCE MORE GENEROUS, THEN I GET THE BENEFIT OF EVERY DOLLAR SHE PUTS IN.
HEALTH CARE

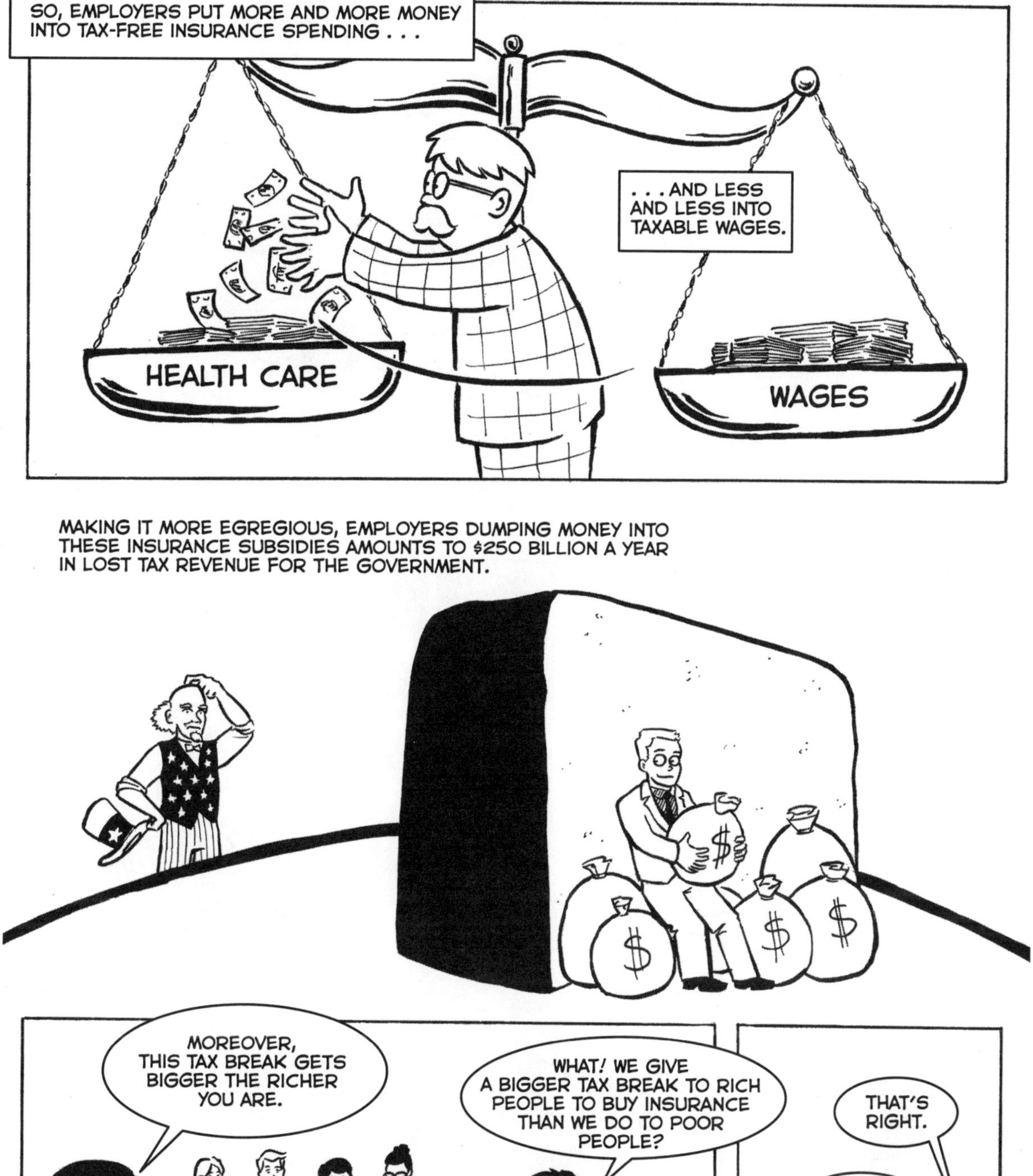

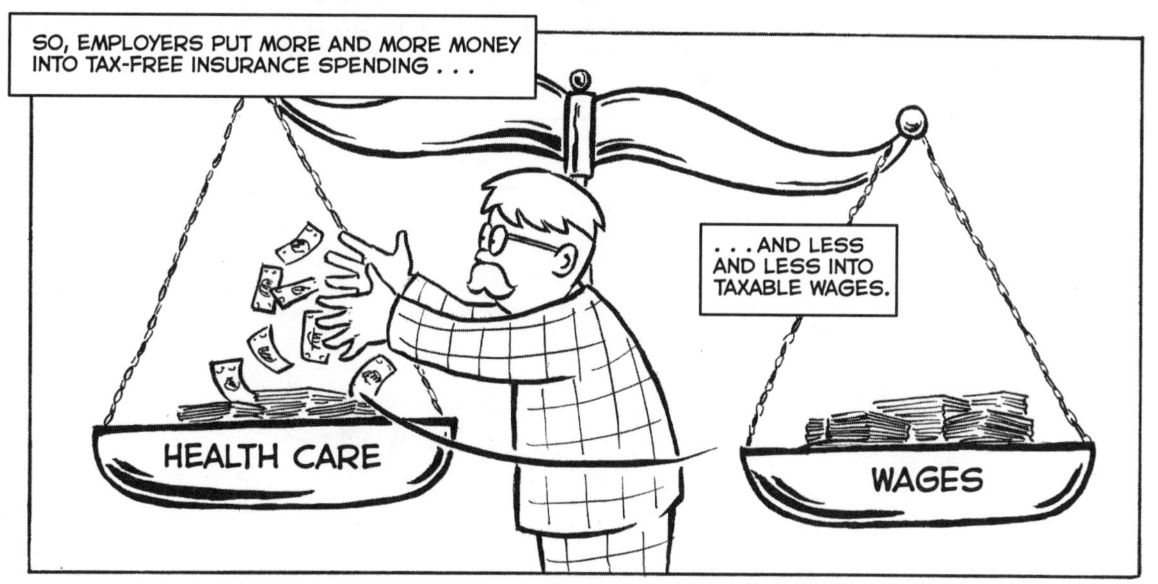
SO, EMPLOYERS PUT MORE AND MORE MONEY INTO TAX-FREE INSURANCE SPENDING . . .
. . . AND LESS AND LESS INTO TAXABLE WAGES.
HEALTH CARE
WAGES

MAKING IT MORE EGREGIOUS, EMPLOYERS DUMPING MONEY INTO THESE INSURANCE SUBSIDIES AMOUNTS TO $250 BILLION A YEAR IN LOST TAX REVENUE FOR THE GOVERNMENT.

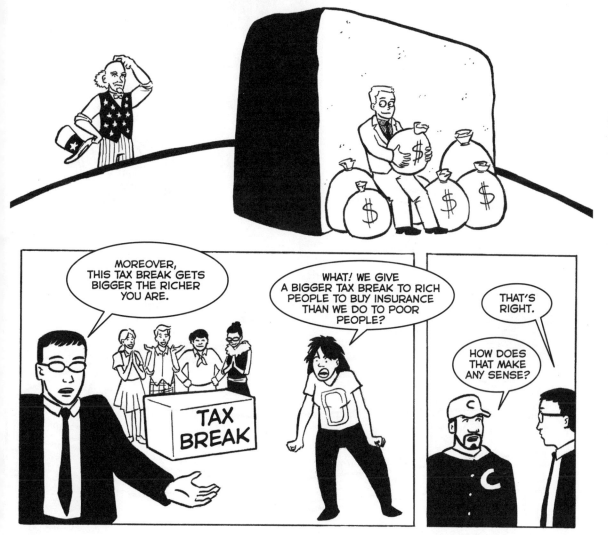

MOREOVER, THIS TAX BREAK GETS BIGGER THE RICHER YOU ARE.

TAX BREAK

WHAT! WE GIVE A BIGGER TAX BREAK TO RICH PEOPLE TO BUY INSURANCE THAN WE DO TO POOR PEOPLE?

THAT'S RIGHT.

HOW DOES THAT MAKE ANY SENSE?

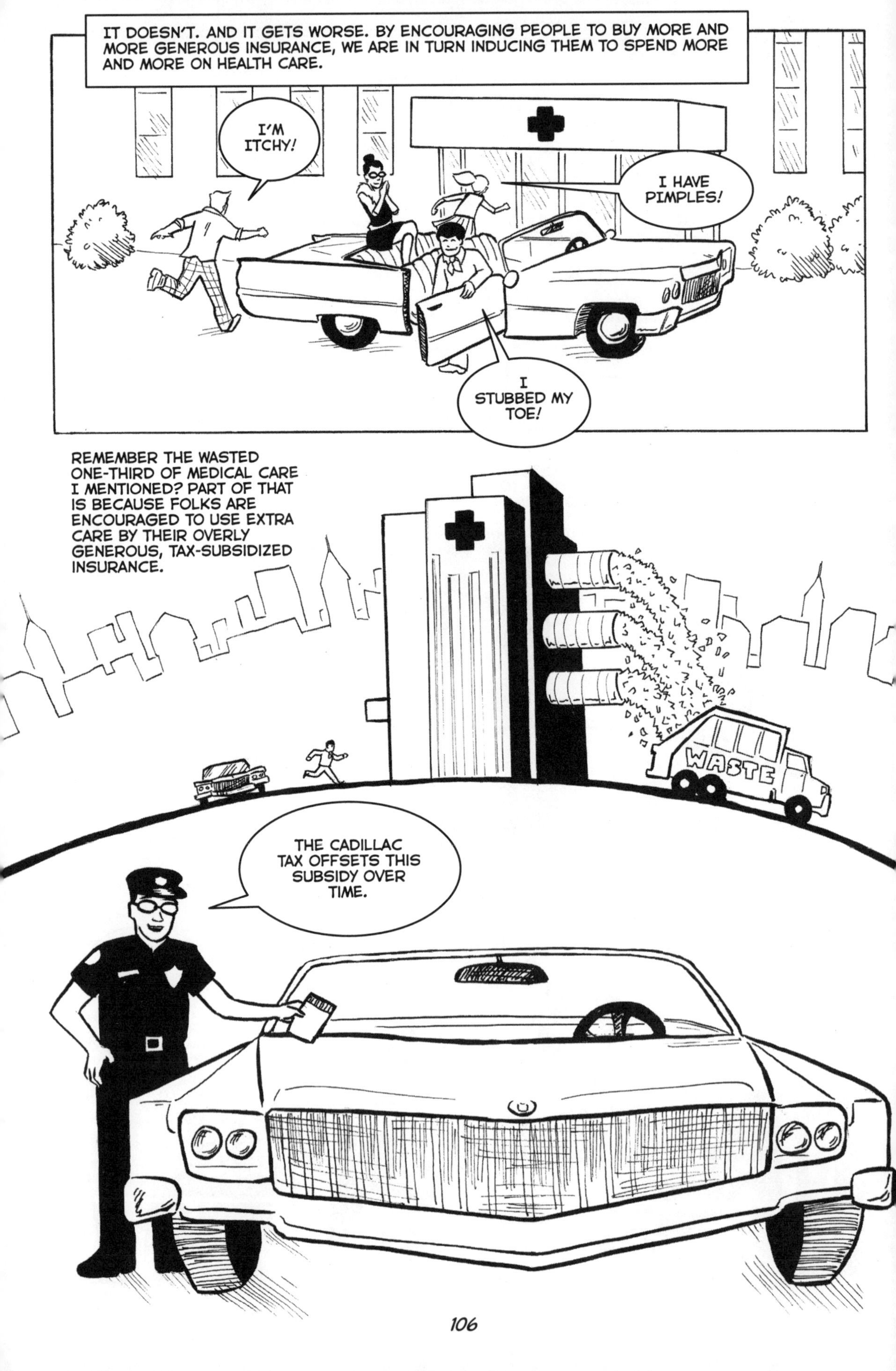
IT DOESN'T. AND IT GETS WORSE. BY ENCOURAGING PEOPLE TO BUY MORE AND MORE GENEROUS INSURANCE, WE ARE IN TURN INDUCING THEM TO SPEND MORE AND MORE ON HEALTH CARE.
I'M ITCHY!
I HAVE PIMPLES!
I STUBBED MY TOE!
REMEMBER THE WASTED ONE-THIRD OF MEDICAL CARE I MENTIONED? PART OF THAT IS BECAUSE FOLKS ARE ENCOURAGED TO USE EXTRA CARE BY THEIR OVERLY GENEROUS, TAX-SUBSIDIZED INSURANCE.
WASTE
THE CADILLAC TAX OFFSETS THIS SUBSIDY OVER TIME.

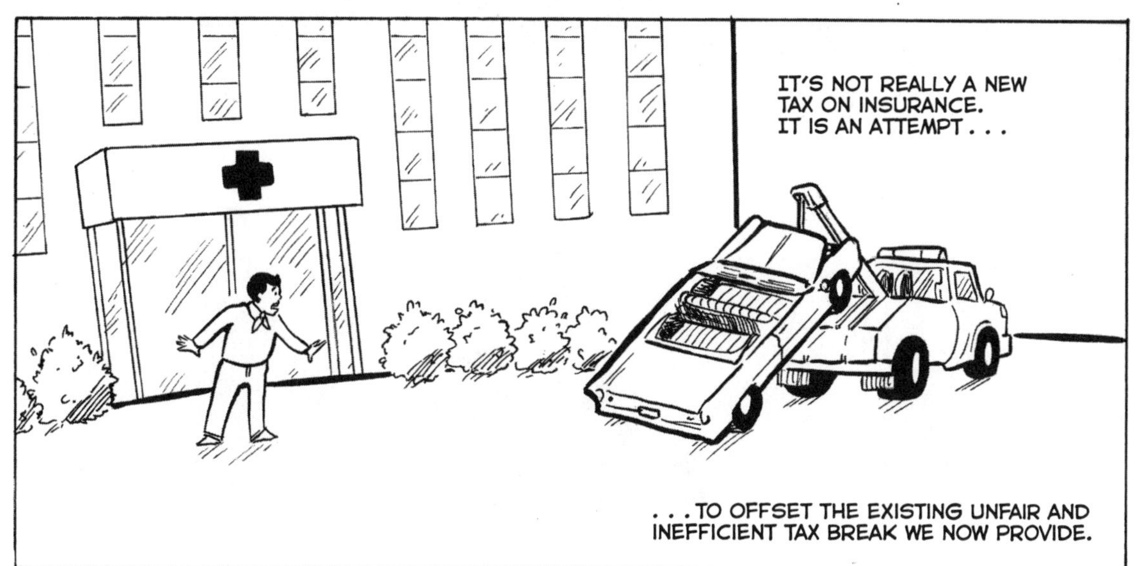

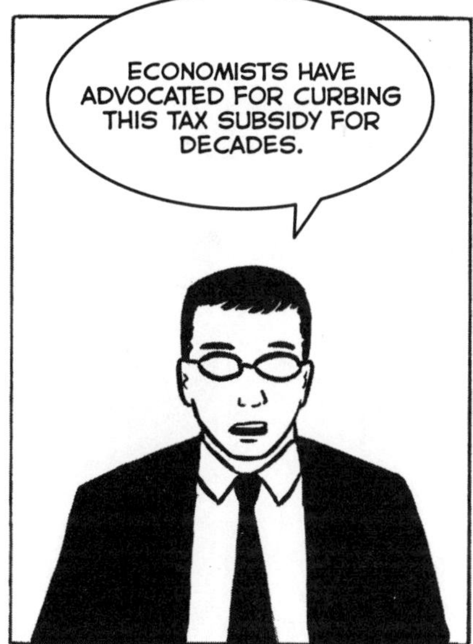

IT IS THE MOST OBVIOUS WAY TO REDUCE INEFFICIENT MEDICAL SPENDING BY NO LONGER SUBSIDIZING INDIVIDUALS WHO BUY OVERLY GENEROUS INSURANCE. THE ACA ACHIEVES THAT GOAL FOR THE FIRST TIME.

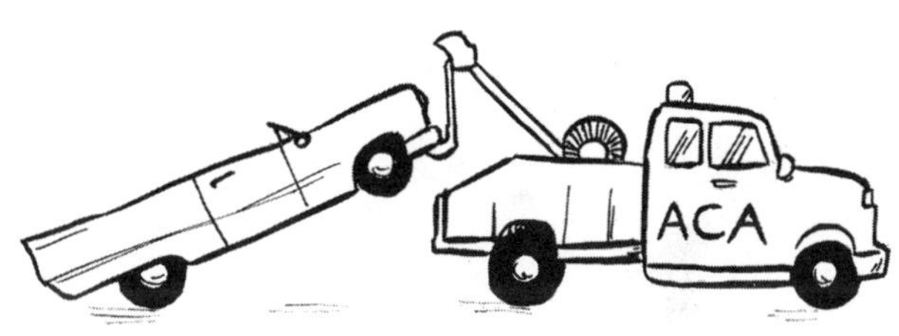

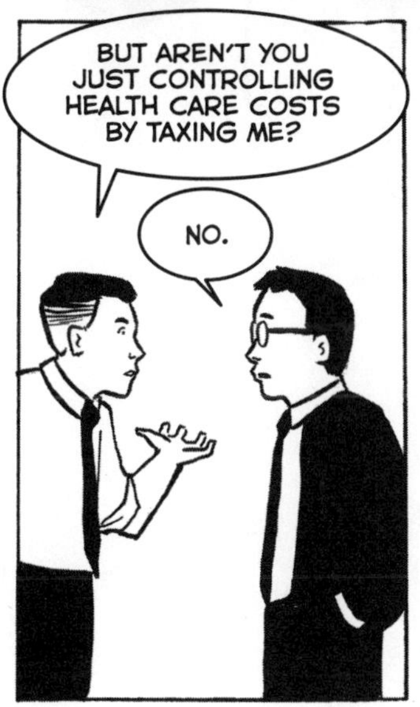

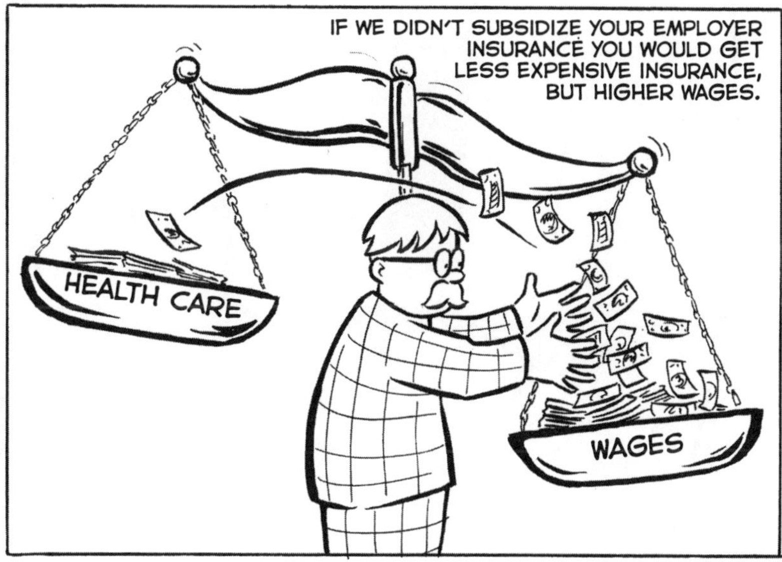

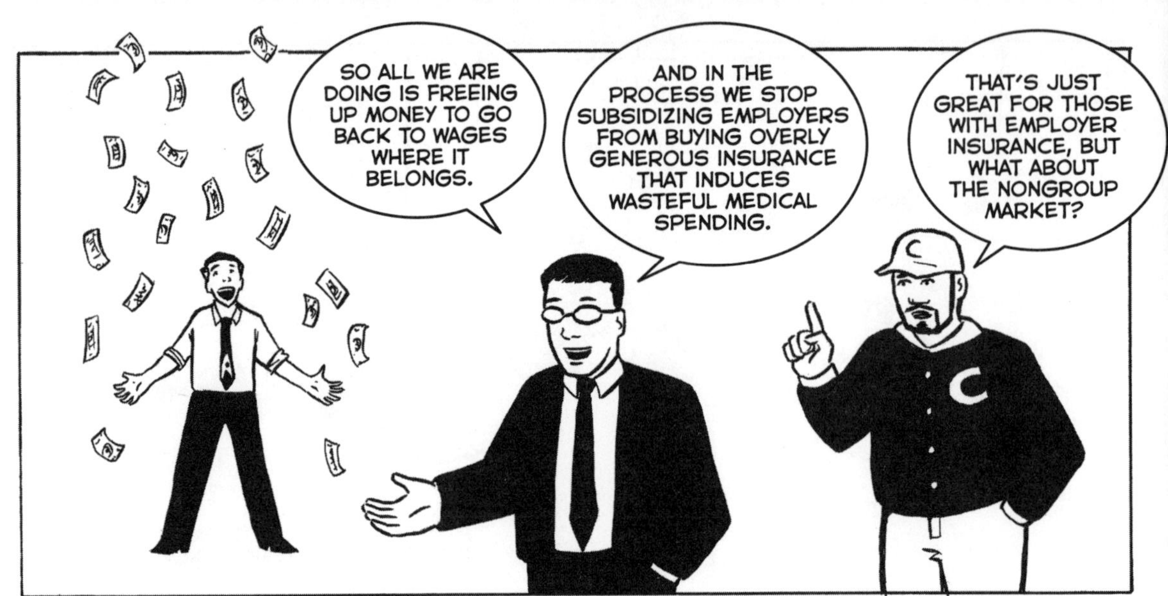
SO ALL WE ARE DOING IS FREEING UP MONEY TO GO BACK TO WAGES WHERE IT BELONGS.
AND IN THE PROCESS WE STOP SUBSIDIZING EMPLOYERS FROM BUYING OVERLY GENEROUS INSURANCE THAT INDUCES WASTEFUL MEDICAL SPENDING.
THAT'S JUST GREAT FOR THOSE WITH EMPLOYER INSURANCE, BUT WHAT ABOUT THE NONGROUP MARKET?

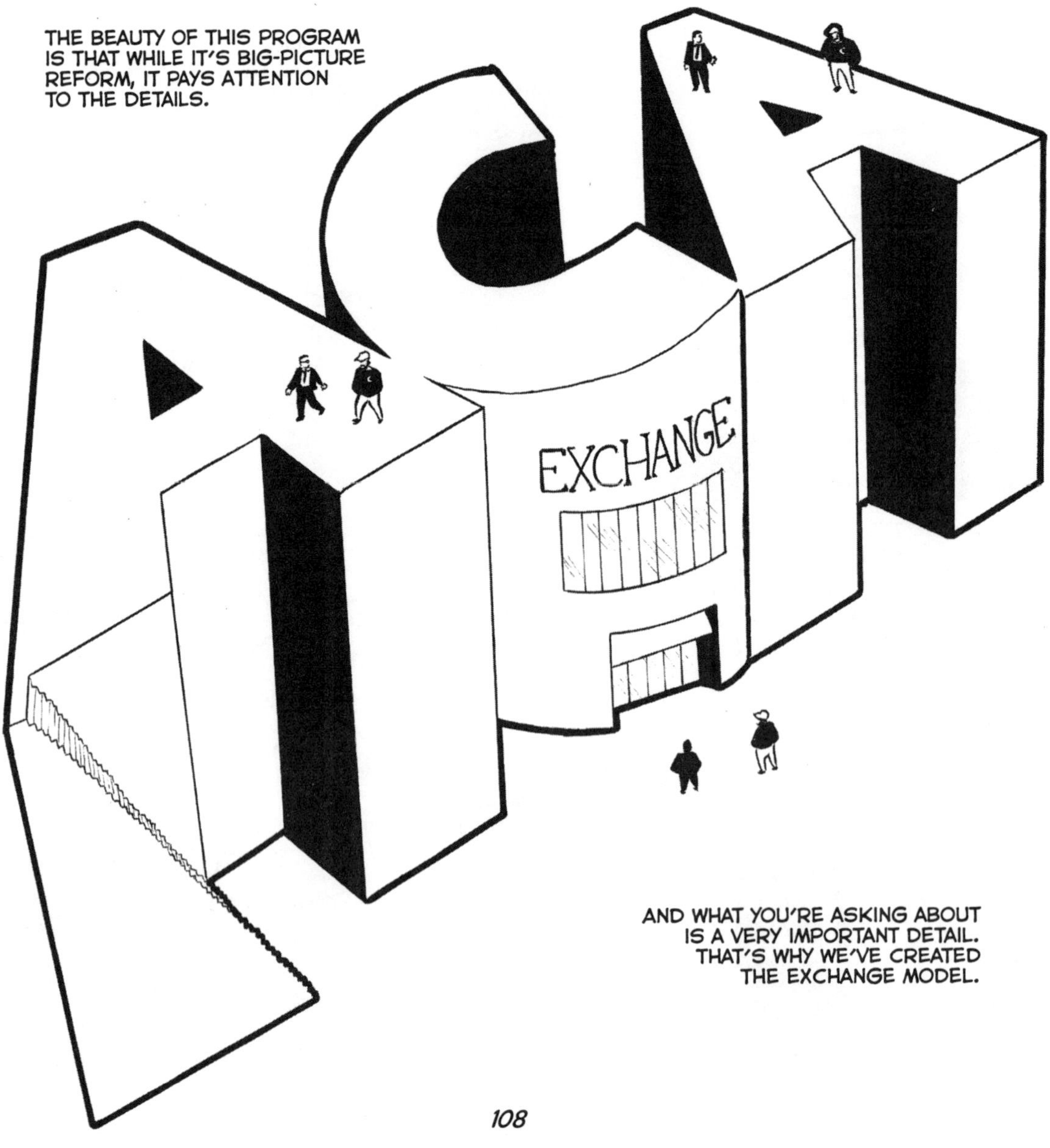

THE BEAUTY OF THIS PROGRAM IS THAT WHILE IT'S BIG-PICTURE REFORM, IT PAYS ATTENTION TO THE DETAILS.

EXCHANGE

AND WHAT YOU'RE ASKING ABOUT IS A VERY IMPORTANT DETAIL. THAT'S WHY WE'VE CREATED THE EXCHANGE MODEL.

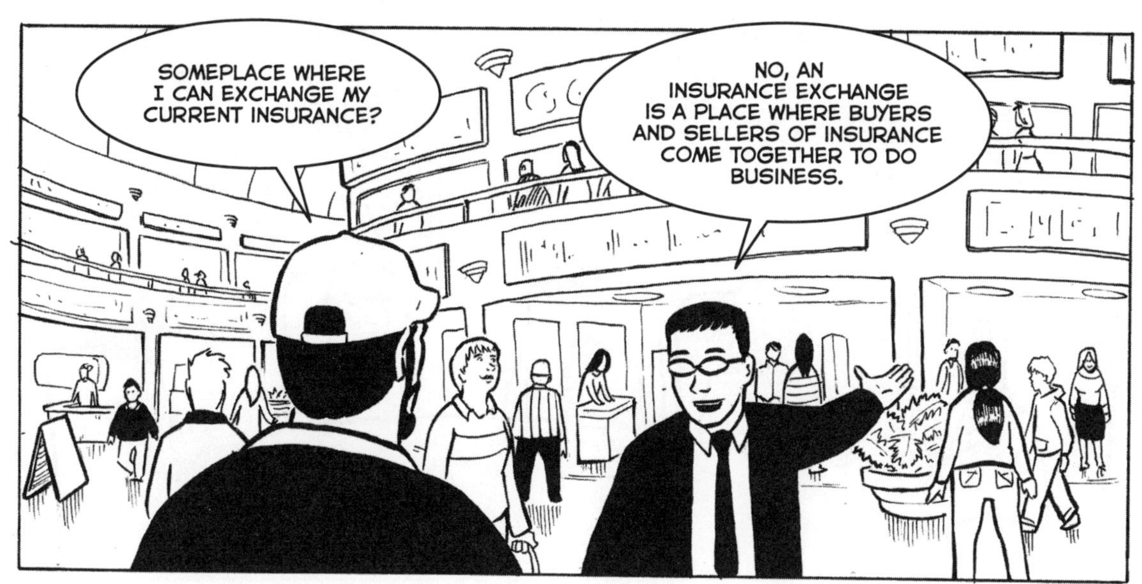
SOMEPLACE WHERE I CAN EXCHANGE MY CURRENT INSURANCE?
NO, AN INSURANCE EXCHANGE IS A PLACE WHERE BUYERS AND SELLERS OF INSURANCE COME TOGETHER TO DO BUSINESS.

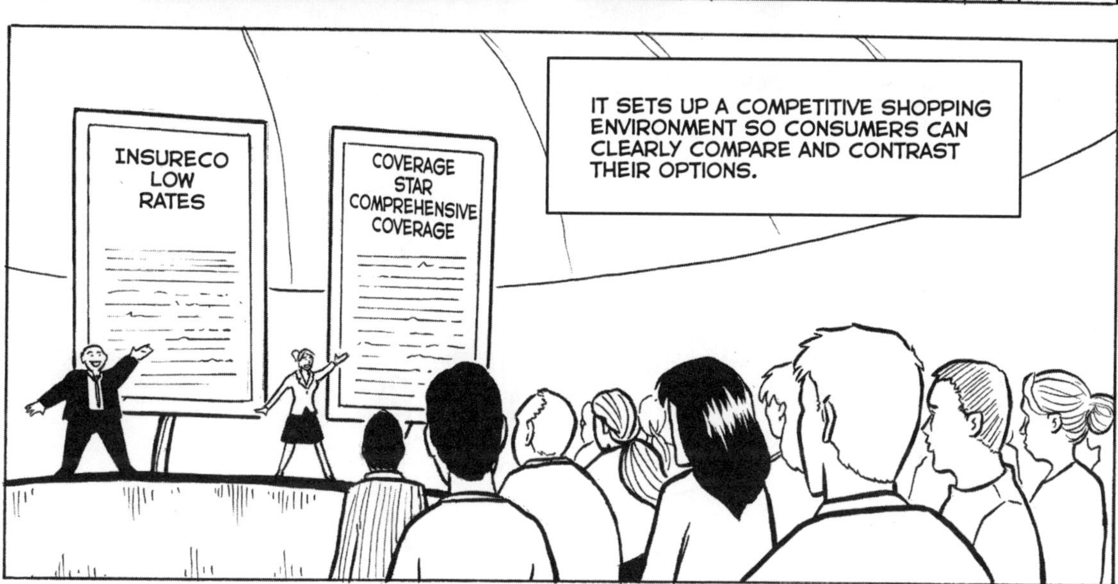
IT SETS UP A COMPETITIVE SHOPPING ENVIRONMENT SO CONSUMERS CAN CLEARLY COMPARE AND CONTRAST THEIR OPTIONS.
INSURECO LOW RATES
COVERAGE STAR COMPREHENSIVE COVERAGE

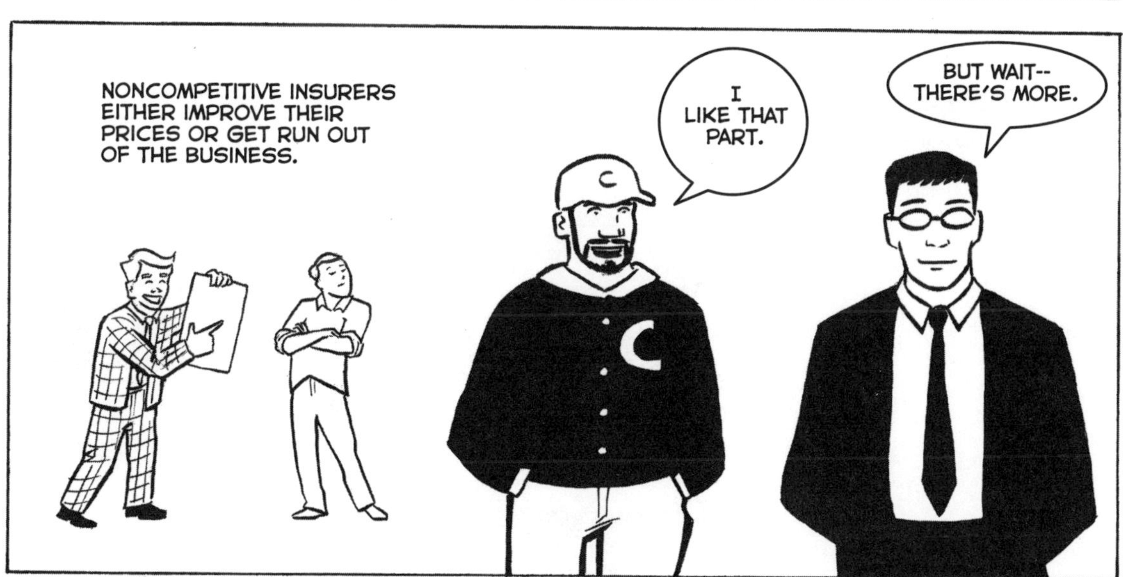
NONCOMPETITIVE INSURERS EITHER IMPROVE THEIR PRICES OR GET RUN OUT OF THE BUSINESS.
I LIKE THAT PART.
BUT WAIT-- THERE'S MORE.

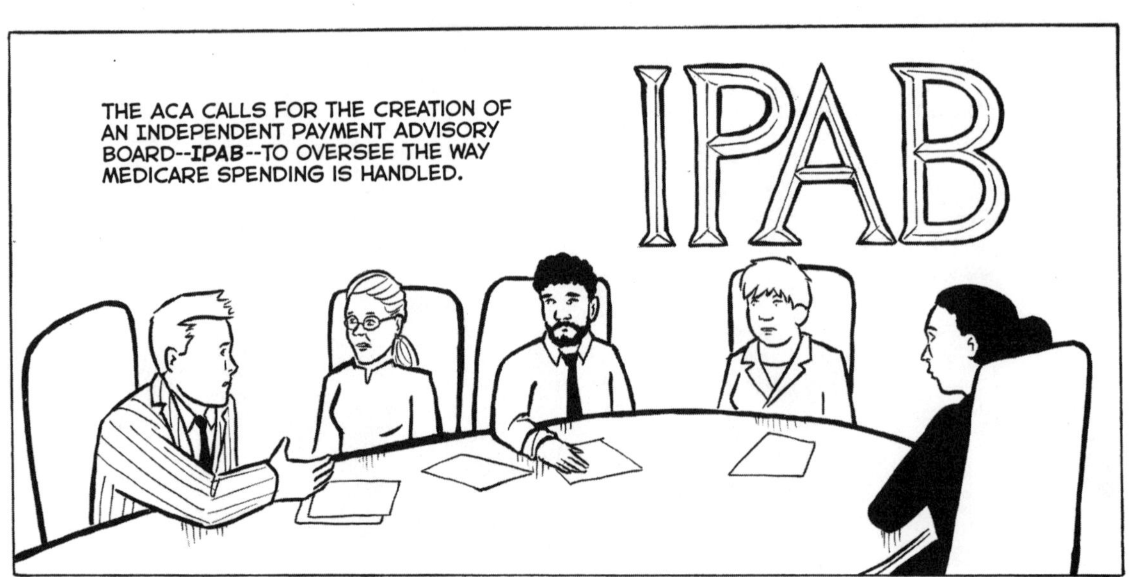
THE ACA CALLS FOR THE CREATION OF AN INDEPENDENT PAYMENT ADVISORY BOARD--IPAB--TO OVERSEE THE WAY MEDICARE SPENDING IS HANDLED.
IPAB

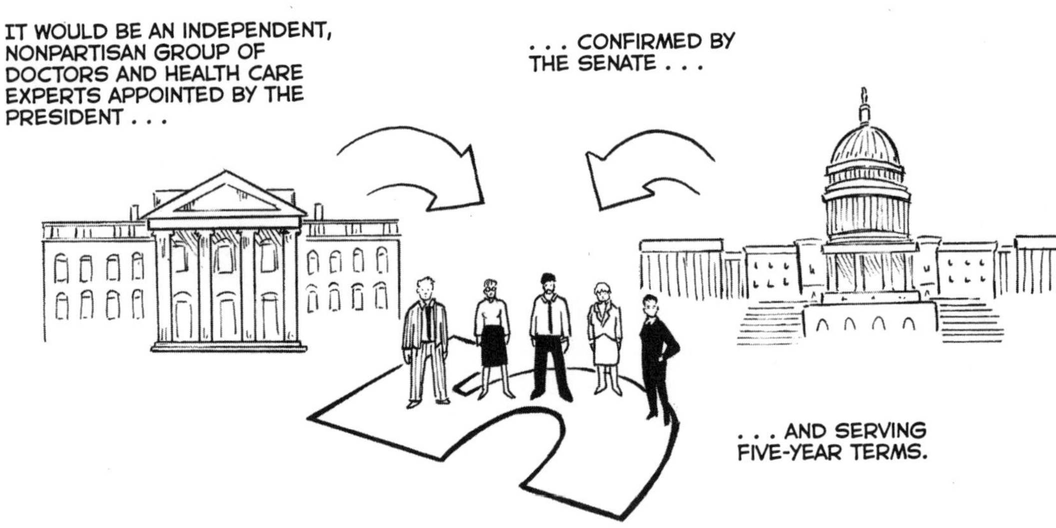
IT WOULD BE AN INDEPENDENT, NONPARTISAN GROUP OF DOCTORS AND HEALTH CARE EXPERTS APPOINTED BY THE PRESIDENT . . .
. . . CONFIRMED BY THE SENATE . . .
. . . AND SERVING FIVE-YEAR TERMS.

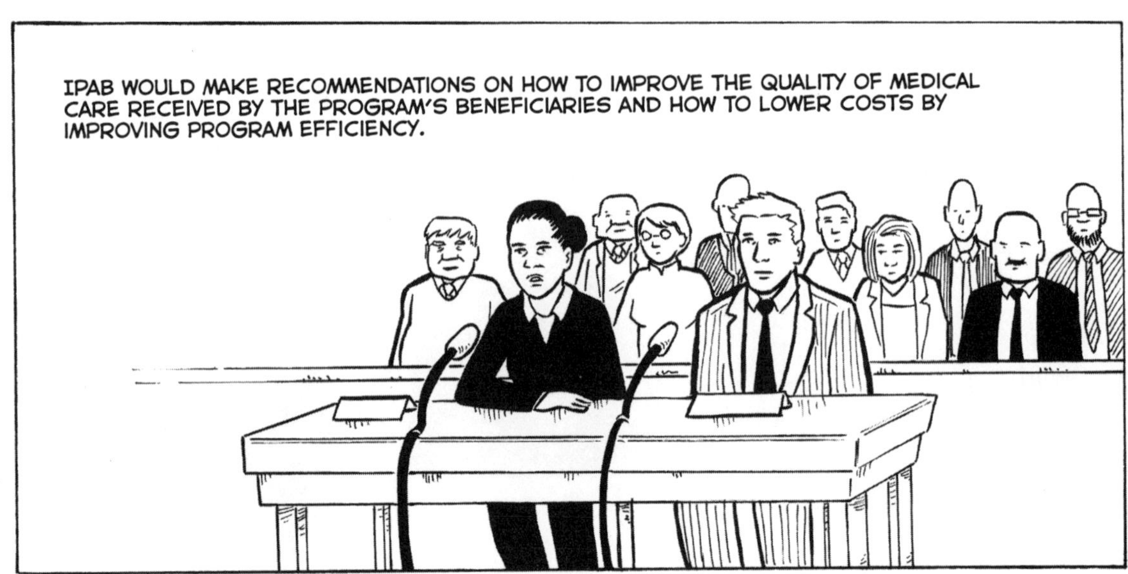
IPAB WOULD MAKE RECOMMENDATIONS ON HOW TO IMPROVE THE QUALITY OF MEDICAL CARE RECEIVED BY THE PROGRAM'S BENEFICIARIES AND HOW TO LOWER COSTS BY IMPROVING PROGRAM EFFICIENCY.

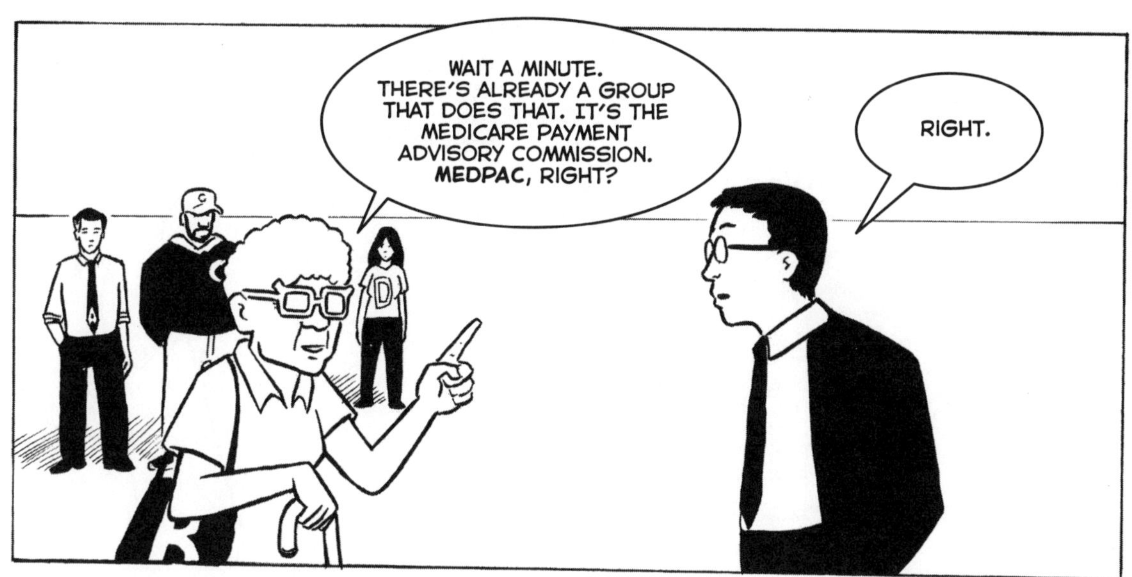
WAIT A MINUTE.
THERE'S ALREADY A GROUP THAT DOES THAT. IT'S THE MEDICARE PAYMENT ADVISORY COMMISSION. MEDPAC, RIGHT?
RIGHT.

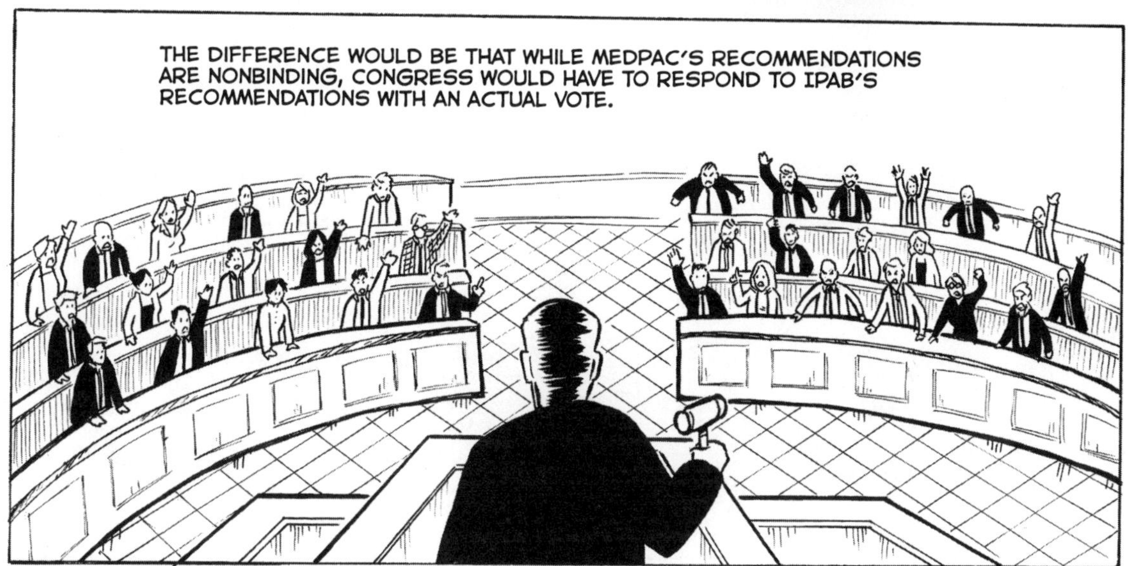
THE DIFFERENCE WOULD BE THAT WHILE MEDPAC'S RECOMMENDATIONS ARE NONBINDING, CONGRESS WOULD HAVE TO RESPOND TO IPAB'S RECOMMENDATIONS WITH AN ACTUAL VOTE.

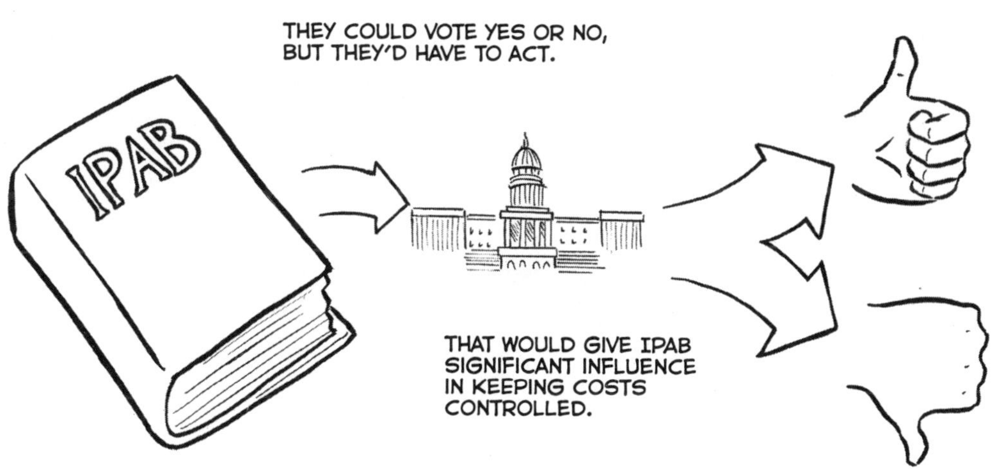
THEY COULD VOTE YES OR NO, BUT THEY'D HAVE TO ACT.
IPAB
THAT WOULD GIVE IPAB SIGNIFICANT INFLUENCE IN KEEPING COSTS CONTROLLED.

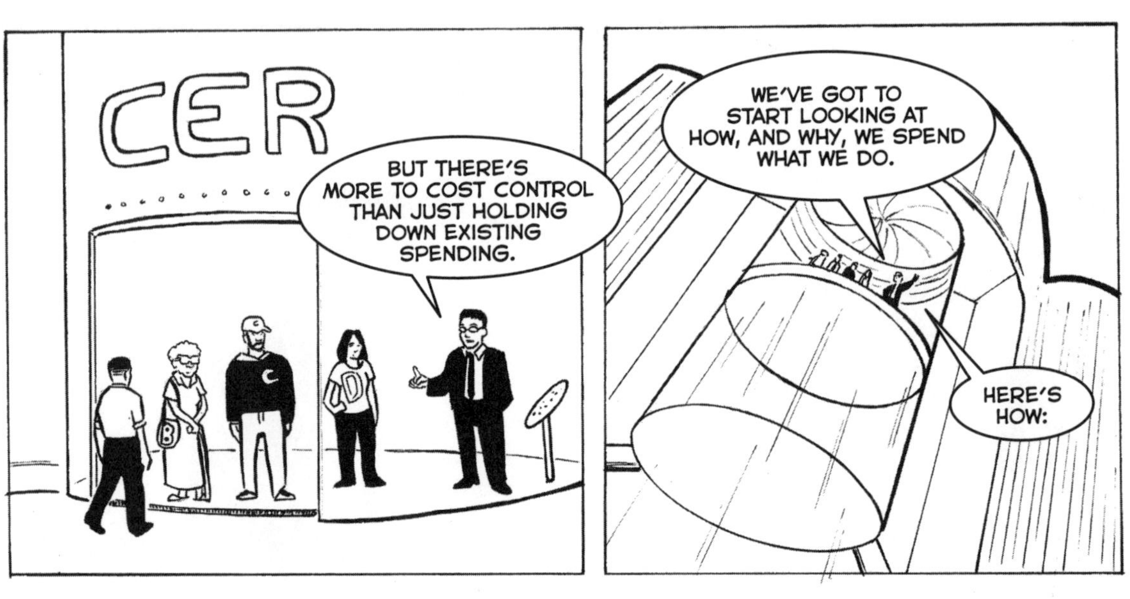
CER
BUT THERE'S MORE TO COST CONTROL THAN JUST HOLDING DOWN EXISTING SPENDING.
WE'VE GOT TO START LOOKING AT HOW, AND WHY, WE SPEND WHAT WE DO.
HERE'S HOW:

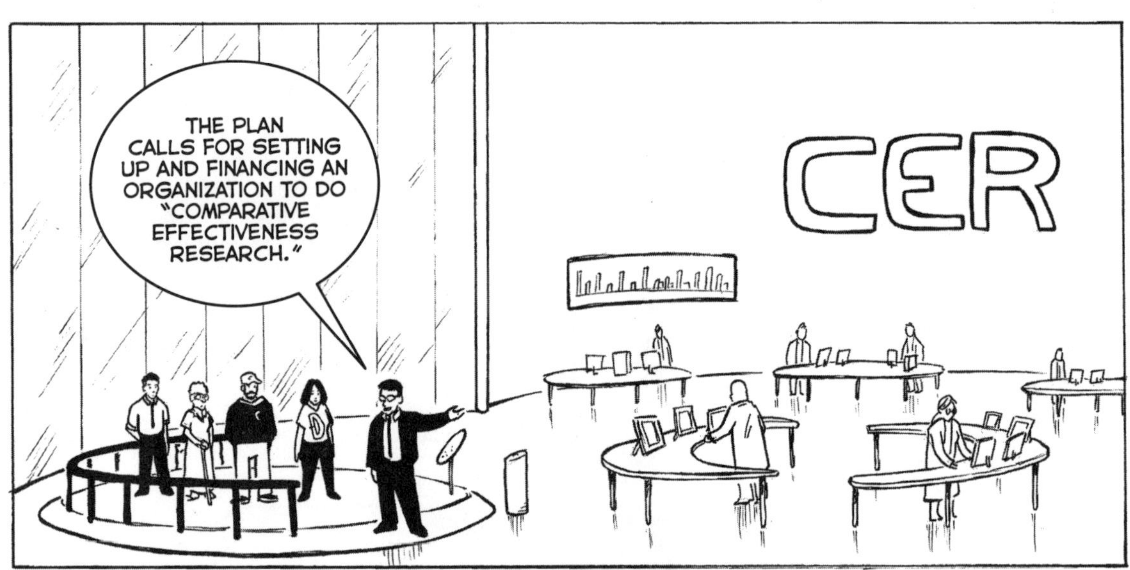
THE PLAN CALLS FOR SETTING UP AND FINANCING AN ORGANIZATION TO DO "COMPARATIVE EFFECTIVENESS RESEARCH."
CER

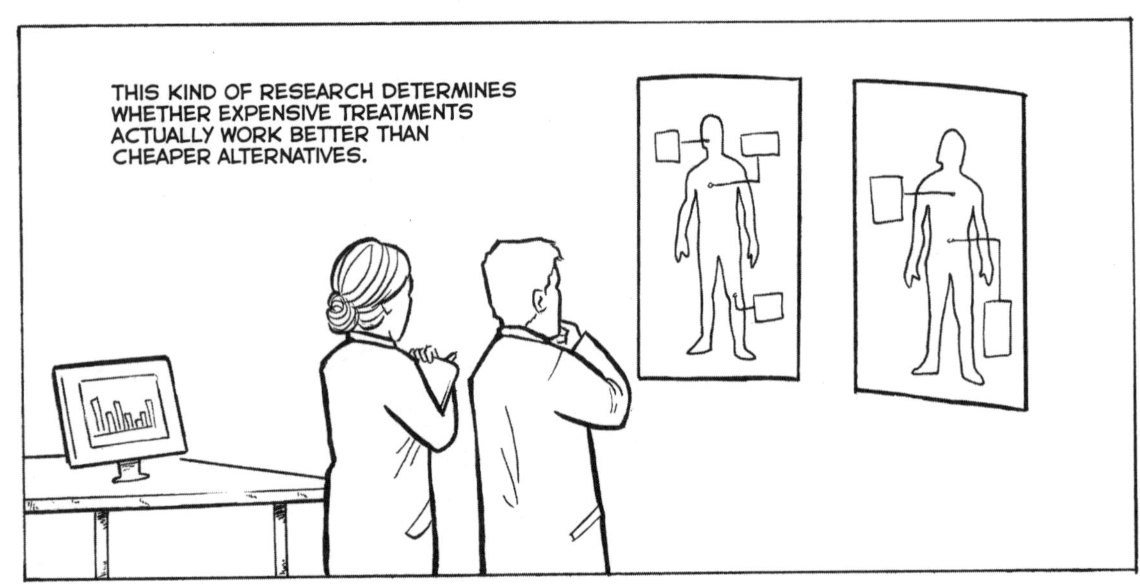
THIS KIND OF RESEARCH DETERMINES WHETHER EXPENSIVE TREATMENTS ACTUALLY WORK BETTER THAN CHEAPER ALTERNATIVES.

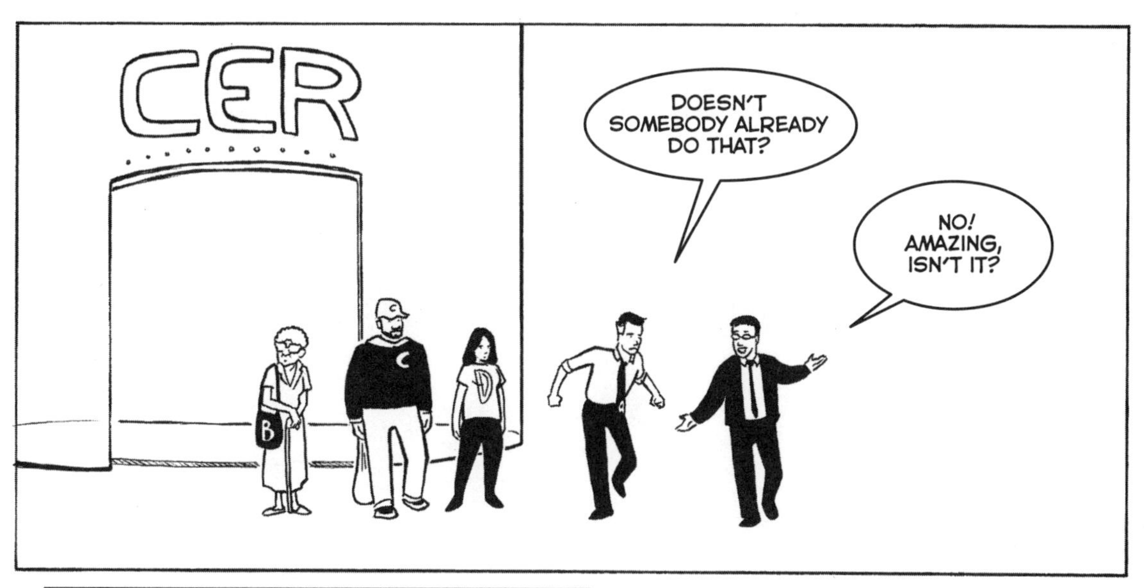
CER
DOESN'T SOMEBODY ALREADY DO THAT?
NO! AMAZING, ISN'T IT?

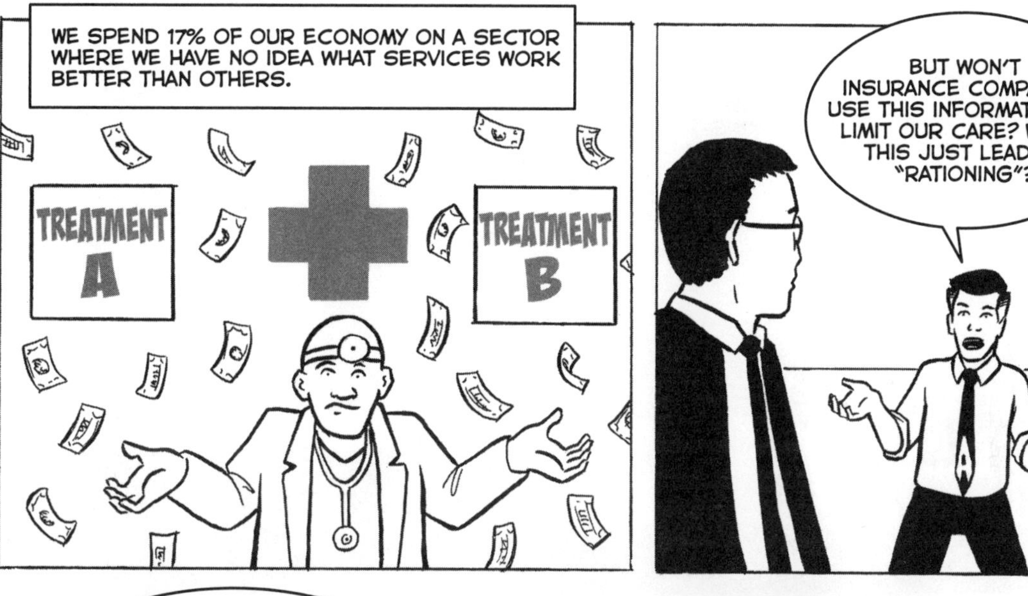
WE SPEND 17% OF OUR ECONOMY ON A SECTOR WHERE WE HAVE NO IDEA WHAT SERVICES WORK BETTER THAN OTHERS.
TREATMENT A
TREATMENT B
BUT WON'T INSURANCE COMPANIES USE THIS INFORMATION TO LIMIT OUR CARE? WON'T THIS JUST LEAD TO "RATIONING"?

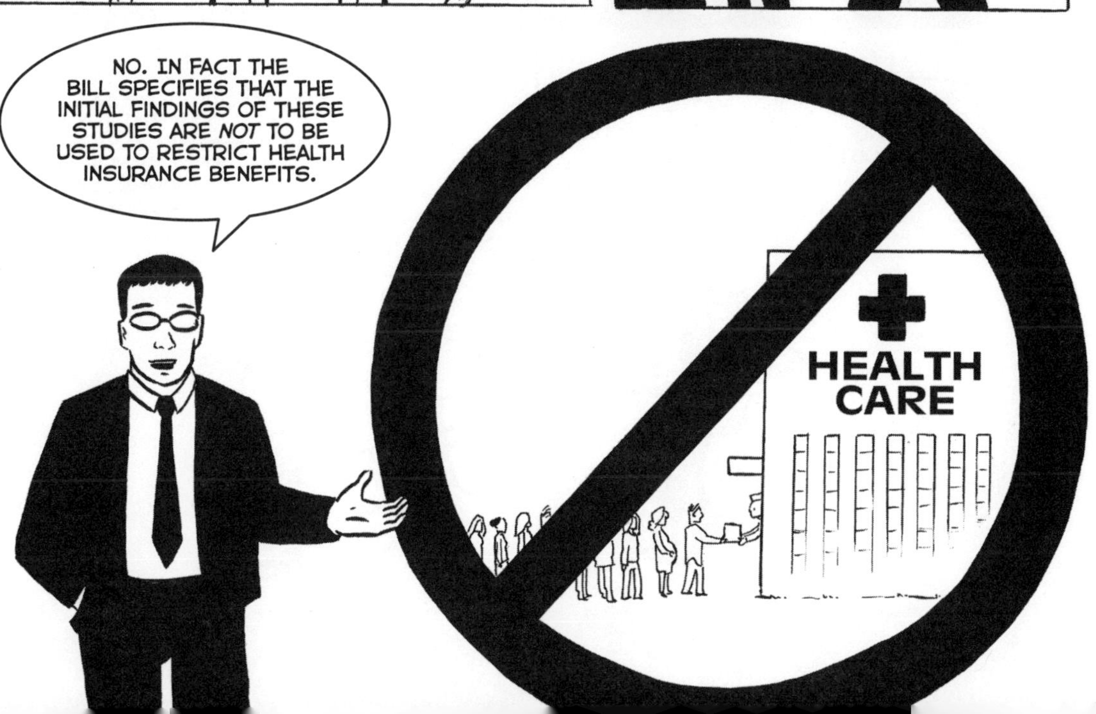
NO. IN FACT THE BILL SPECIFIES THAT THE INITIAL FINDINGS OF THESE STUDIES ARE *NOT* TO BE USED TO RESTRICT HEALTH INSURANCE BENEFITS.
HEALTH CARE

IF WE DEVELOP CONVINCING-ENOUGH EVIDENCE ON WHAT WORKS AND WHAT DOESN'T, WE CAN DEVELOP A NATIONAL CONSENSUS ON WHAT TO DO ABOUT WASTEFUL SERVICES.

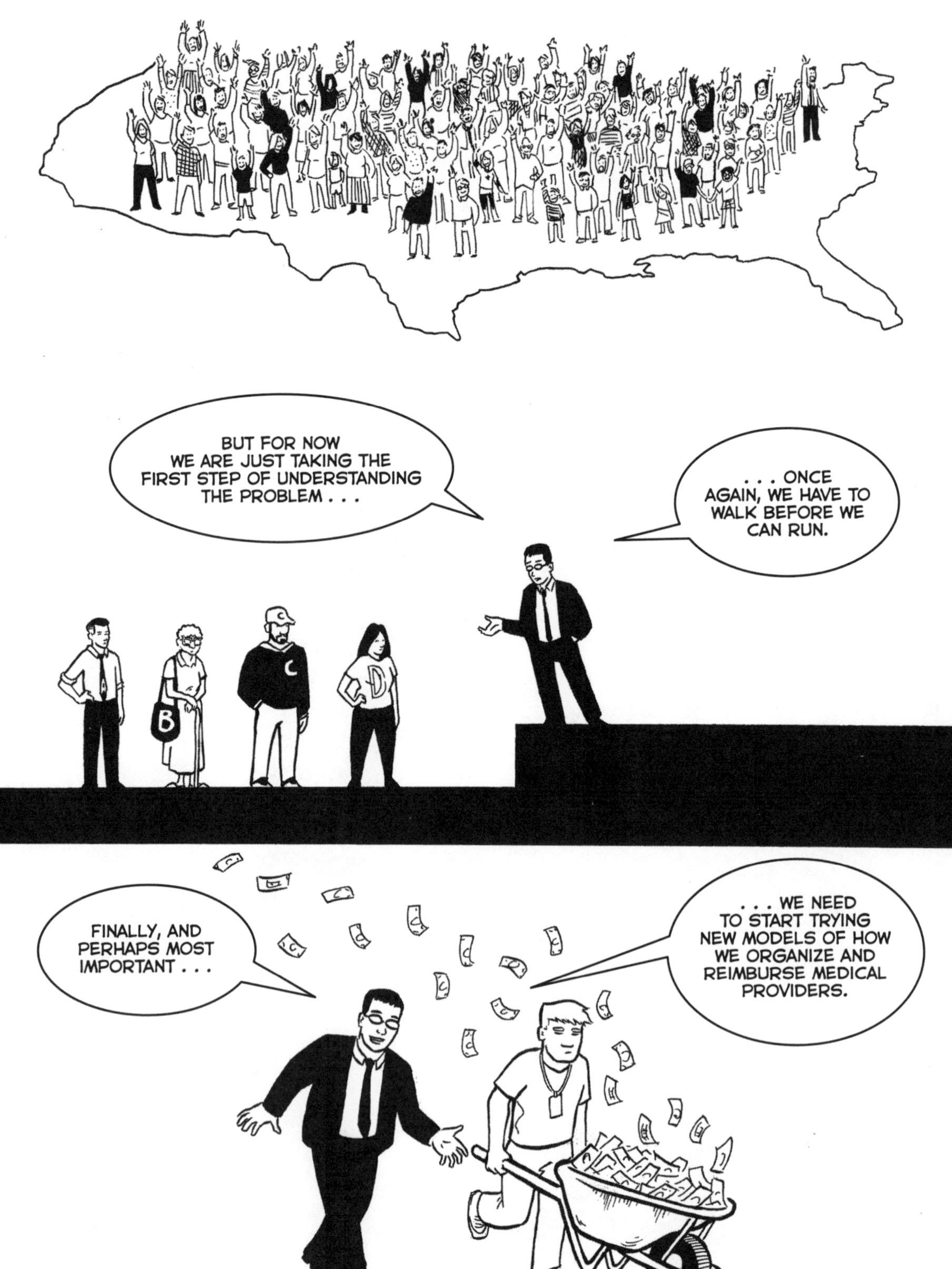
BUT FOR NOW WE ARE JUST TAKING THE FIRST STEP OF UNDERSTANDING THE PROBLEM . . .
. . . ONCE AGAIN, WE HAVE TO WALK BEFORE WE CAN RUN.
FINALLY, AND PERHAPS MOST IMPORTANT . . .
. . . WE NEED TO START TRYING NEW MODELS OF HOW WE ORGANIZE AND REIMBURSE MEDICAL PROVIDERS.

THE CURRENT "FEE FOR SERVICE" REIMBURSEMENT SYSTEM BREEDS OVERUSE BY REWARDING PHYSICIANS BASED ON *HOW MUCH* CARE THEY DELIVER. THE MORE SERVICES A DOCTOR PROVIDES, THE MORE MONEY THEY MAKE.

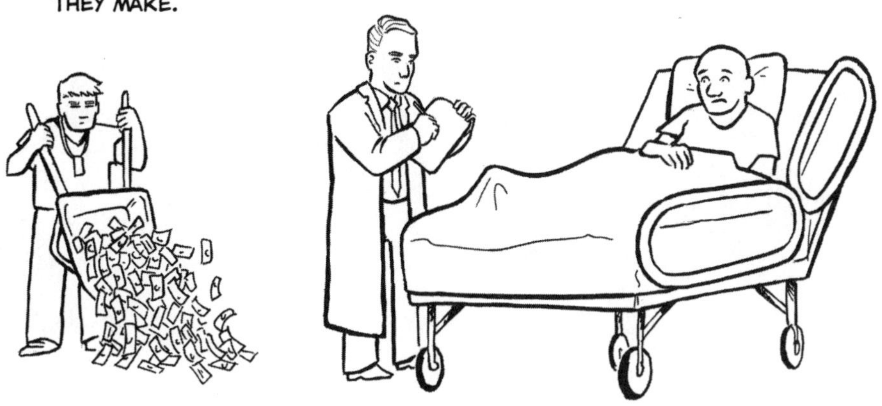

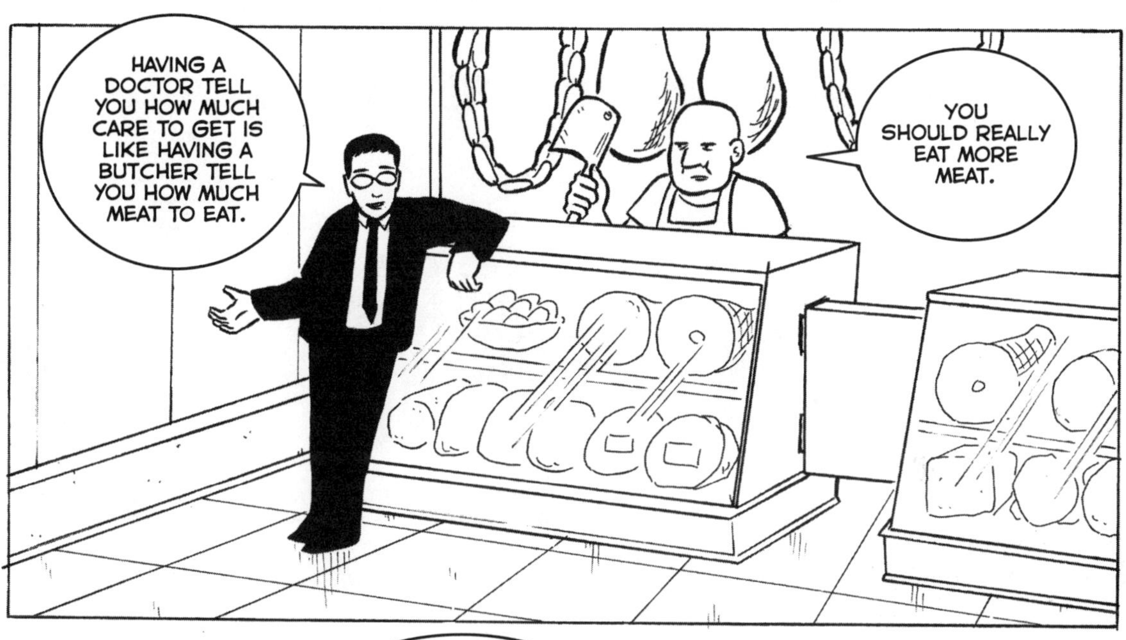

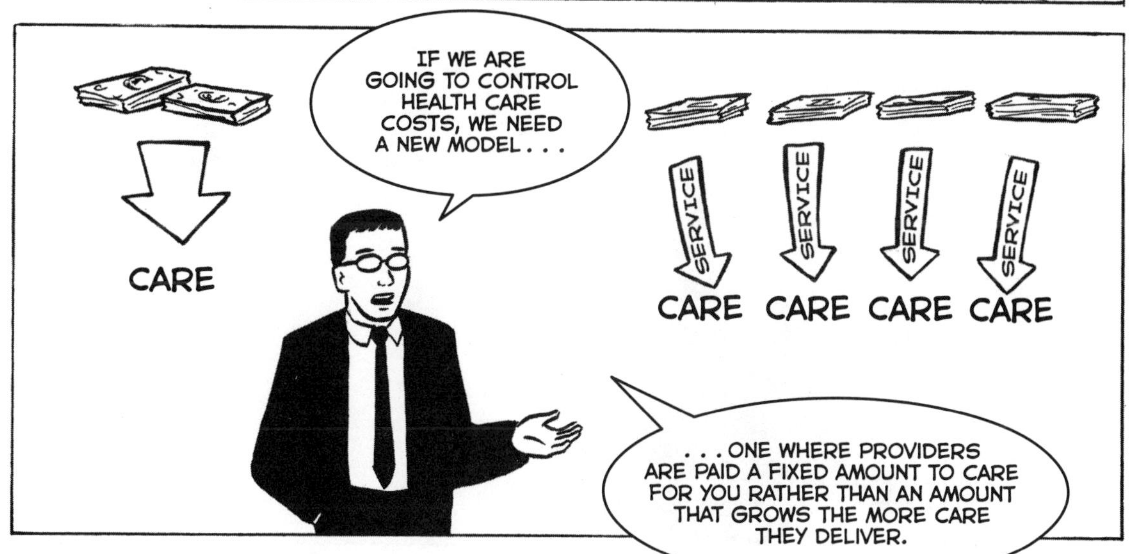

HAVING A DOCTOR TELL YOU HOW MUCH CARE TO GET IS LIKE HAVING A BUTCHER TELL YOU HOW MUCH MEAT TO EAT.
YOU SHOULD REALLY EAT MORE MEAT.

CARE
IF WE ARE GOING TO CONTROL HEALTH CARE COSTS, WE NEED A NEW MODEL . . .
SERVICE
SERVICE
SERVICE
SERVICE
CARE CARE CARE CARE
. . . ONE WHERE PROVIDERS ARE PAID A FIXED AMOUNT TO CARE FOR YOU RATHER THAN AN AMOUNT THAT GROWS THE MORE CARE THEY DELIVER.

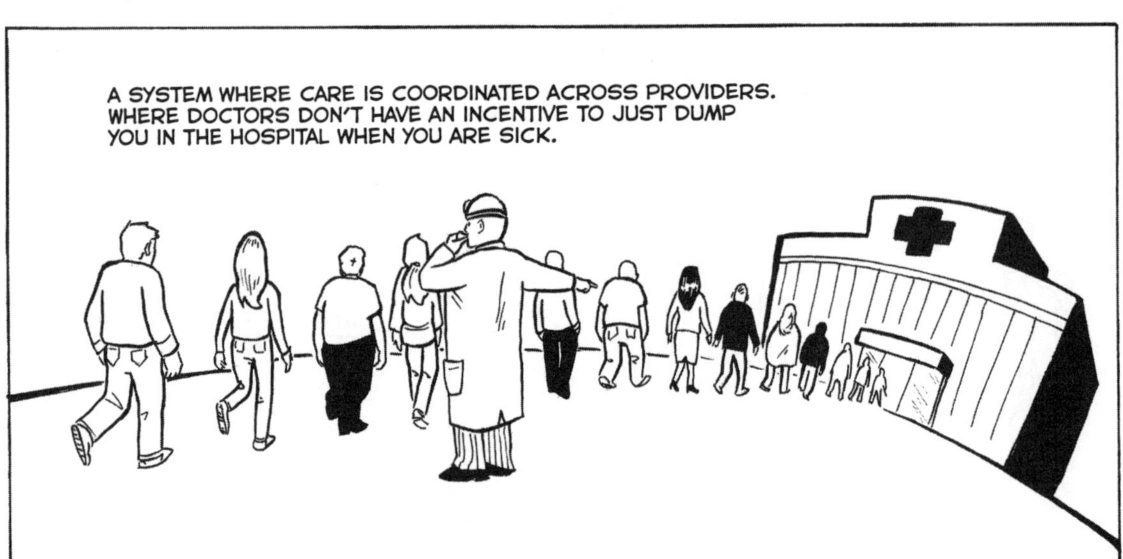
A SYSTEM WHERE CARE IS COORDINATED ACROSS PROVIDERS. WHERE DOCTORS DON'T HAVE AN INCENTIVE TO JUST DUMP YOU IN THE HOSPITAL WHEN YOU ARE SICK.

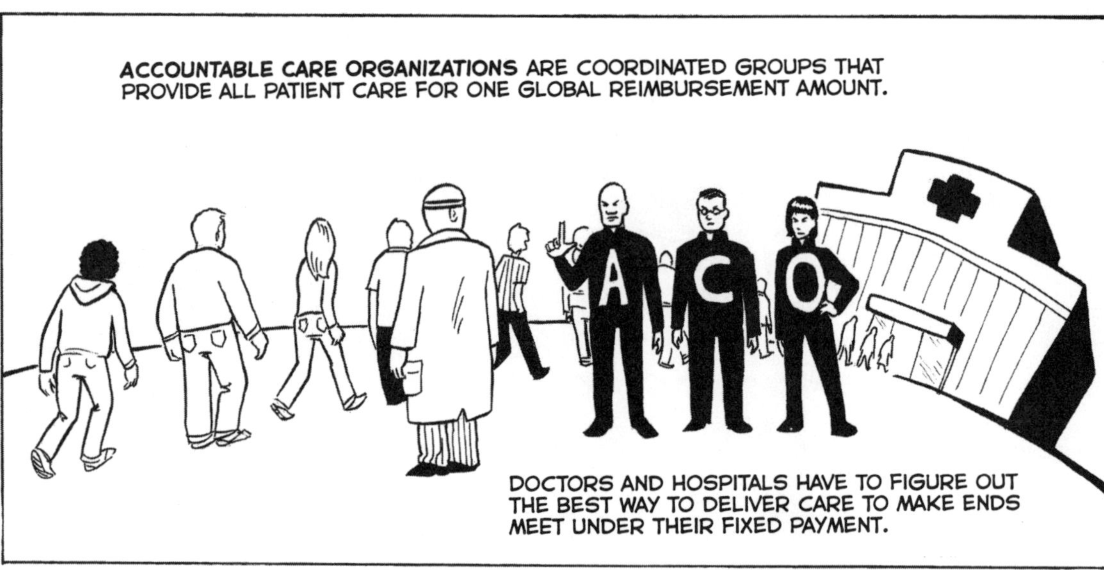
ACCOUNTABLE CARE ORGANIZATIONS ARE COORDINATED GROUPS THAT PROVIDE ALL PATIENT CARE FOR ONE GLOBAL REIMBURSEMENT AMOUNT.
A C O
DOCTORS AND HOSPITALS HAVE TO FIGURE OUT THE BEST WAY TO DELIVER CARE TO MAKE ENDS MEET UNDER THEIR FIXED PAYMENT.

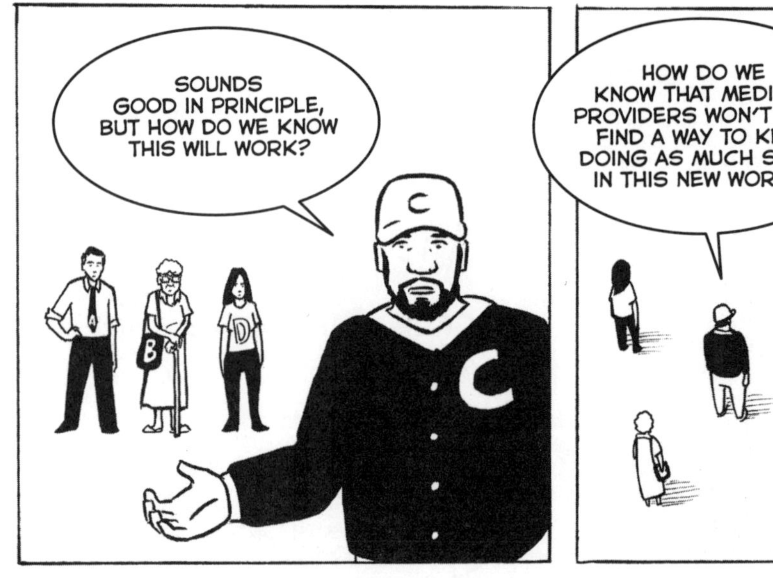
SOUNDS GOOD IN PRINCIPLE, BUT HOW DO WE KNOW THIS WILL WORK?
C
A
B
D
C

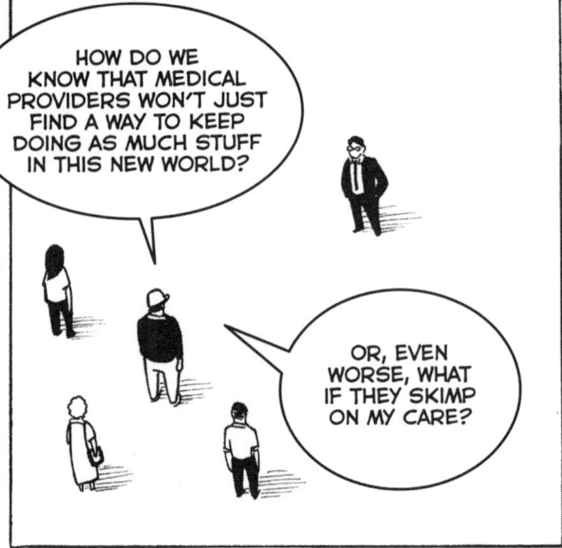
HOW DO WE KNOW THAT MEDICAL PROVIDERS WON'T JUST FIND A WAY TO KEEP DOING AS MUCH STUFF IN THIS NEW WORLD?
OR, EVEN WORSE, WHAT IF THEY SKIMP ON MY CARE?

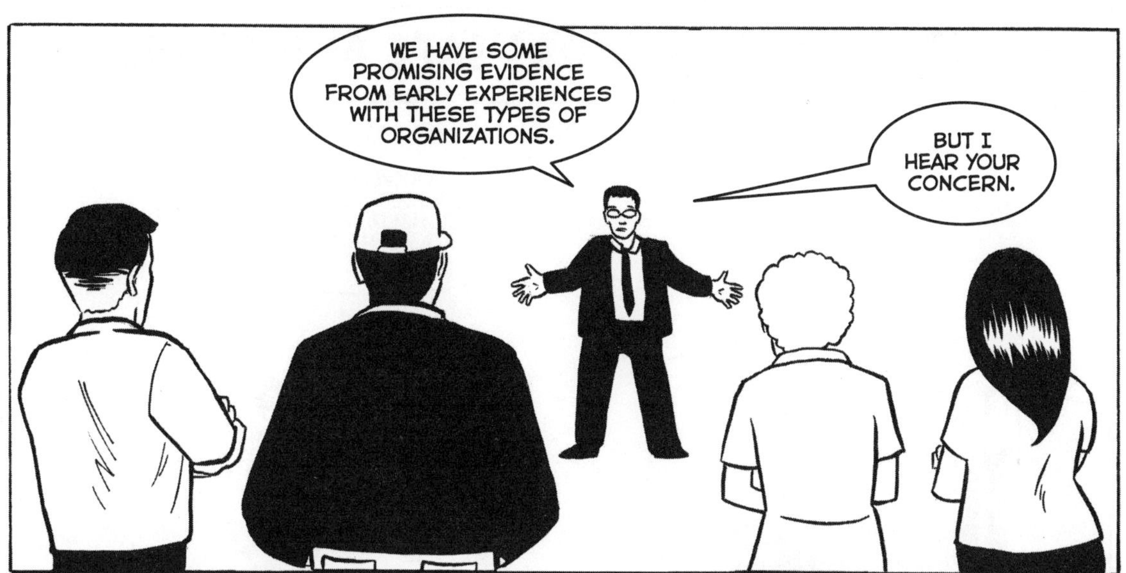
WE HAVE SOME PROMISING EVIDENCE FROM EARLY EXPERIENCES WITH THESE TYPES OF ORGANIZATIONS.
BUT I HEAR YOUR CONCERN.

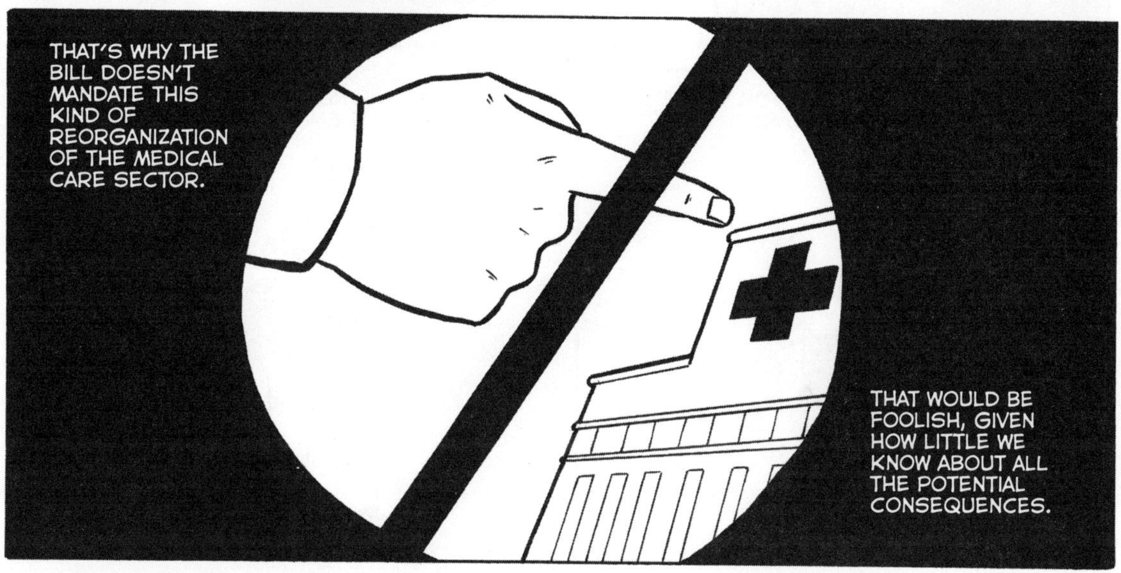

RATHER, THE BILL SETS UP PILOT PROGRAMS OR ALTERNATIVE WAYS TO REIMBURSE AND REORGANIZE MEDICAL PROVIDERS. AS WE LEARN HOW BEST TO CHANGE THE STRUCTURE OF OUR MEDICAL SYSTEM, WE WILL CONTROL COSTS WITHOUT SACRIFICING PATIENT HEALTH.

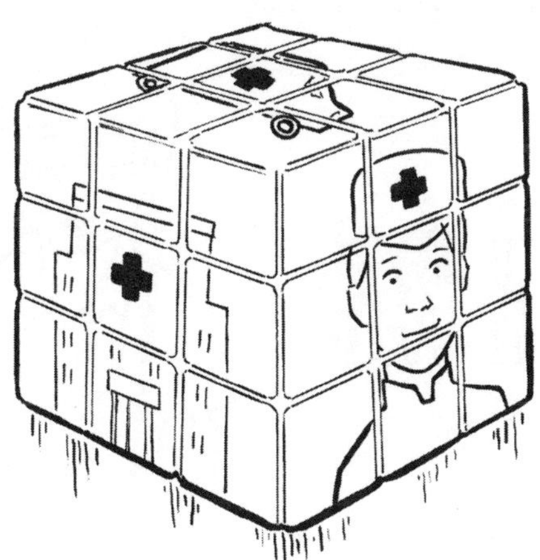

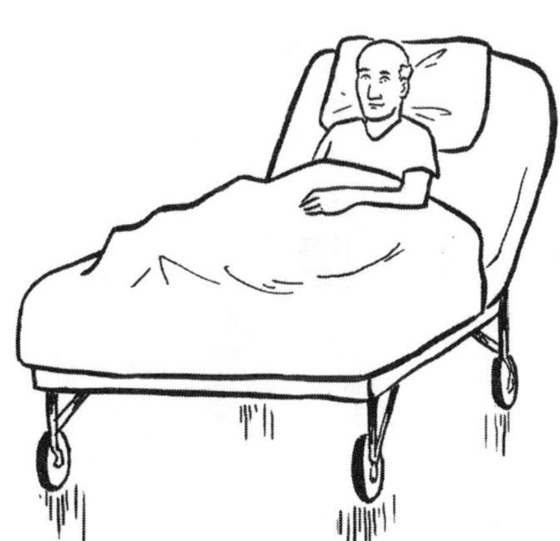

CHAPTER 11 KEEPING SENIORS SAFE AND SOUND

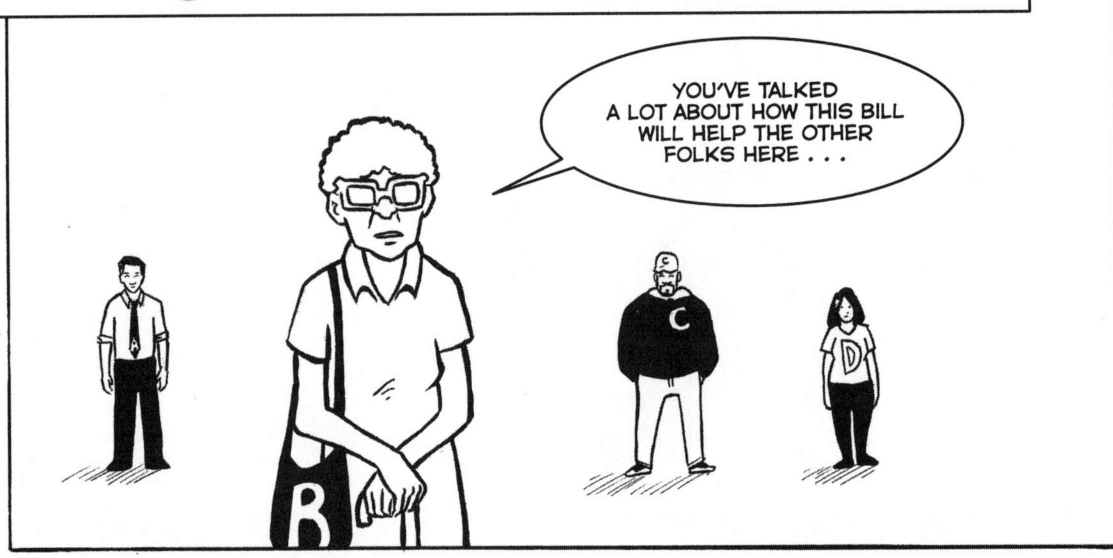
YOU'VE TALKED A LOT ABOUT HOW THIS BILL WILL HELP THE OTHER FOLKS HERE . . .

. . . LOWERING COSTS FOR THOSE WITH EMPLOYER INSURANCE . . .

. . . FIXING THE NONGROUP MARKET FOR THOSE WITHOUT EMPLOYER INSURANCE . . .

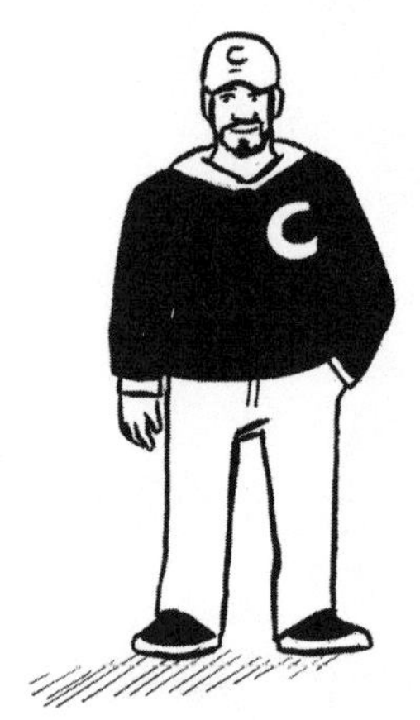

. . . AND MAKING INSURANCE AFFORDABLE FOR THE UNINSURED.

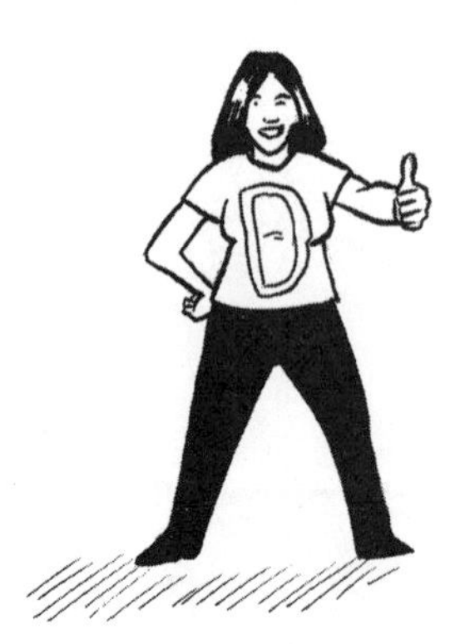

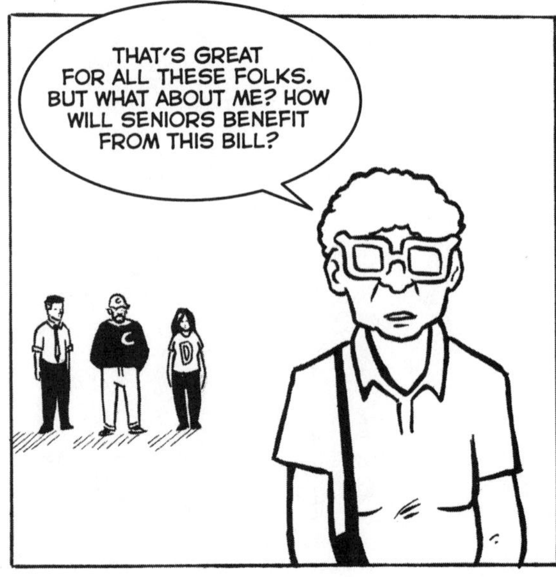
THAT'S GREAT FOR ALL THESE FOLKS. BUT WHAT ABOUT ME? HOW WILL SENIORS BENEFIT FROM THIS BILL?

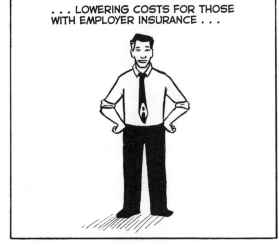

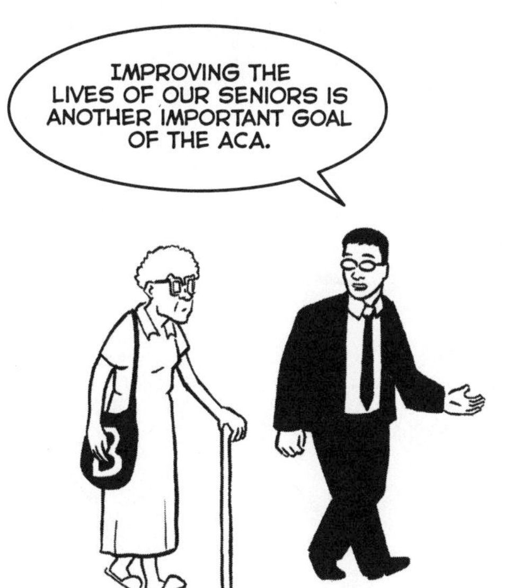
IMPROVING THE LIVES OF OUR SENIORS IS ANOTHER IMPORTANT GOAL OF THE ACA.

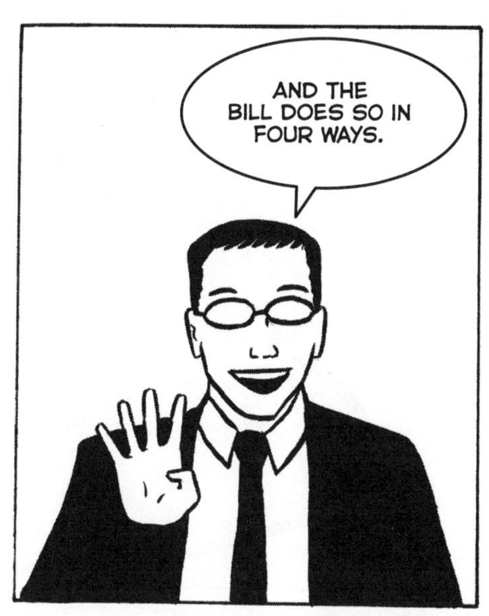
AND THE BILL DOES SO IN FOUR WAYS.

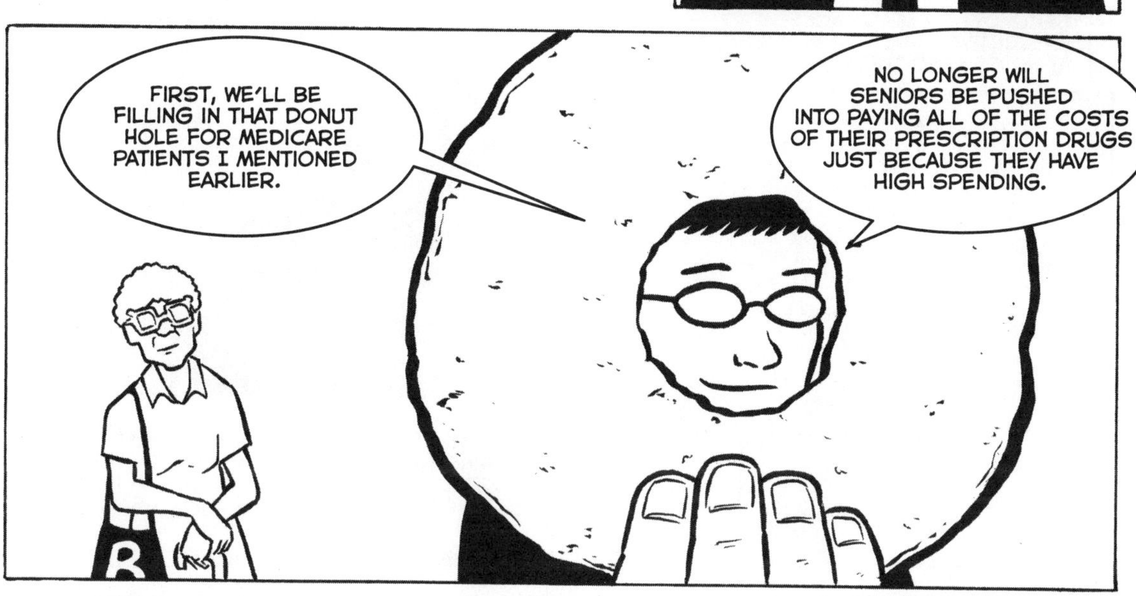
FIRST, WE'LL BE FILLING IN THAT DONUT HOLE FOR MEDICARE PATIENTS I MENTIONED EARLIER.
NO LONGER WILL SENIORS BE PUSHED INTO PAYING ALL OF THE COSTS OF THEIR PRESCRIPTION DRUGS JUST BECAUSE THEY HAVE HIGH SPENDING.

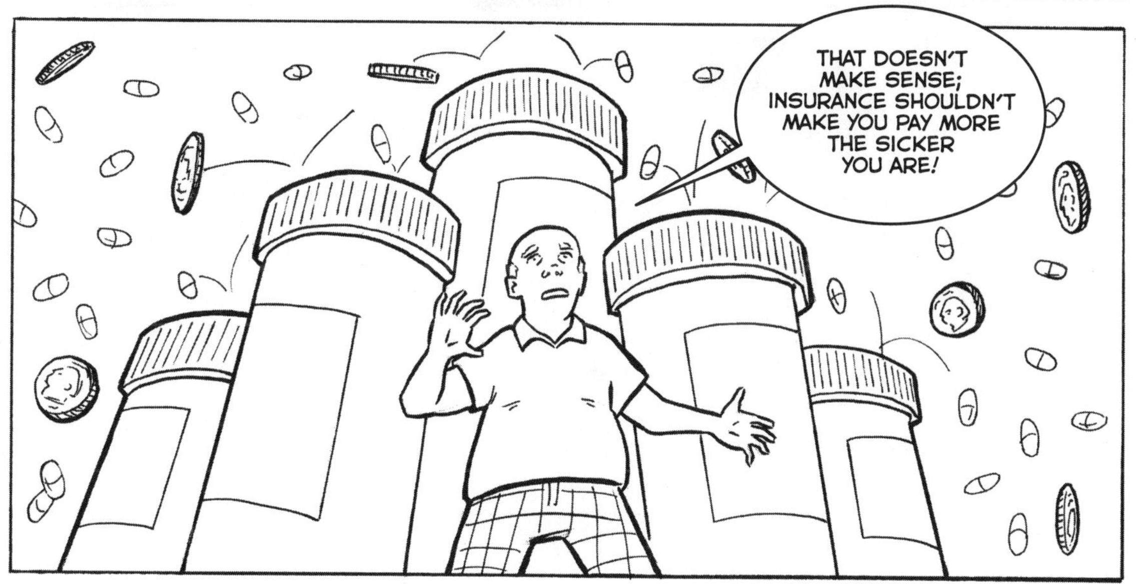
THAT DOESN'T MAKE SENSE; INSURANCE SHOULDN'T MAKE YOU PAY MORE THE SICKER YOU ARE!

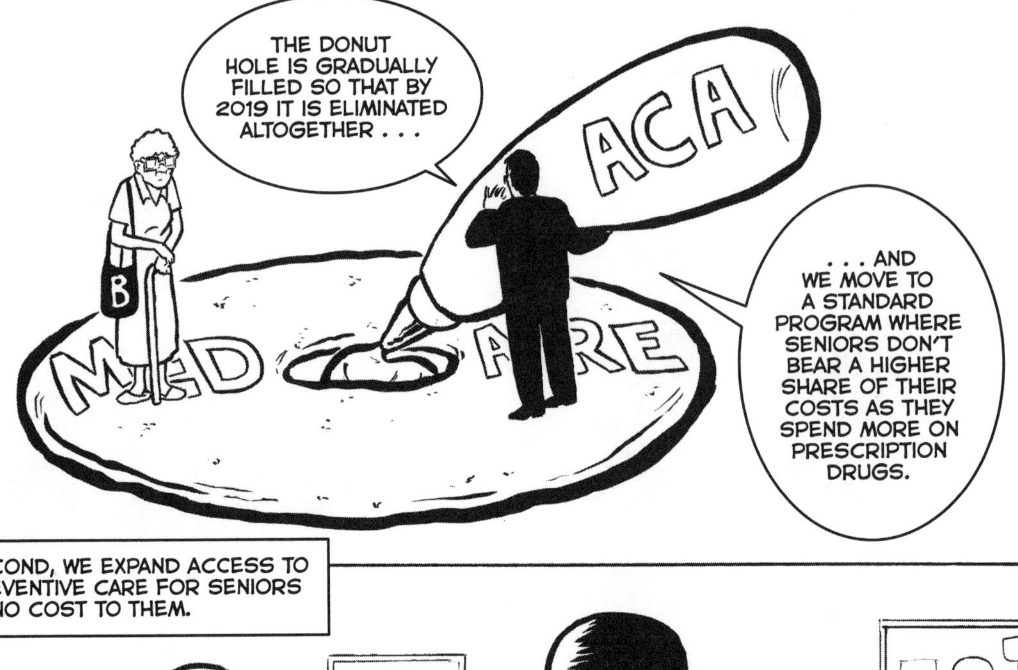
THE DONUT HOLE IS GRADUALLY FILLED SO THAT BY 2019 IT IS ELIMINATED ALTOGETHER . . .
ACA
B
. . . AND WE MOVE TO A STANDARD PROGRAM WHERE SENIORS DON'T BEAR A HIGHER SHARE OF THEIR COSTS AS THEY SPEND MORE ON PRESCRIPTION DRUGS.

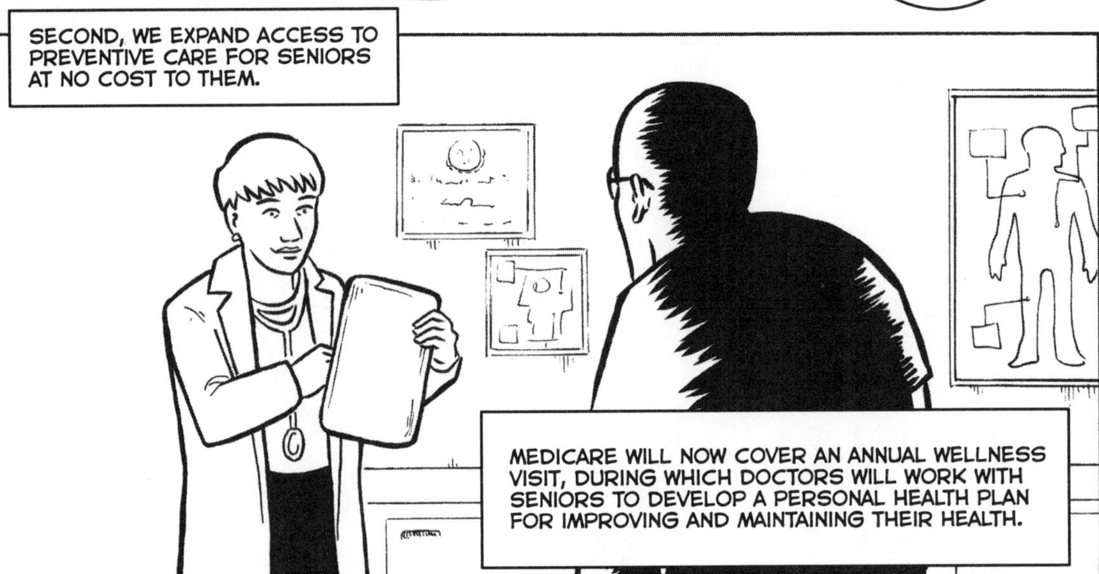
SECOND, WE EXPAND ACCESS TO PREVENTIVE CARE FOR SENIORS AT NO COST TO THEM.
MEDICARE WILL NOW COVER AN ANNUAL WELLNESS VISIT, DURING WHICH DOCTORS WILL WORK WITH SENIORS TO DEVELOP A PERSONAL HEALTH PLAN FOR IMPROVING AND MAINTAINING THEIR HEALTH.

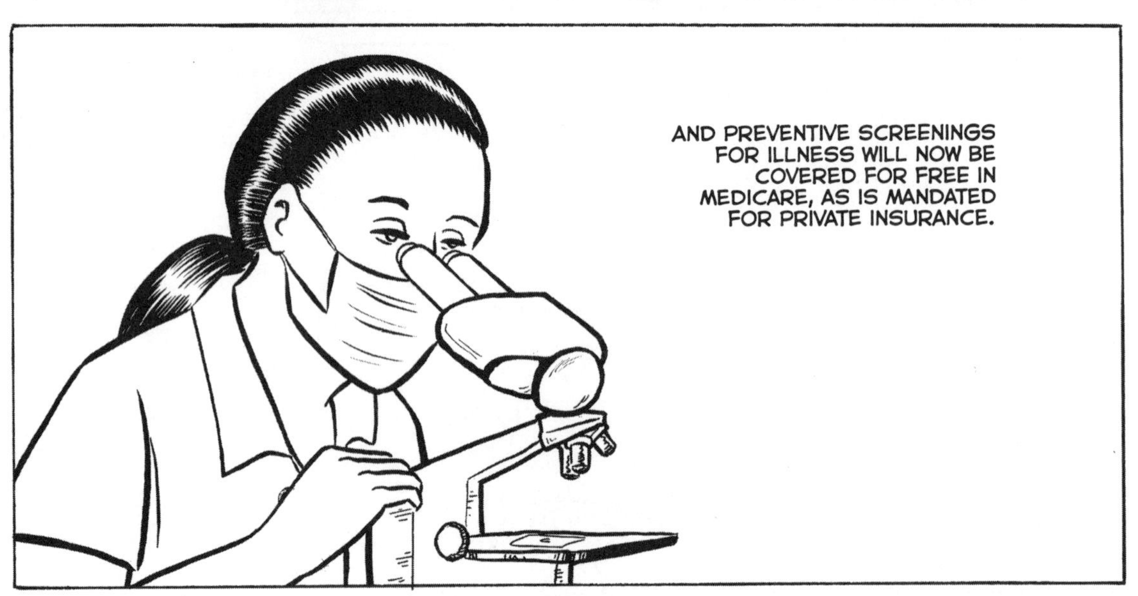
AND PREVENTIVE SCREENINGS FOR ILLNESS WILL NOW BE COVERED FOR FREE IN MEDICARE, AS IS MANDATED FOR PRIVATE INSURANCE.

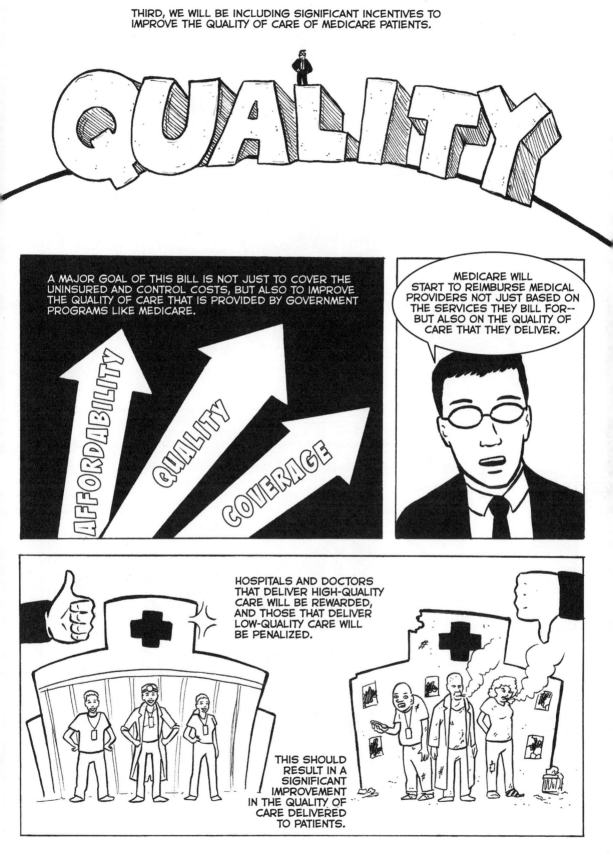

THIRD, WE WILL BE INCLUDING SIGNIFICANT INCENTIVES TO IMPROVE THE QUALITY OF CARE OF MEDICARE PATIENTS.

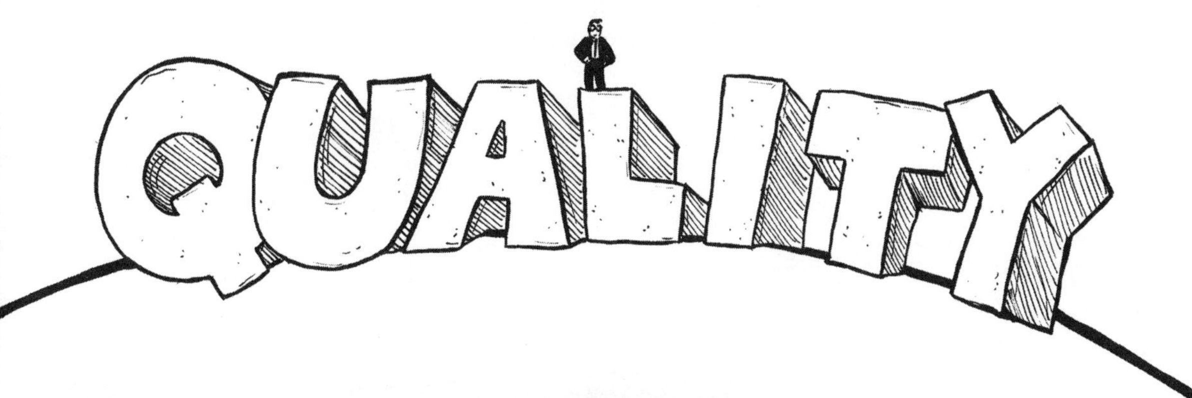

A MAJOR GOAL OF THIS BILL IS NOT JUST TO COVER THE UNINSURED AND CONTROL COSTS, BUT ALSO TO IMPROVE THE QUALITY OF CARE THAT IS PROVIDED BY GOVERNMENT PROGRAMS LIKE MEDICARE.

AFFORDABILITY

QUALITY

COVERAGE

MEDICARE WILL START TO REIMBURSE MEDICAL PROVIDERS NOT JUST BASED ON THE SERVICES THEY BILL FOR-- BUT ALSO ON THE QUALITY OF CARE THAT THEY DELIVER.

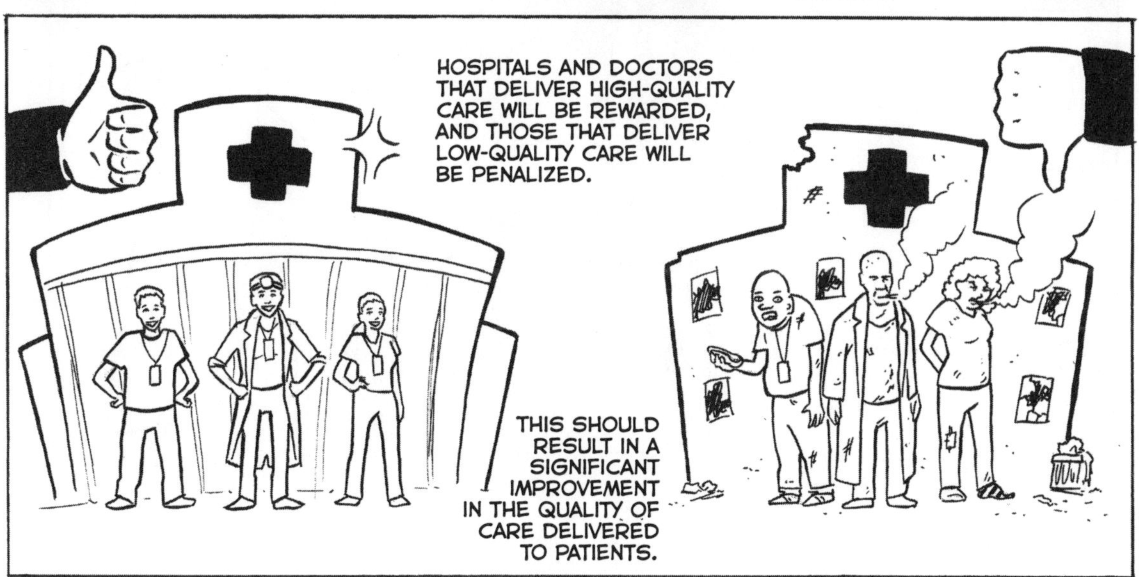

HOSPITALS AND DOCTORS THAT DELIVER HIGH-QUALITY CARE WILL BE REWARDED, AND THOSE THAT DELIVER LOW-QUALITY CARE WILL BE PENALIZED.
THIS SHOULD RESULT IN A SIGNIFICANT IMPROVEMENT IN THE QUALITY OF CARE DELIVERED TO PATIENTS.

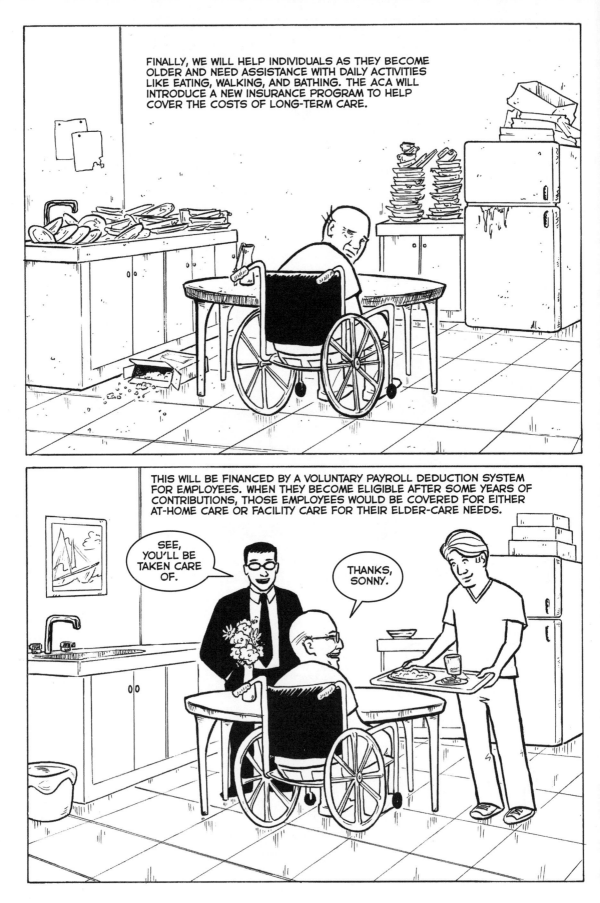

FINALLY, WE WILL HELP INDIVIDUALS AS THEY BECOME OLDER AND NEED ASSISTANCE WITH DAILY ACTIVITIES LIKE EATING, WALKING, AND BATHING. THE ACA WILL INTRODUCE A NEW INSURANCE PROGRAM TO HELP COVER THE COSTS OF LONG-TERM CARE.

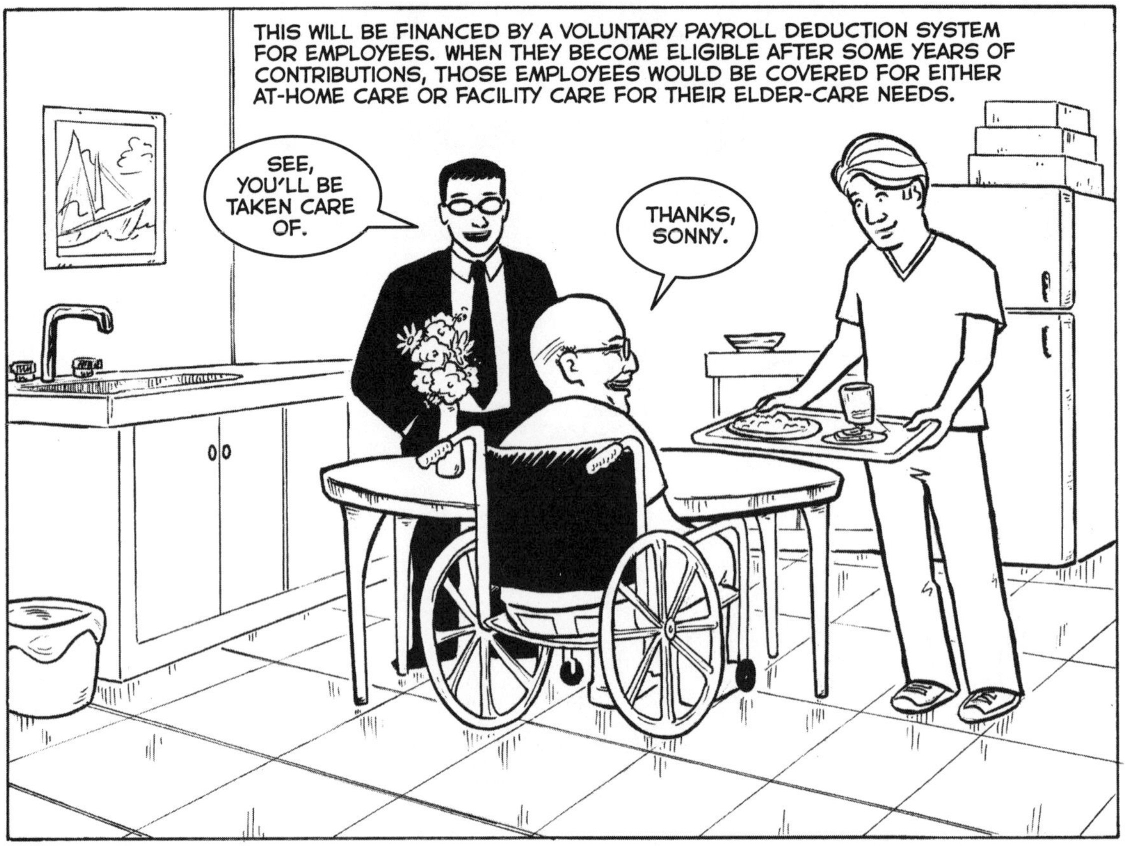

THIS WILL BE FINANCED BY A VOLUNTARY PAYROLL DEDUCTION SYSTEM FOR EMPLOYEES. WHEN THEY BECOME ELIGIBLE AFTER SOME YEARS OF CONTRIBUTIONS, THOSE EMPLOYEES WOULD BE COVERED FOR EITHER AT-HOME CARE OR FACILITY CARE FOR THEIR ELDER-CARE NEEDS.

SEE, YOU'LL BE TAKEN CARE OF.

THANKS, SONNY.

CHAPTER 12 GOOD THINGS ON THE HORIZON

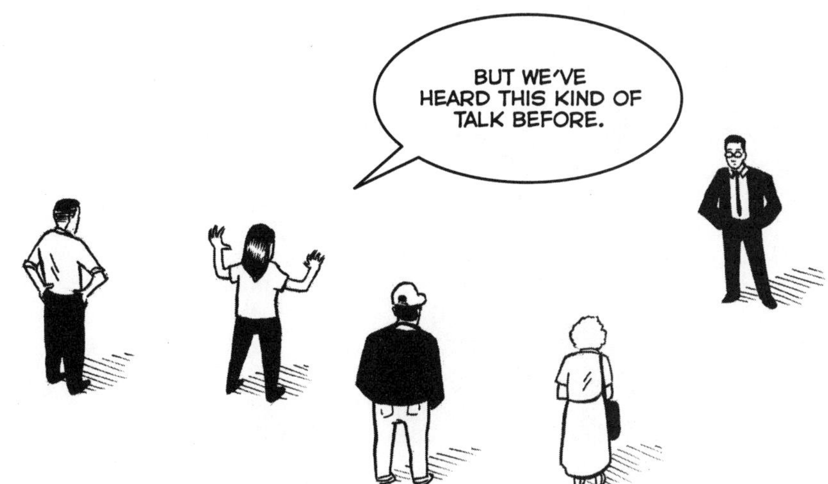
BUT WE'VE HEARD THIS KIND OF TALK BEFORE.

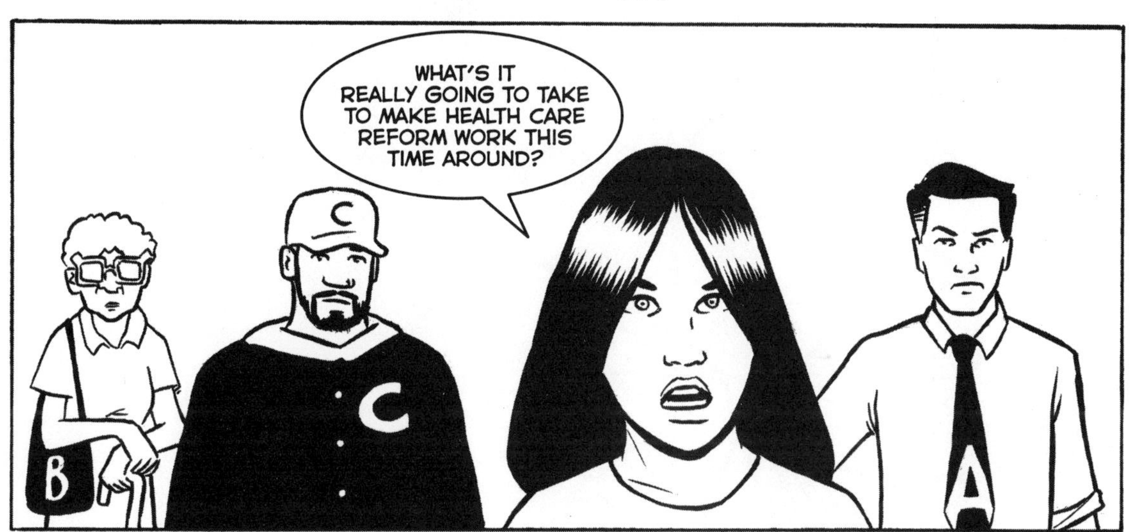
WHAT'S IT REALLY GOING TO TAKE TO MAKE HEALTH CARE REFORM WORK THIS TIME AROUND?
C
B
C
A

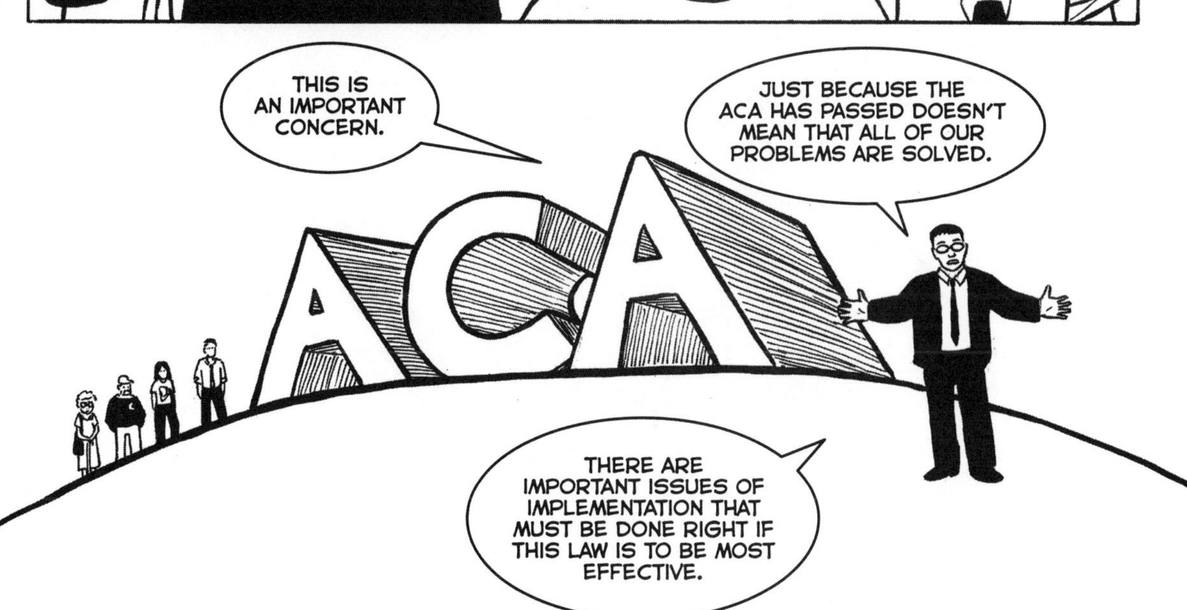

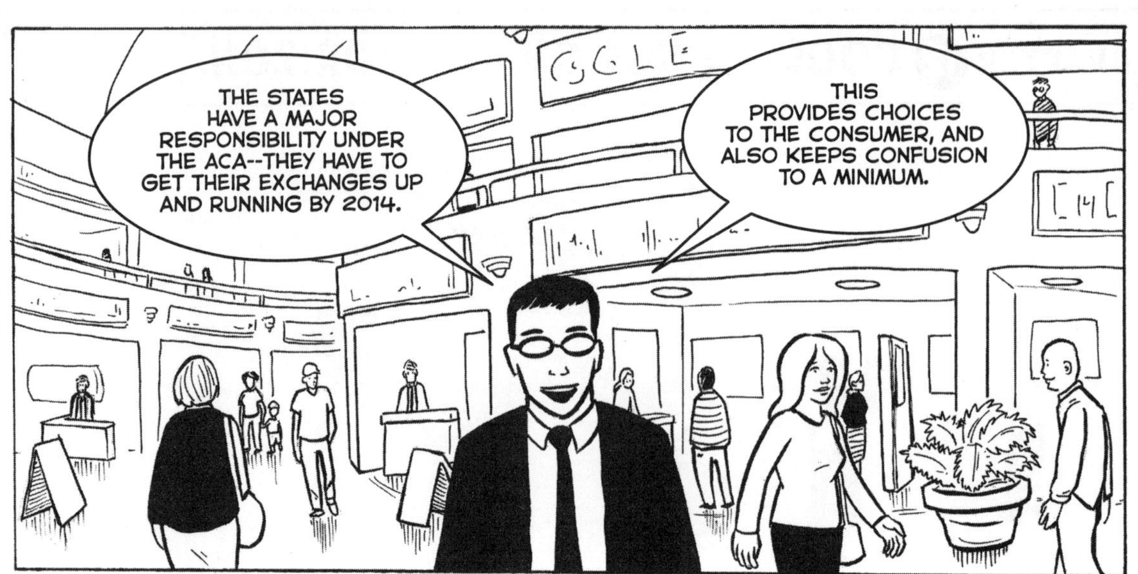
THE STATES HAVE A MAJOR RESPONSIBILITY UNDER THE ACA--THEY HAVE TO GET THEIR EXCHANGES UP AND RUNNING BY 2014.
THIS PROVIDES CHOICES TO THE CONSUMER, AND ALSO KEEPS CONFUSION TO A MINIMUM.

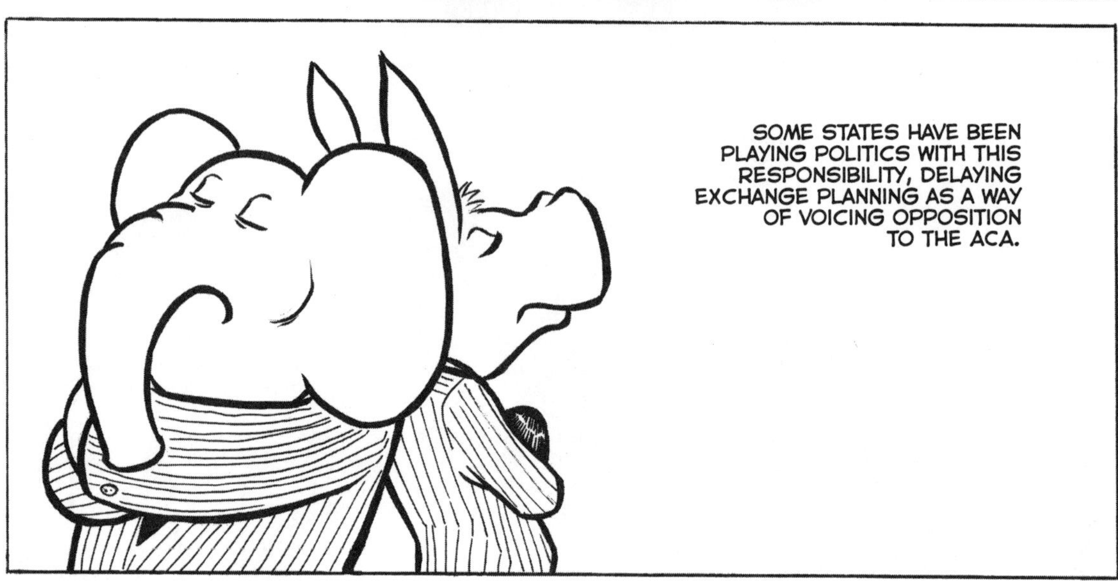
SOME STATES HAVE BEEN PLAYING POLITICS WITH THIS RESPONSIBILITY, DELAYING EXCHANGE PLANNING AS A WAY OF VOICING OPPOSITION TO THE ACA.

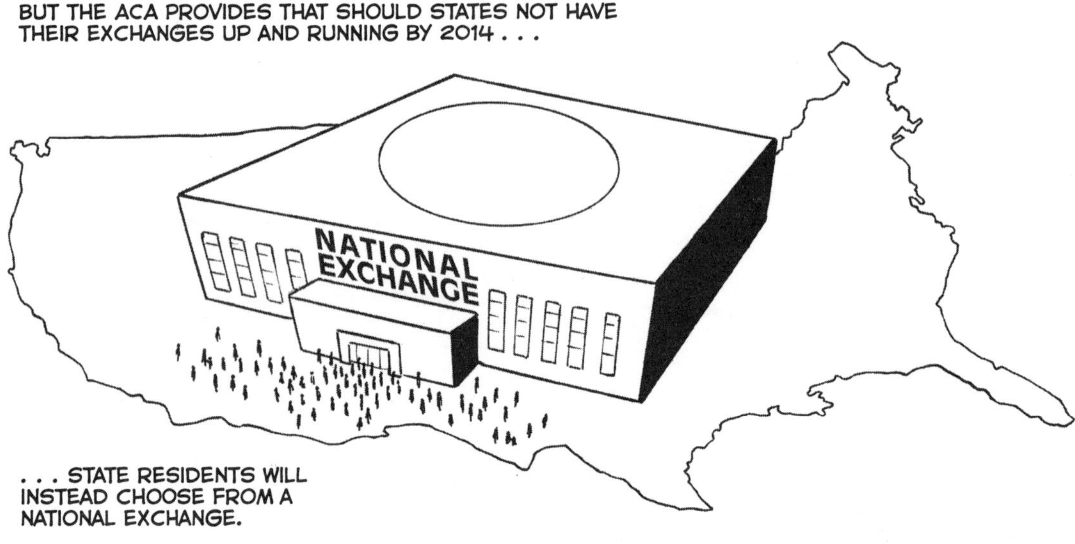
BUT THE ACA PROVIDES THAT SHOULD STATES NOT HAVE THEIR EXCHANGES UP AND RUNNING BY 2014 . . .
NATIONAL EXCHANGE
. . . STATE RESIDENTS WILL INSTEAD CHOOSE FROM A NATIONAL EXCHANGE.

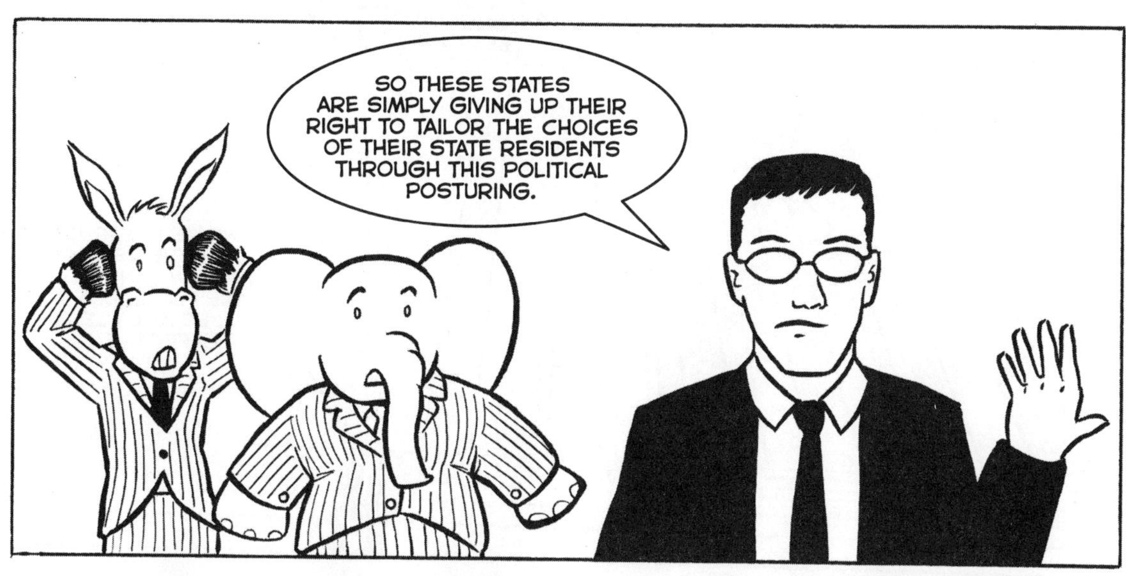
SO THESE STATES ARE SIMPLY GIVING UP THEIR RIGHT TO TAILOR THE CHOICES OF THEIR STATE RESIDENTS THROUGH THIS POLITICAL POSTURING.

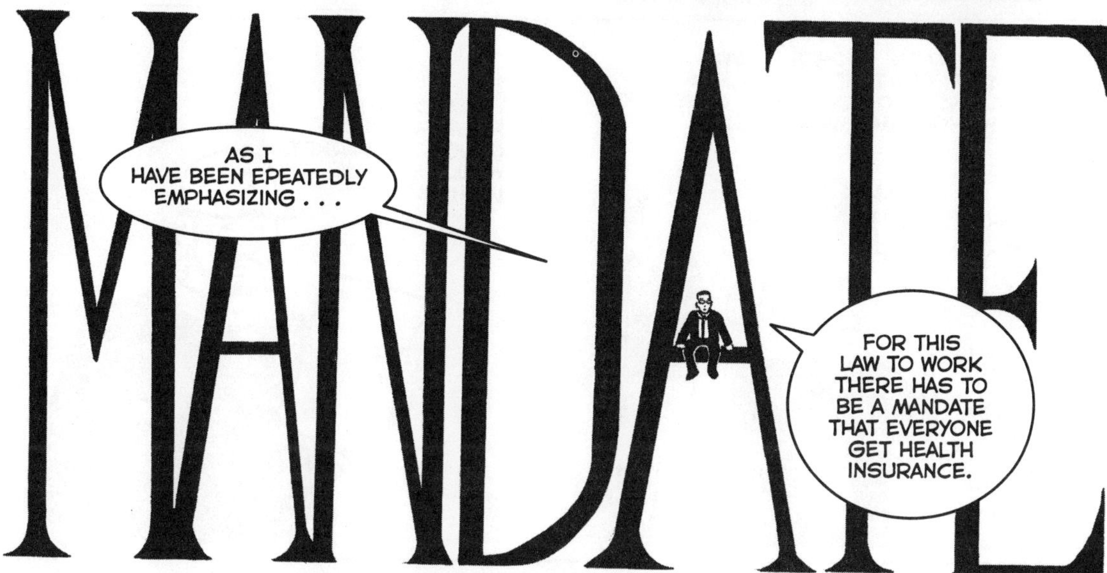
MANDATE
AS I HAVE BEEN EPEATEDLY EMPHASIZING . . .
FOR THIS LAW TO WORK THERE HAS TO BE A MANDATE THAT EVERYONE GET HEALTH INSURANCE.

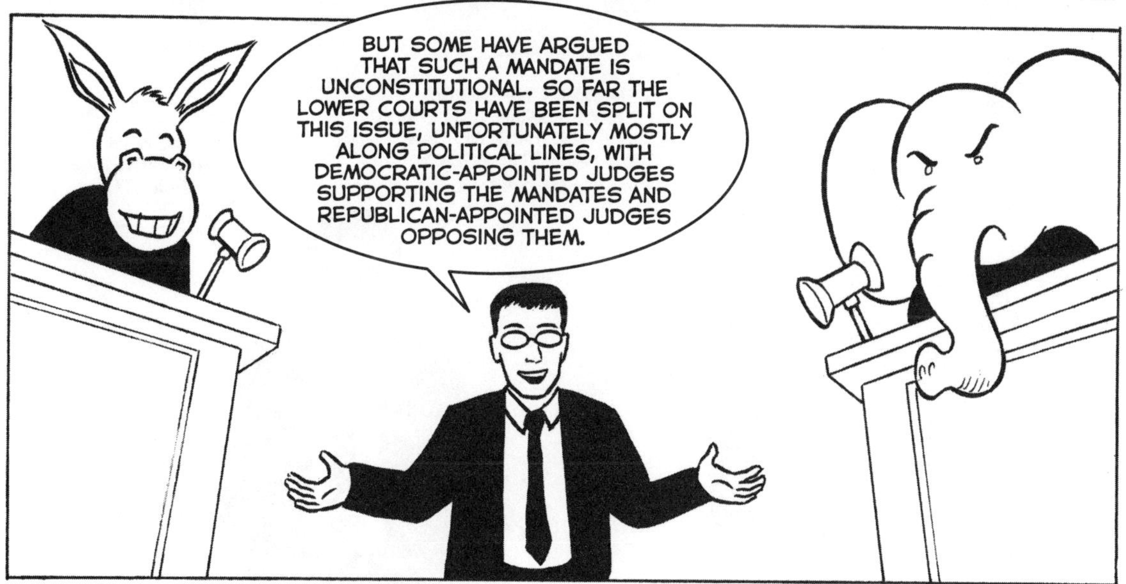
BUT SOME HAVE ARGUED THAT SUCH A MANDATE IS UNCONSTITUTIONAL. SO FAR THE LOWER COURTS HAVE BEEN SPLIT ON THIS ISSUE, UNFORTUNATELY MOSTLY ALONG POLITICAL LINES, WITH DEMOCRATIC-APPOINTED JUDGES SUPPORTING THE MANDATES AND REPUBLICAN-APPOINTED JUDGES OPPOSING THEM.

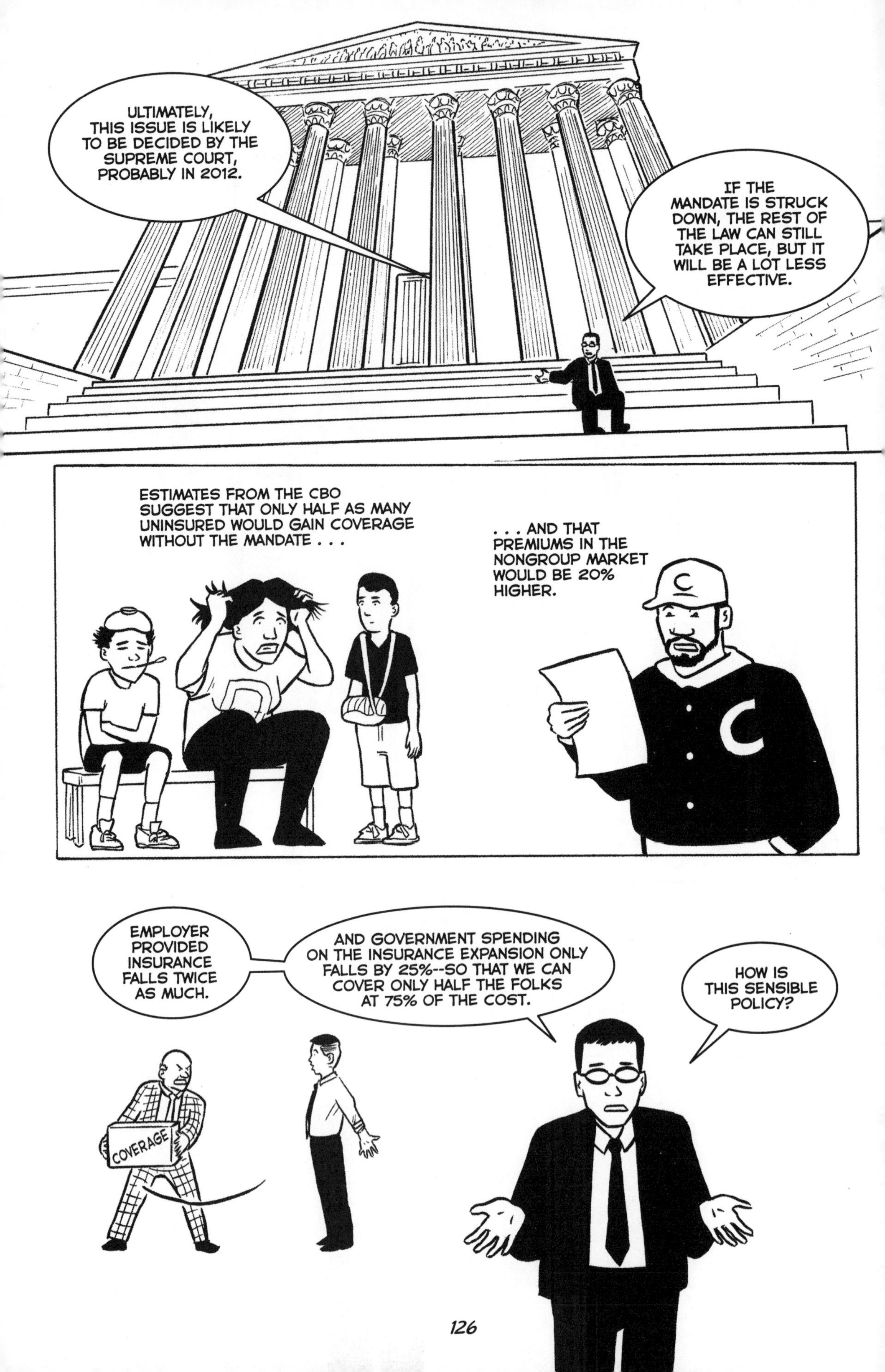

ULTIMATELY, THIS ISSUE IS LIKELY TO BE DECIDED BY THE SUPREME COURT, PROBABLY IN 2012.

IF THE MANDATE IS STRUCK DOWN, THE REST OF THE LAW CAN STILL TAKE PLACE, BUT IT WILL BE A LOT LESS EFFECTIVE.

ESTIMATES FROM THE CBO SUGGEST THAT ONLY HALF AS MANY UNINSURED WOULD GAIN COVERAGE WITHOUT THE MANDATE . . .

. . . AND THAT PREMIUMS IN THE NONGROUP MARKET WOULD BE 20% HIGHER.

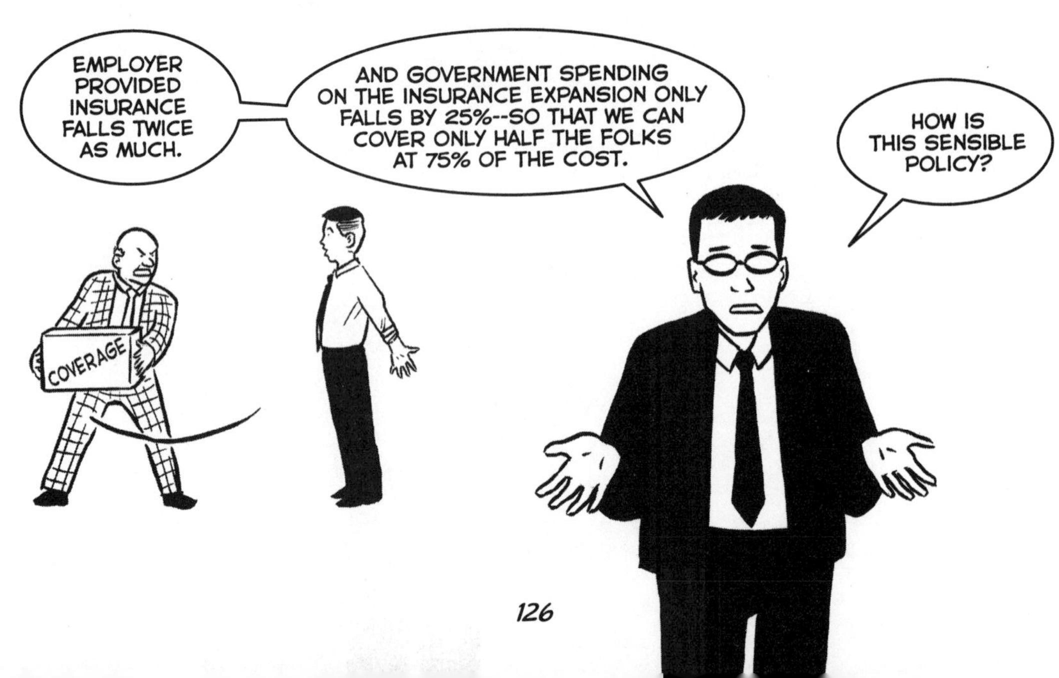
EMPLOYER PROVIDED INSURANCE FALLS TWICE AS MUCH.
AND GOVERNMENT SPENDING ON THE INSURANCE EXPANSION ONLY FALLS BY 25%--SO THAT WE CAN COVER ONLY HALF THE FOLKS AT 75% OF THE COST.
HOW IS THIS SENSIBLE POLICY?
COVERAGE

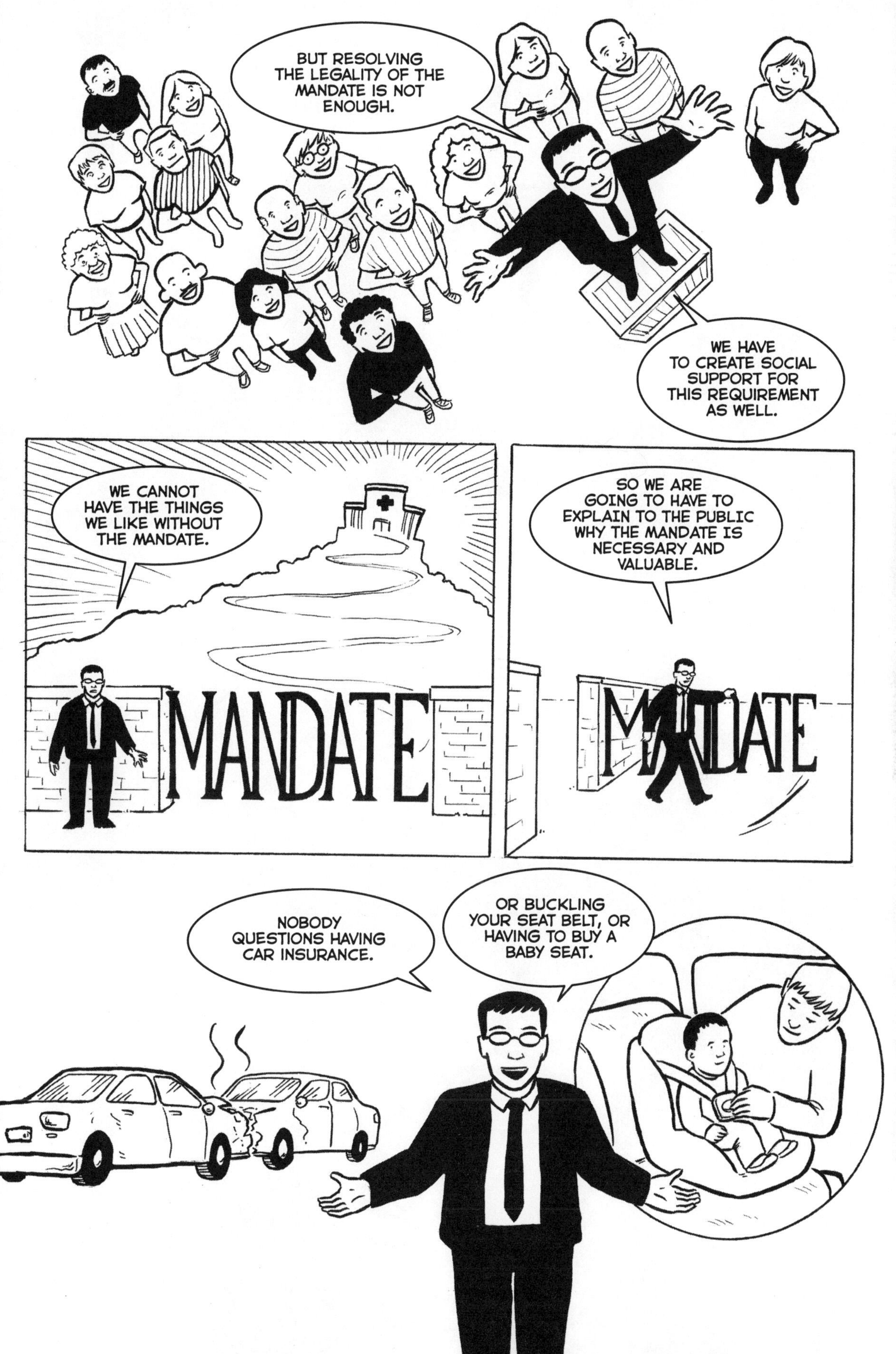
BUT RESOLVING THE LEGALITY OF THE MANDATE IS NOT ENOUGH.
WE HAVE TO CREATE SOCIAL SUPPORT FOR THIS REQUIREMENT AS WELL.
WE CANNOT HAVE THE THINGS WE LIKE WITHOUT THE MANDATE.
MANDATE
SO WE ARE GOING TO HAVE TO EXPLAIN TO THE PUBLIC WHY THE MANDATE IS NECESSARY AND VALUABLE.
MANDATE
NOBODY QUESTIONS HAVING CAR INSURANCE.
OR BUCKLING YOUR SEAT BELT, OR HAVING TO BUY A BABY SEAT.

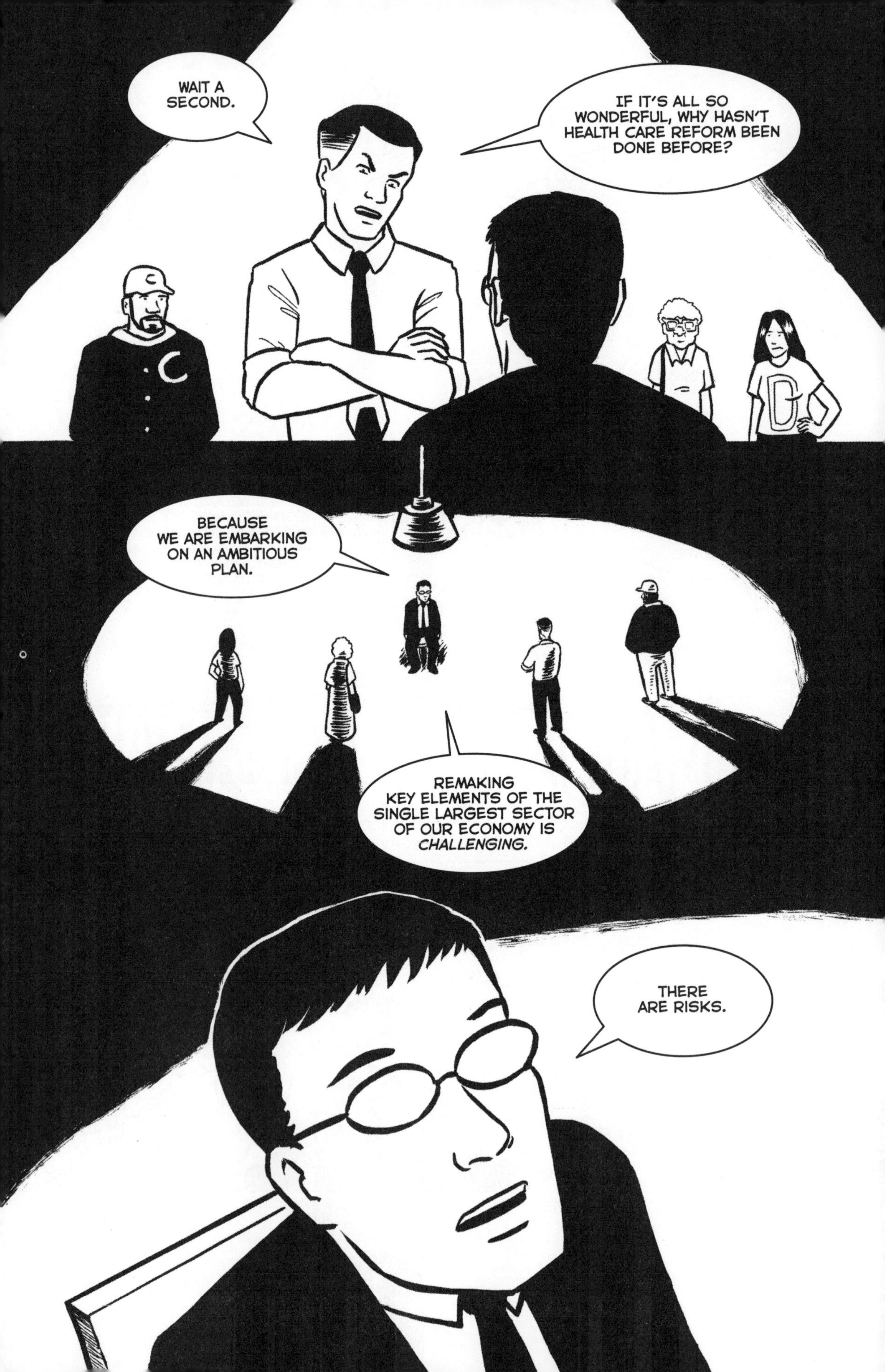
WAIT A SECOND.
IF IT'S ALL SO WONDERFUL, WHY HASN'T HEALTH CARE REFORM BEEN DONE BEFORE?
BECAUSE WE ARE EMBARKING ON AN AMBITIOUS PLAN.
REMAKING KEY ELEMENTS OF THE SINGLE LARGEST SECTOR OF OUR ECONOMY IS *CHALLENGING.*
THERE ARE RISKS.

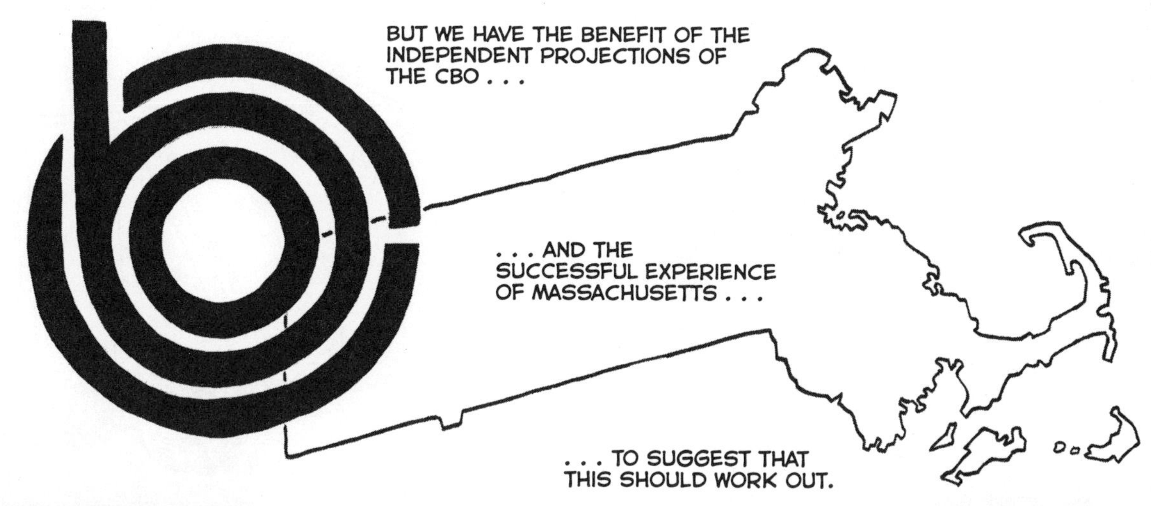
BUT WE HAVE THE BENEFIT OF THE INDEPENDENT PROJECTIONS OF THE CBO . . .
. . . AND THE SUCCESSFUL EXPERIENCE OF MASSACHUSETTS . . .
. . . TO SUGGEST THAT THIS SHOULD WORK OUT.

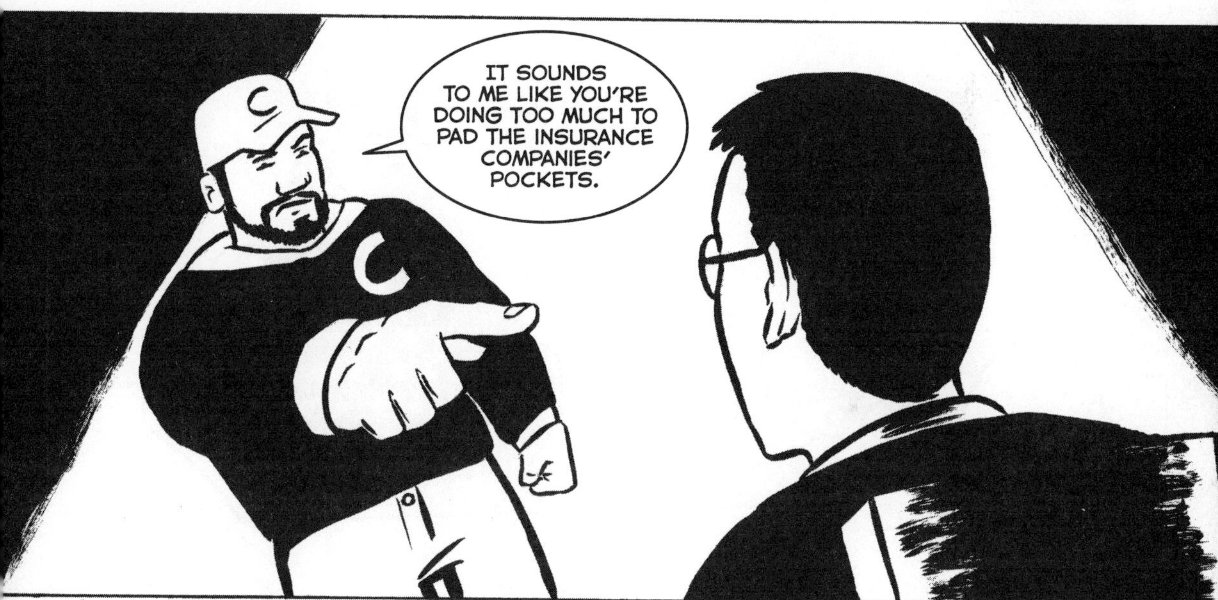
IT SOUNDS TO ME LIKE YOU'RE DOING TOO MUCH TO PAD THE INSURANCE COMPANIES' POCKETS.

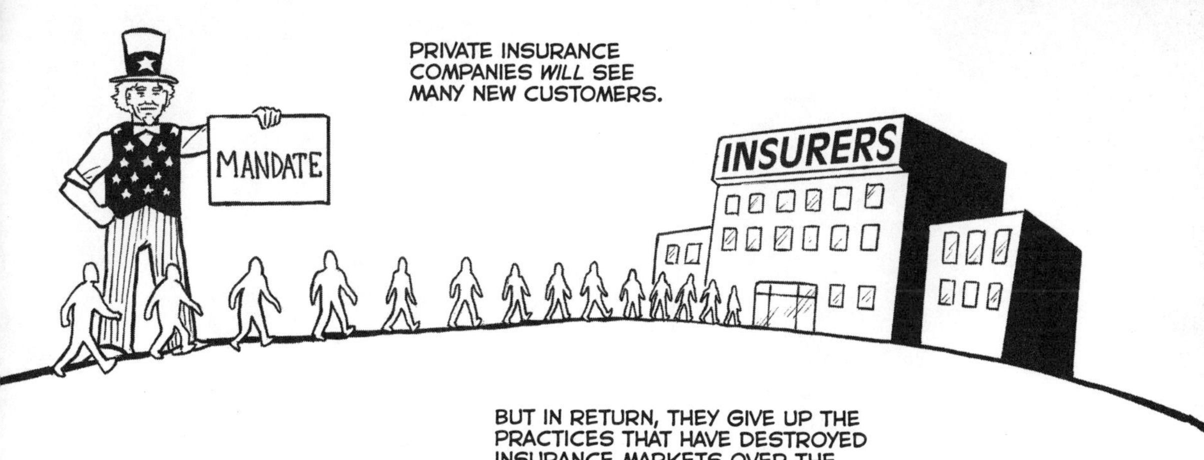
PRIVATE INSURANCE COMPANIES *WILL* SEE MANY NEW CUSTOMERS.
MANDATE
INSURERS
BUT IN RETURN, THEY GIVE UP THE PRACTICES THAT HAVE DESTROYED INSURANCE MARKETS OVER THE PAST 50 YEARS.

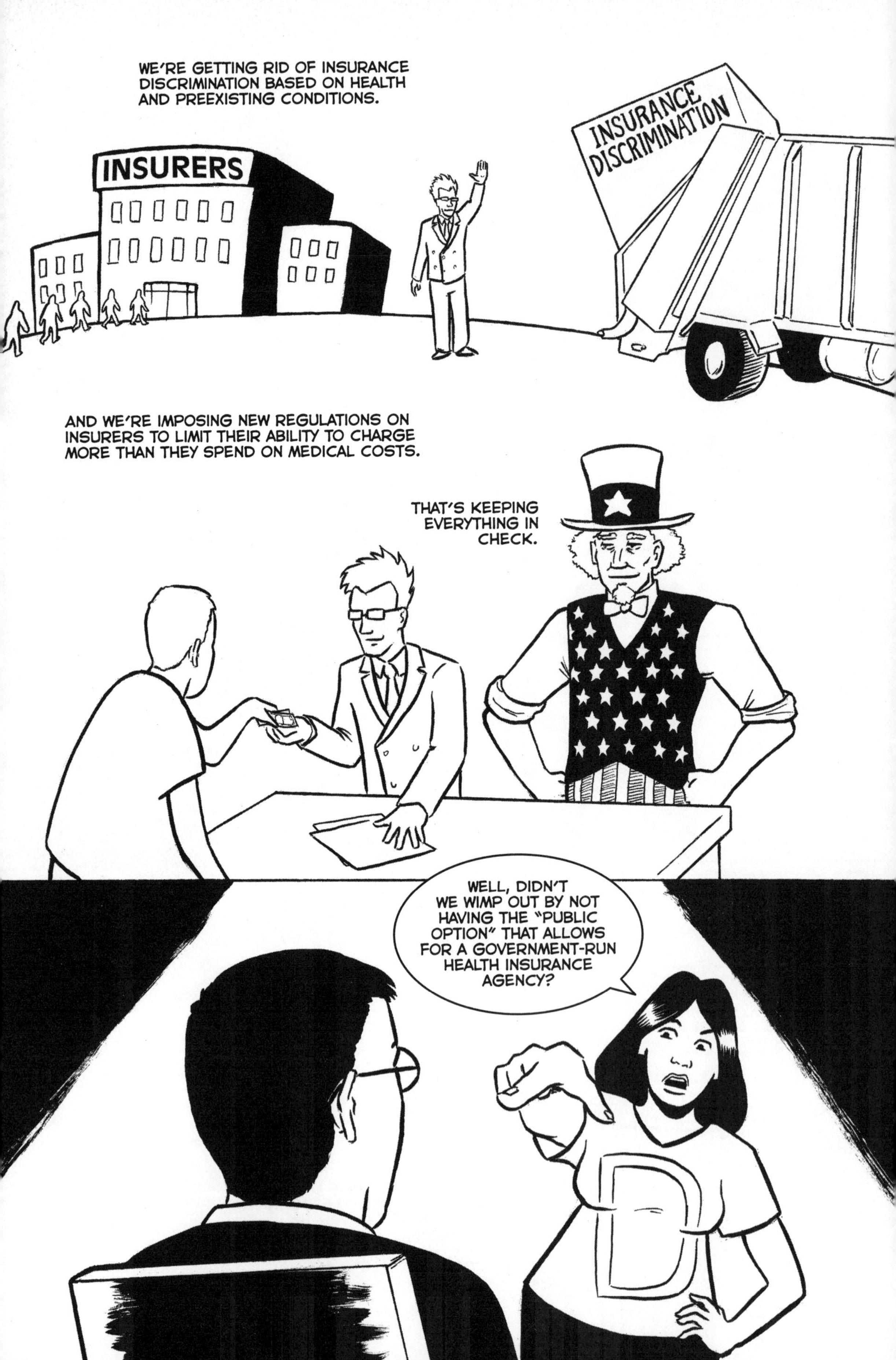
WE'RE GETTING RID OF INSURANCE DISCRIMINATION BASED ON HEALTH AND PREEXISTING CONDITIONS.
INSURERS
INSURANCE DISCRIMINATION
AND WE'RE IMPOSING NEW REGULATIONS ON INSURERS TO LIMIT THEIR ABILITY TO CHARGE MORE THAN THEY SPEND ON MEDICAL COSTS.
THAT'S KEEPING EVERYTHING IN CHECK.
WELL, DIDN'T WE WIMP OUT BY NOT HAVING THE "PUBLIC OPTION" THAT ALLOWS FOR A GOVERNMENT-RUN HEALTH INSURANCE AGENCY?

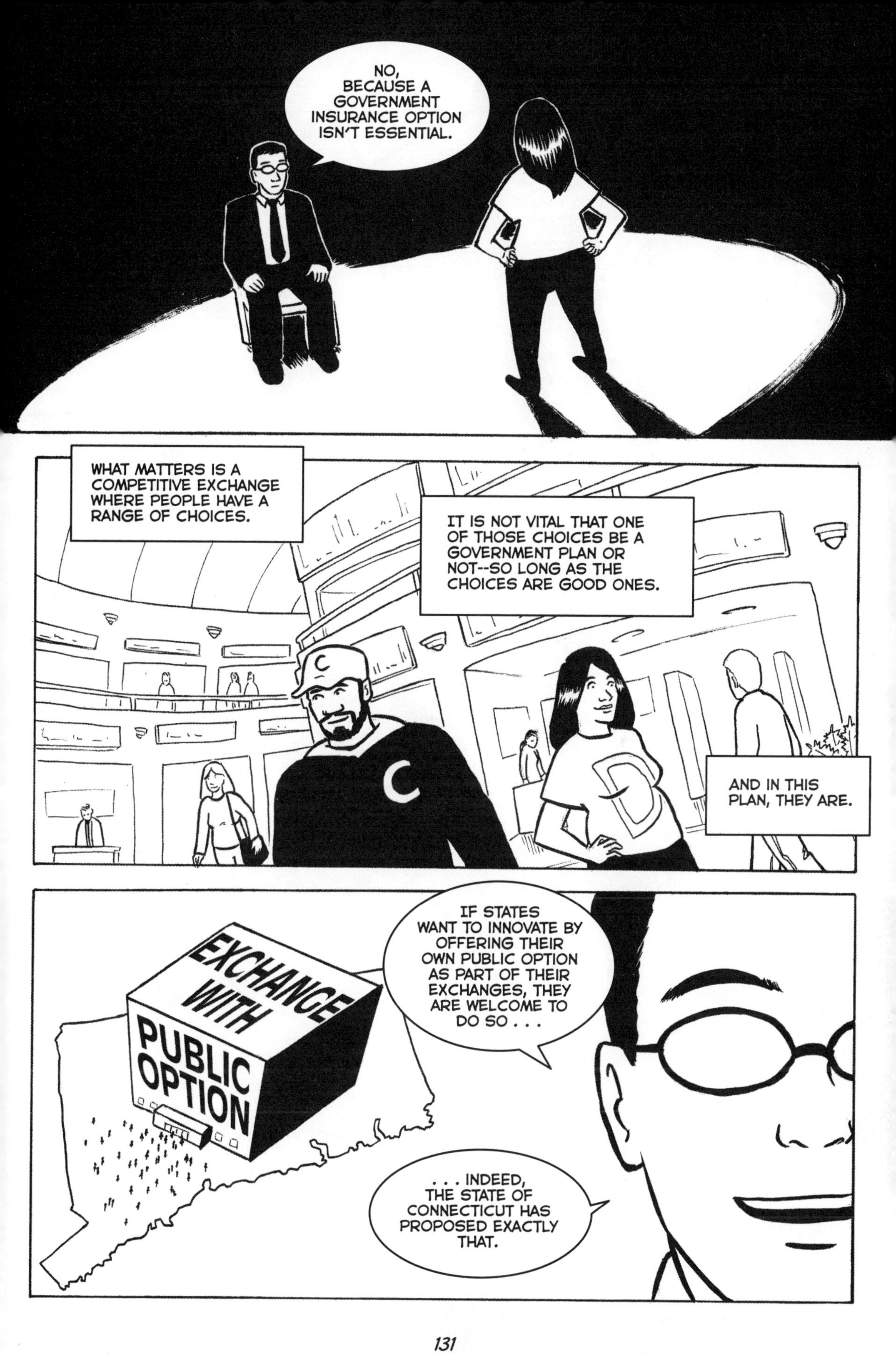

NO, BECAUSE A GOVERNMENT INSURANCE OPTION ISN'T ESSENTIAL.

WHAT MATTERS IS A COMPETITIVE EXCHANGE WHERE PEOPLE HAVE A RANGE OF CHOICES.

IT IS NOT VITAL THAT ONE OF THOSE CHOICES BE A GOVERNMENT PLAN OR NOT--SO LONG AS THE CHOICES ARE GOOD ONES.

AND IN THIS PLAN, THEY ARE.

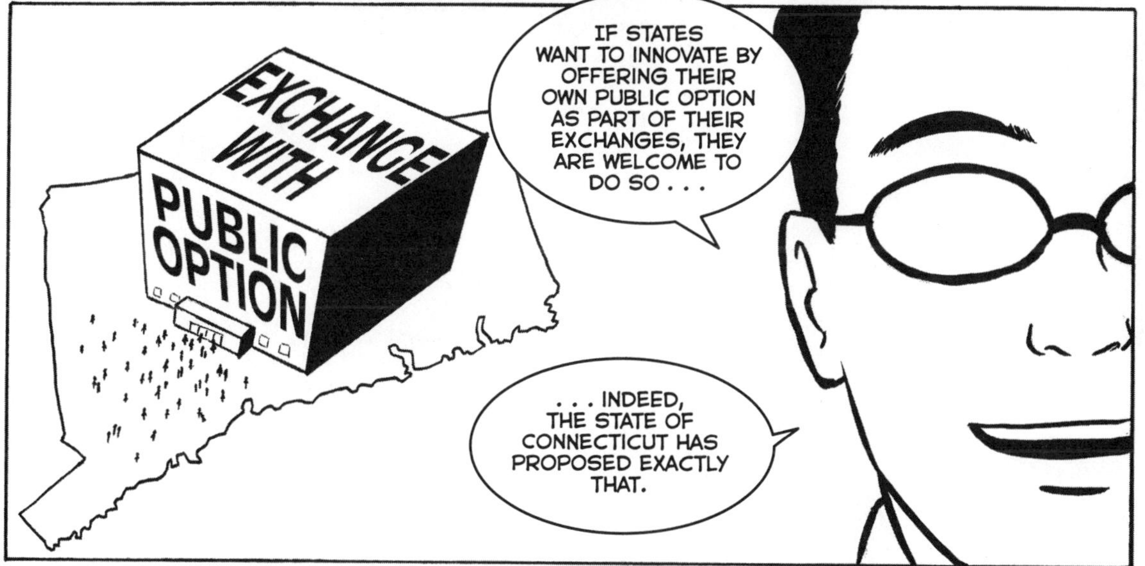
EXCHANGE WITH PUBLIC OPTION
IF STATES WANT TO INNOVATE BY OFFERING THEIR OWN PUBLIC OPTION AS PART OF THEIR EXCHANGES, THEY ARE WELCOME TO DO SO . . .
. . . INDEED, THE STATE OF CONNECTICUT HAS PROPOSED EXACTLY THAT.

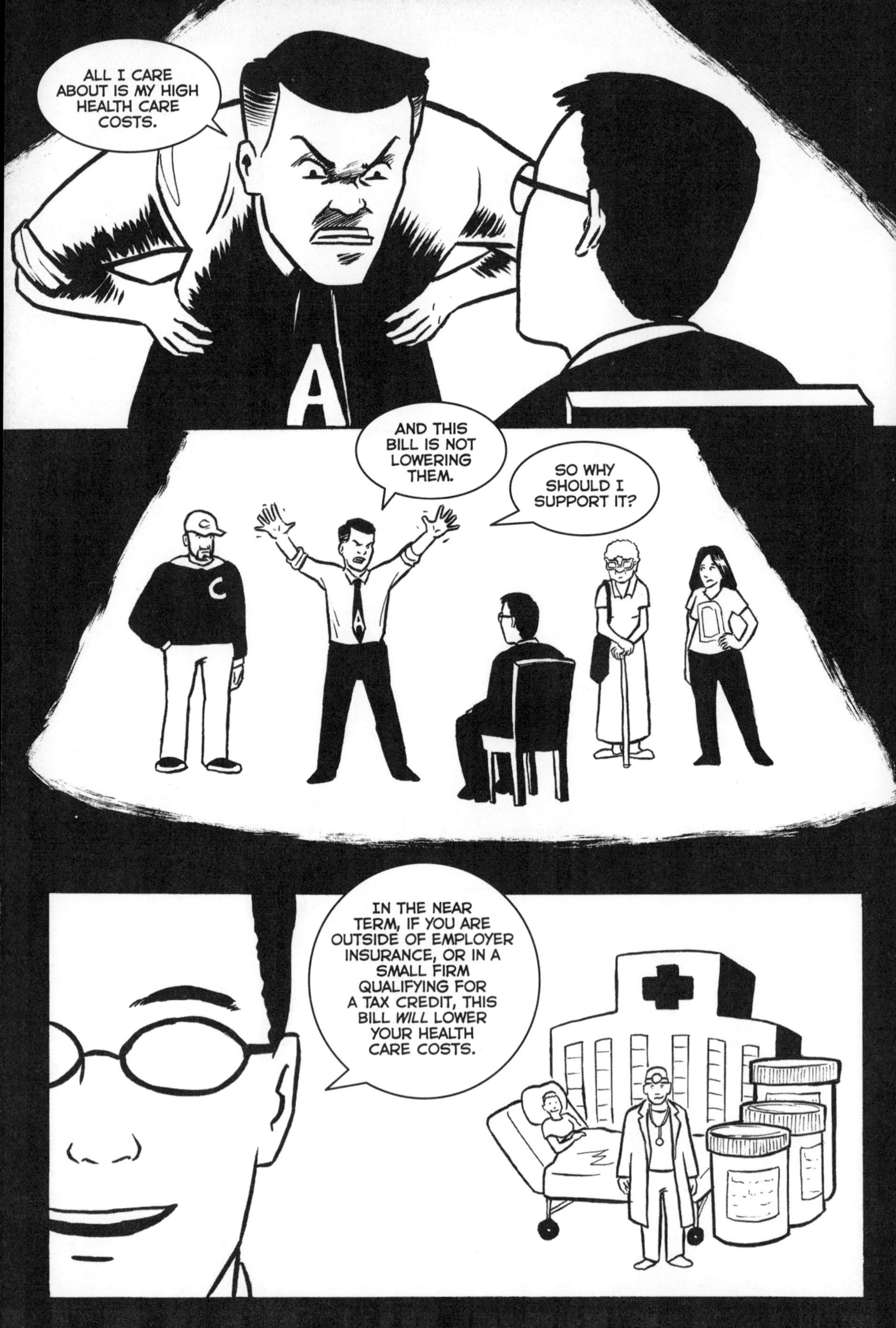
ALL I CARE ABOUT IS MY HIGH HEALTH CARE COSTS.
AND THIS BILL IS NOT LOWERING THEM.
SO WHY SHOULD I SUPPORT IT?
IN THE NEAR TERM, IF YOU ARE OUTSIDE OF EMPLOYER INSURANCE, OR IN A SMALL FIRM QUALIFYING FOR A TAX CREDIT, THIS BILL *WILL* LOWER YOUR HEALTH CARE COSTS.

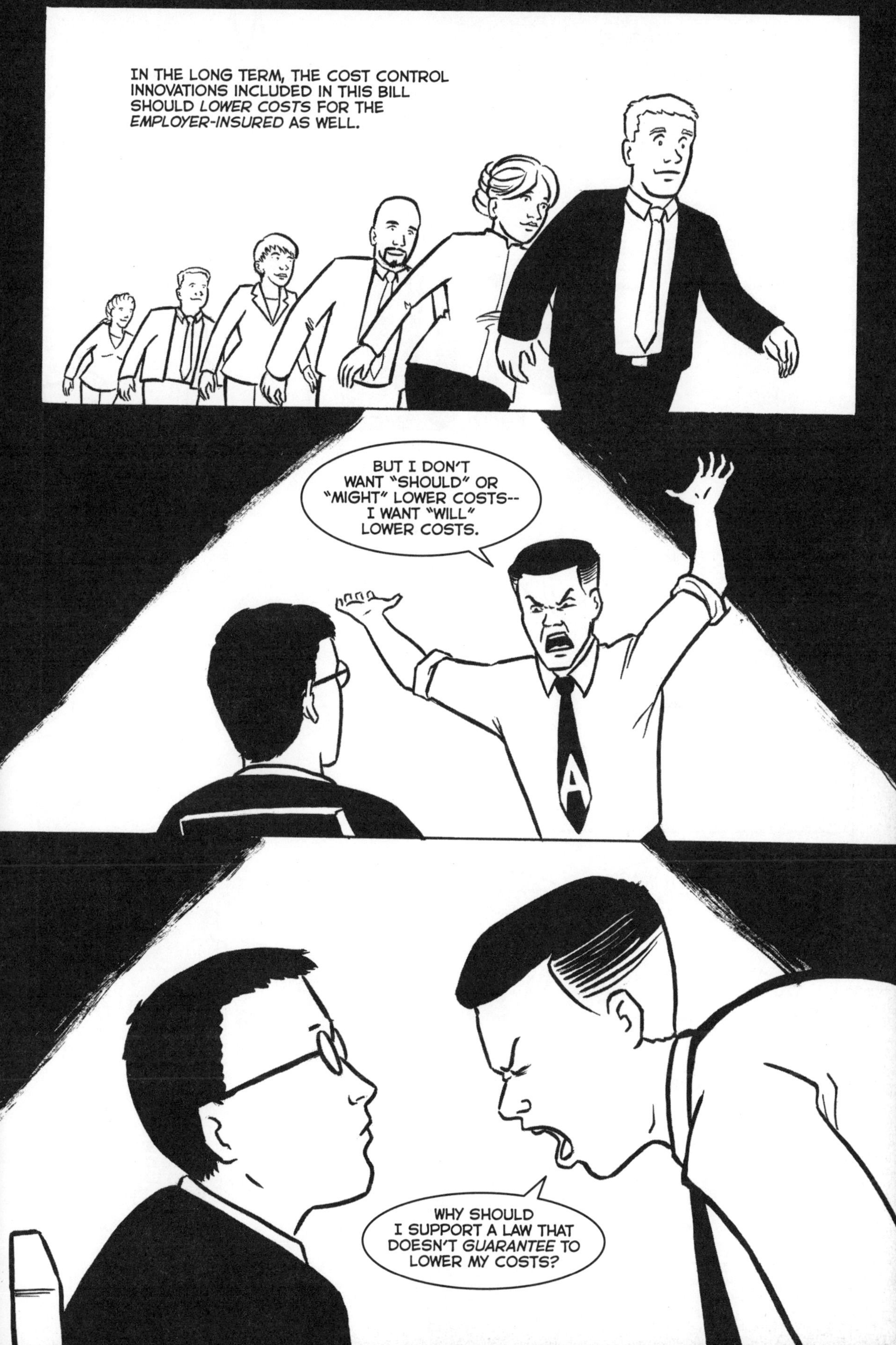
IN THE LONG TERM, THE COST CONTROL INNOVATIONS INCLUDED IN THIS BILL SHOULD *LOWER COSTS* FOR THE *EMPLOYER-INSURED* AS WELL.
BUT I DON'T WANT "SHOULD" OR "MIGHT" LOWER COSTS-- I WANT "WILL" LOWER COSTS.
WHY SHOULD I SUPPORT A LAW THAT DOESN'T *GUARANTEE* TO LOWER MY COSTS?

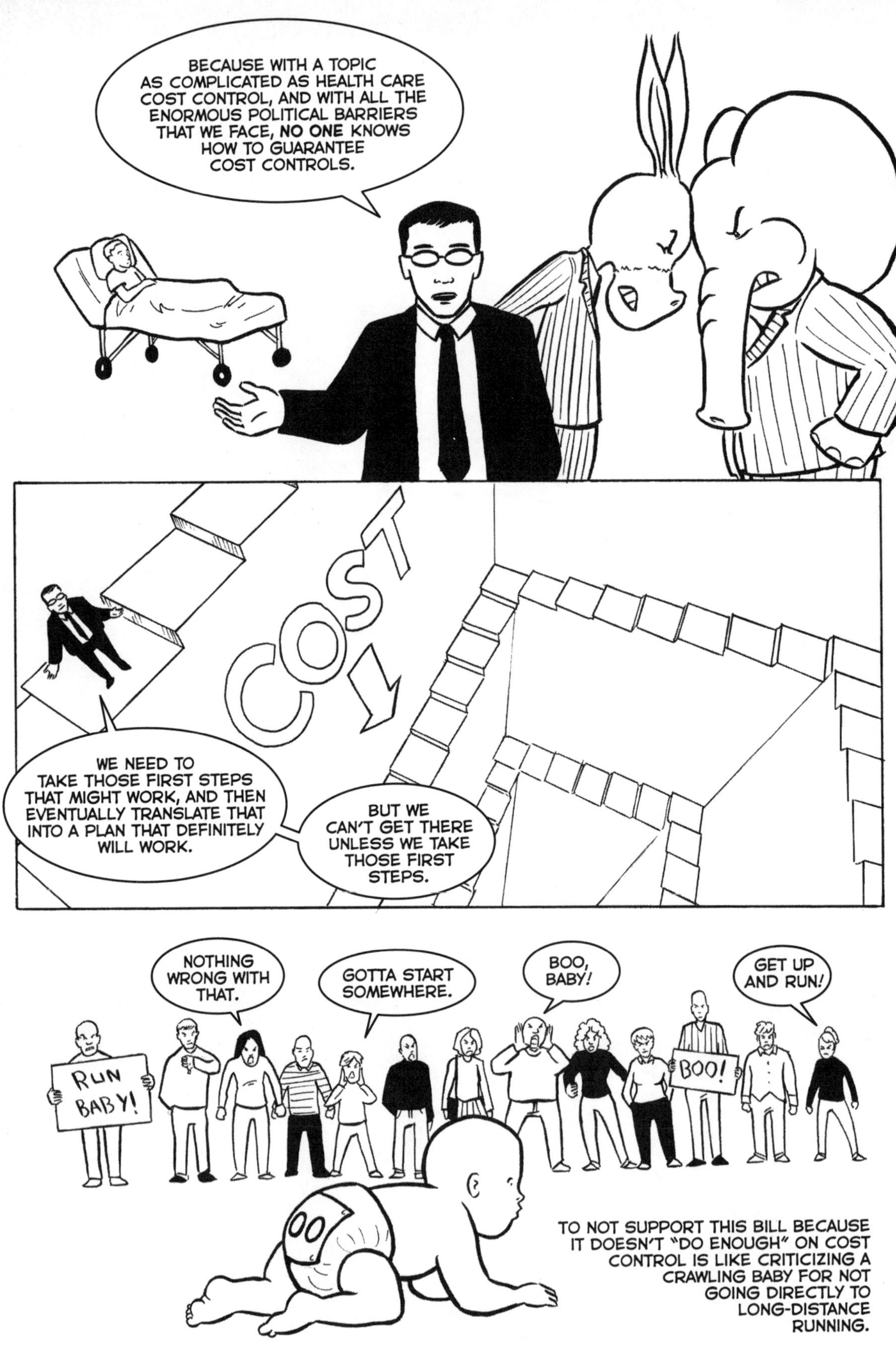
BECAUSE WITH A TOPIC AS COMPLICATED AS HEALTH CARE COST CONTROL, AND WITH ALL THE ENORMOUS POLITICAL BARRIERS THAT WE FACE, **NO ONE** KNOWS HOW TO GUARANTEE COST CONTROLS.
COST
WE NEED TO TAKE THOSE FIRST STEPS THAT MIGHT WORK, AND THEN EVENTUALLY TRANSLATE THAT INTO A PLAN THAT DEFINITELY WILL WORK.
BUT WE CAN'T GET THERE UNLESS WE TAKE THOSE FIRST STEPS.
NOTHING WRONG WITH THAT.
GOTTA START SOMEWHERE.
BOO, BABY!
GET UP AND RUN!
RUN BABY!
BOO!
TO NOT SUPPORT THIS BILL BECAUSE IT DOESN'T "DO ENOUGH" ON COST CONTROL IS LIKE CRITICIZING A CRAWLING BABY FOR NOT GOING DIRECTLY TO LONG-DISTANCE RUNNING.

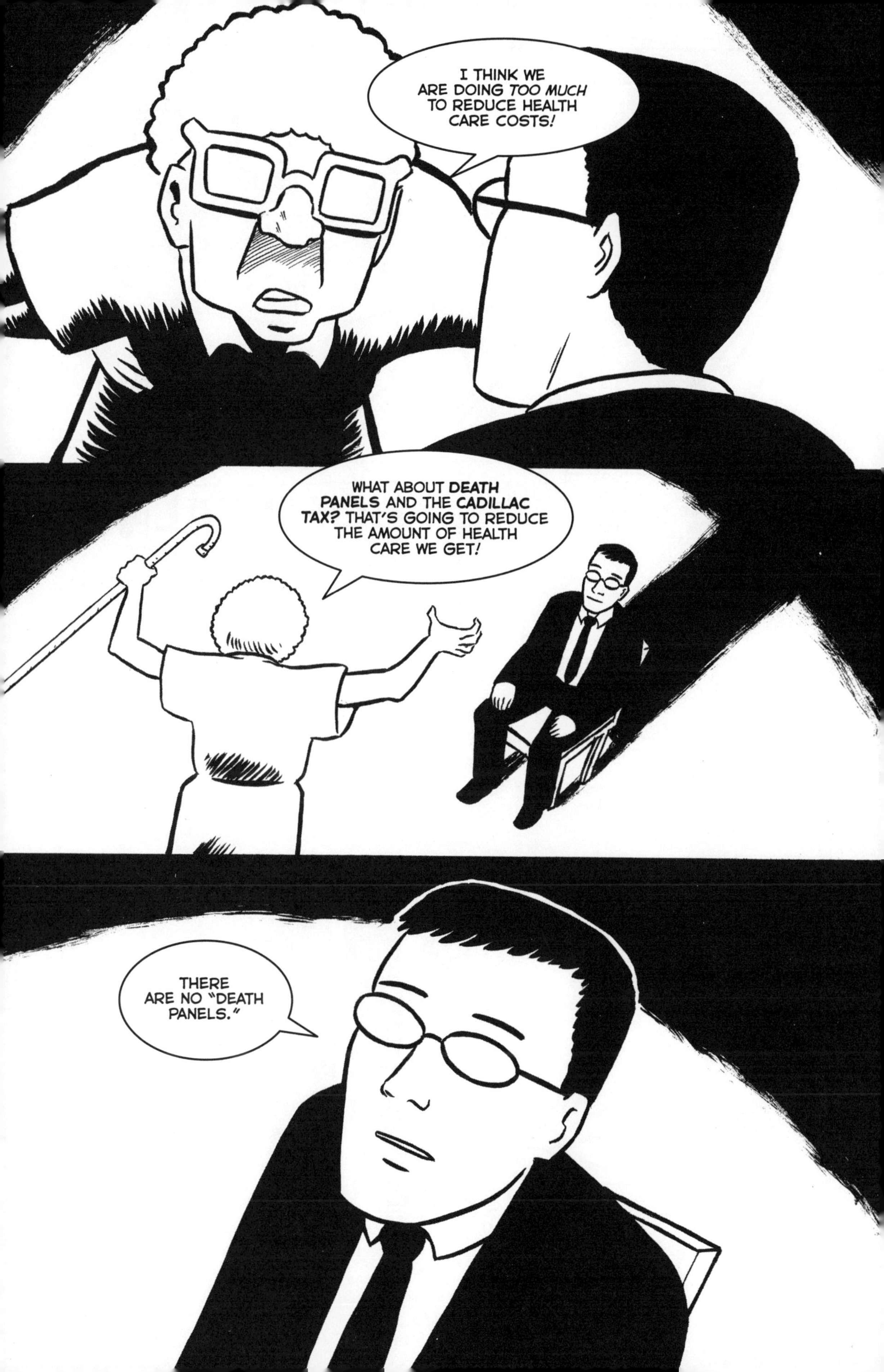
I THINK WE ARE DOING *TOO MUCH* TO REDUCE HEALTH CARE COSTS!
WHAT ABOUT **DEATH PANELS** AND THE **CADILLAC TAX?** THAT'S GOING TO REDUCE THE AMOUNT OF HEALTH CARE WE GET!
THERE ARE NO "DEATH PANELS."

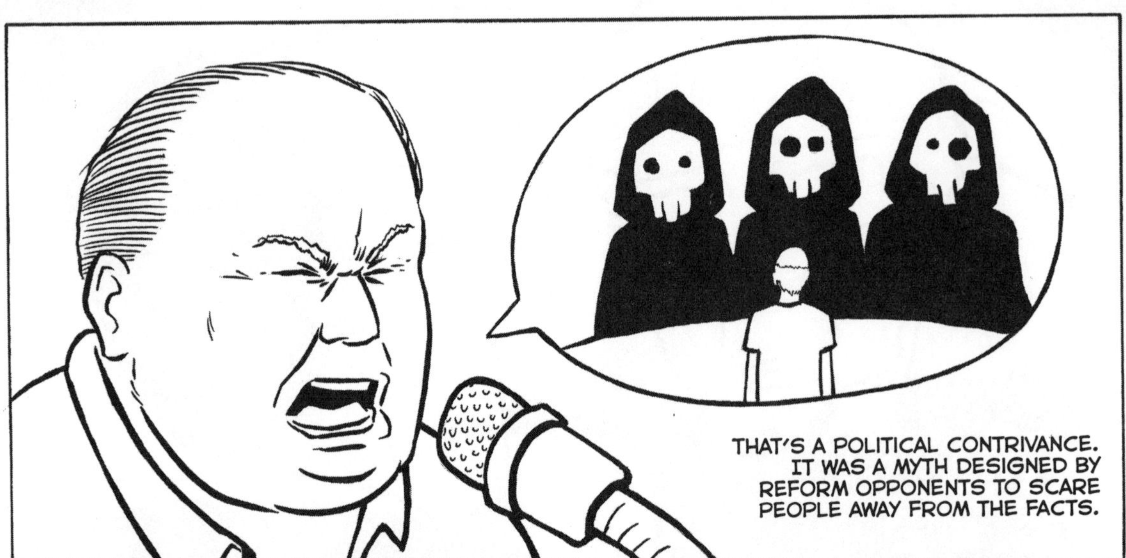
THAT'S A POLITICAL CONTRIVANCE.
IT WAS A MYTH DESIGNED BY
REFORM OPPONENTS TO SCARE
PEOPLE AWAY FROM THE FACTS.

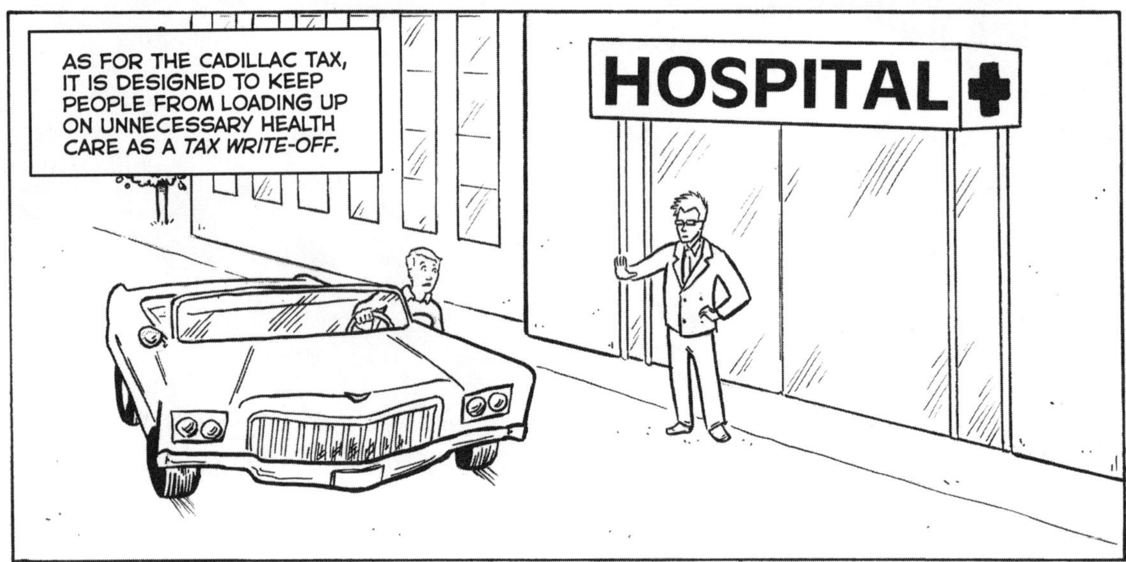
AS FOR THE CADILLAC TAX, IT IS DESIGNED TO KEEP PEOPLE FROM LOADING UP ON UNNECESSARY HEALTH CARE AS A *TAX WRITE-OFF*.
HOSPITAL

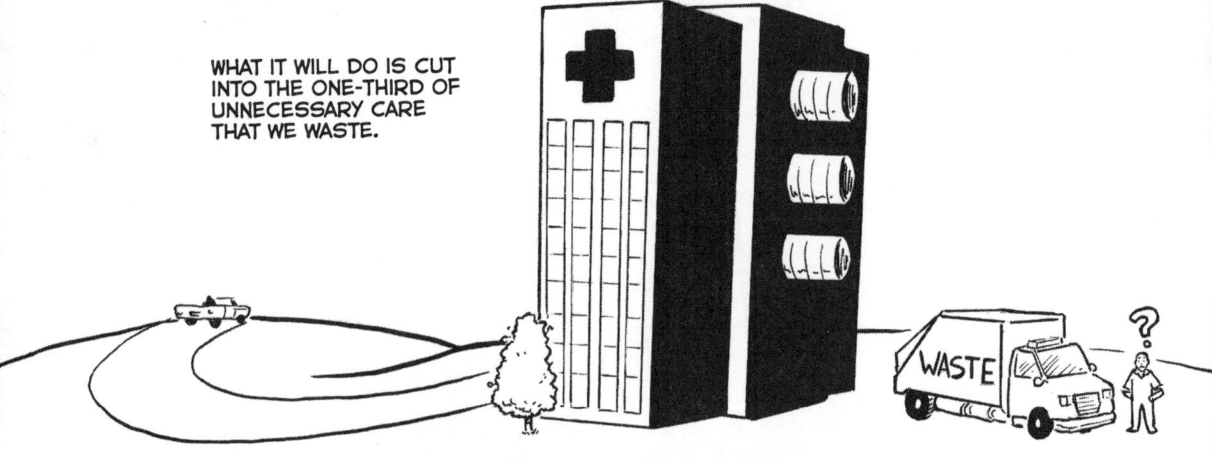
WHAT IT WILL DO IS CUT INTO THE ONE-THIRD OF UNNECESSARY CARE THAT WE WASTE.
WASTE
?

WE'RE WITH YOU ON THAT!

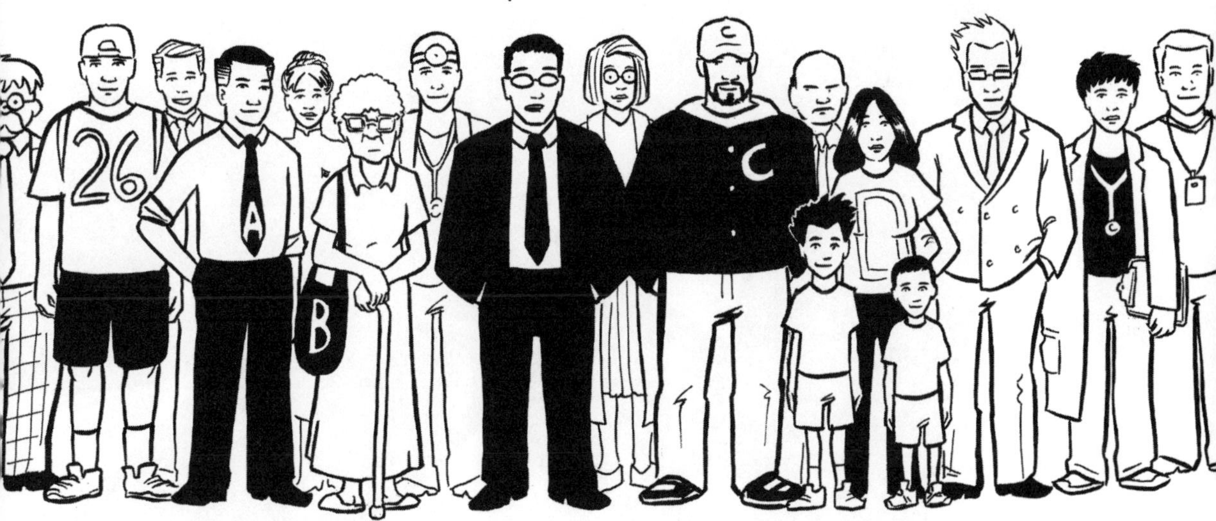
AT THE END OF THE DAY, WHAT EVERYONE WANTS IS A WAY TO MAKE SURE WE'RE TAKEN CARE OF WHEN WE'RE SICK, AND THAT IT DOESN'T RUIN US FINANCIALLY TO GET THAT CARE.
NO ONE DISPUTES THAT.
26
A
B
C
D

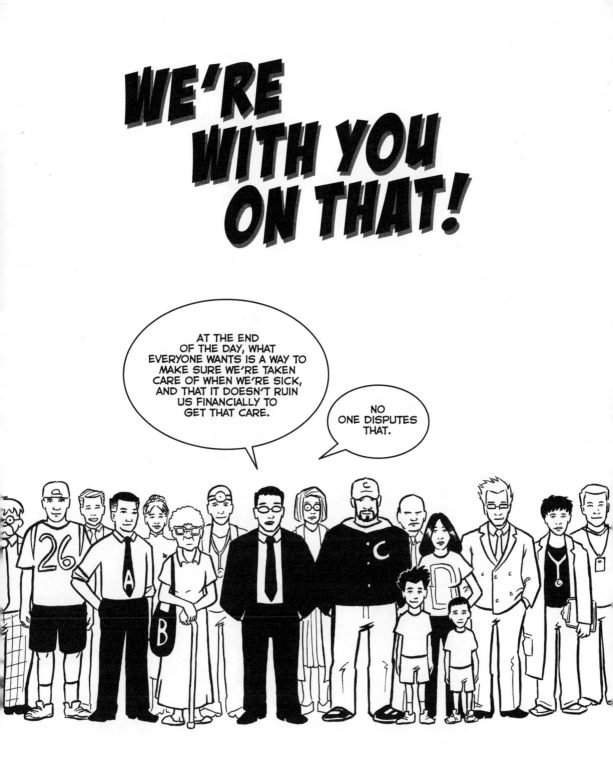

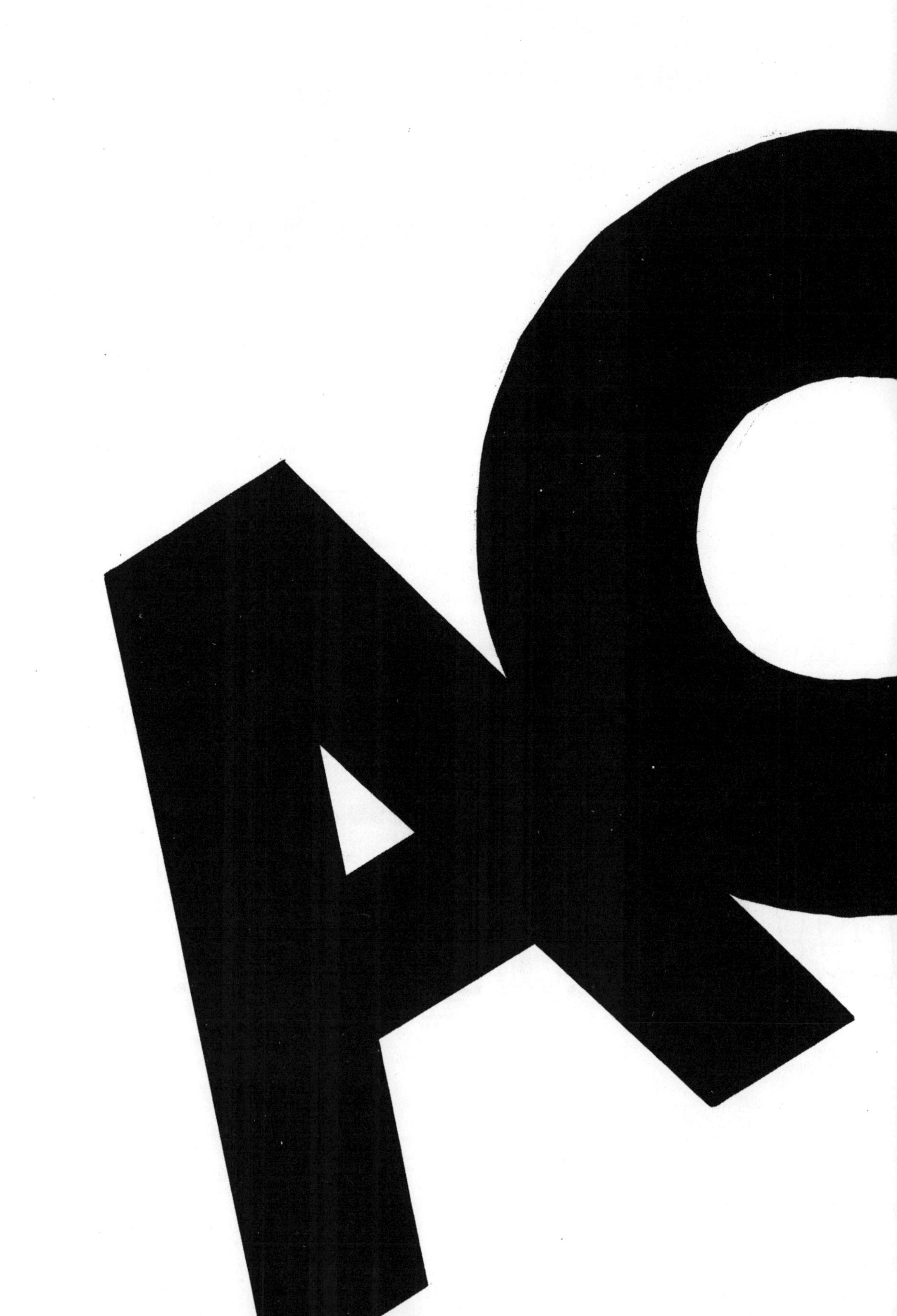

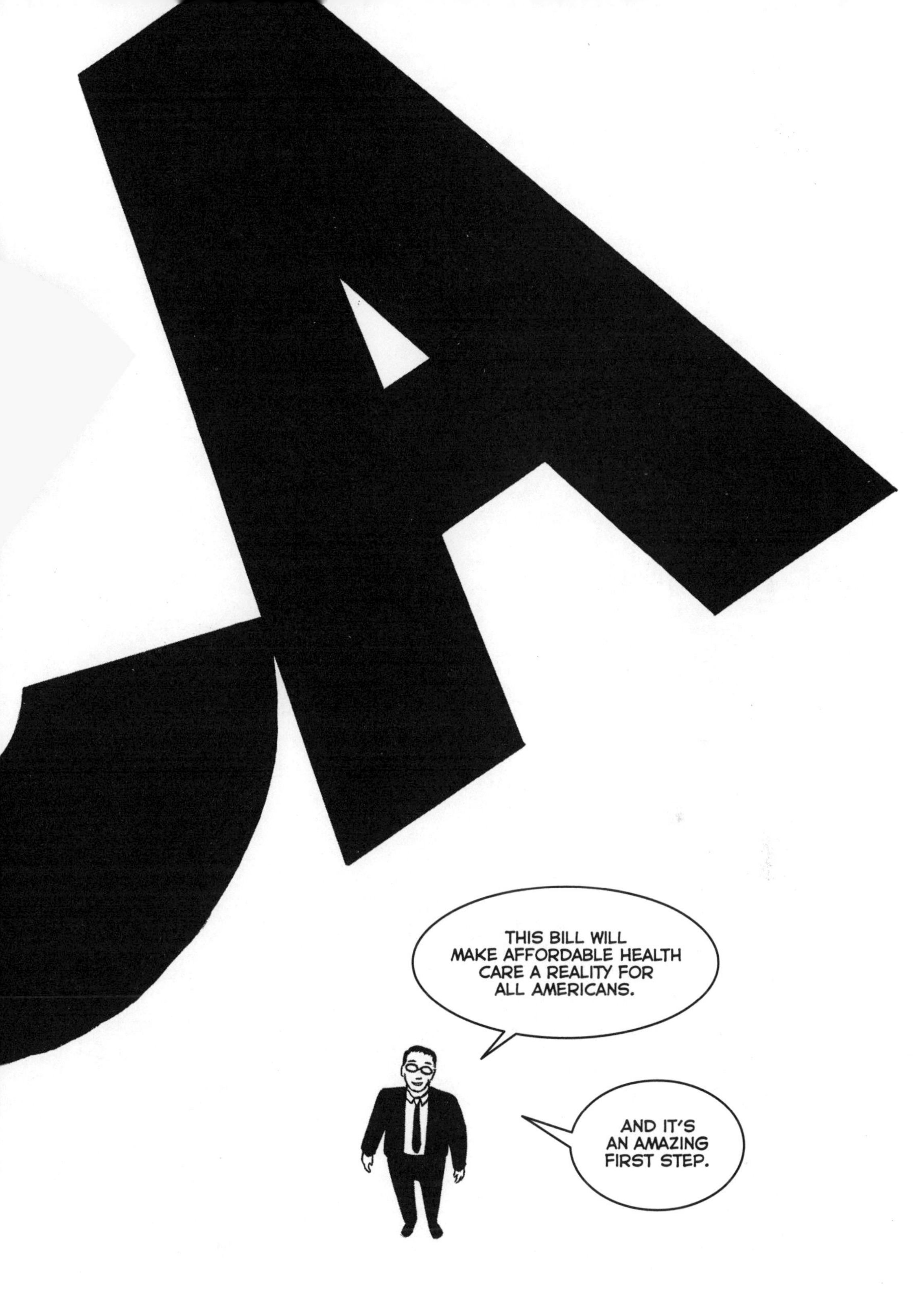
THIS BILL WILL MAKE AFFORDABLE HEALTH CARE A REALITY FOR ALL AMERICANS.
AND IT'S AN AMAZING FIRST STEP.

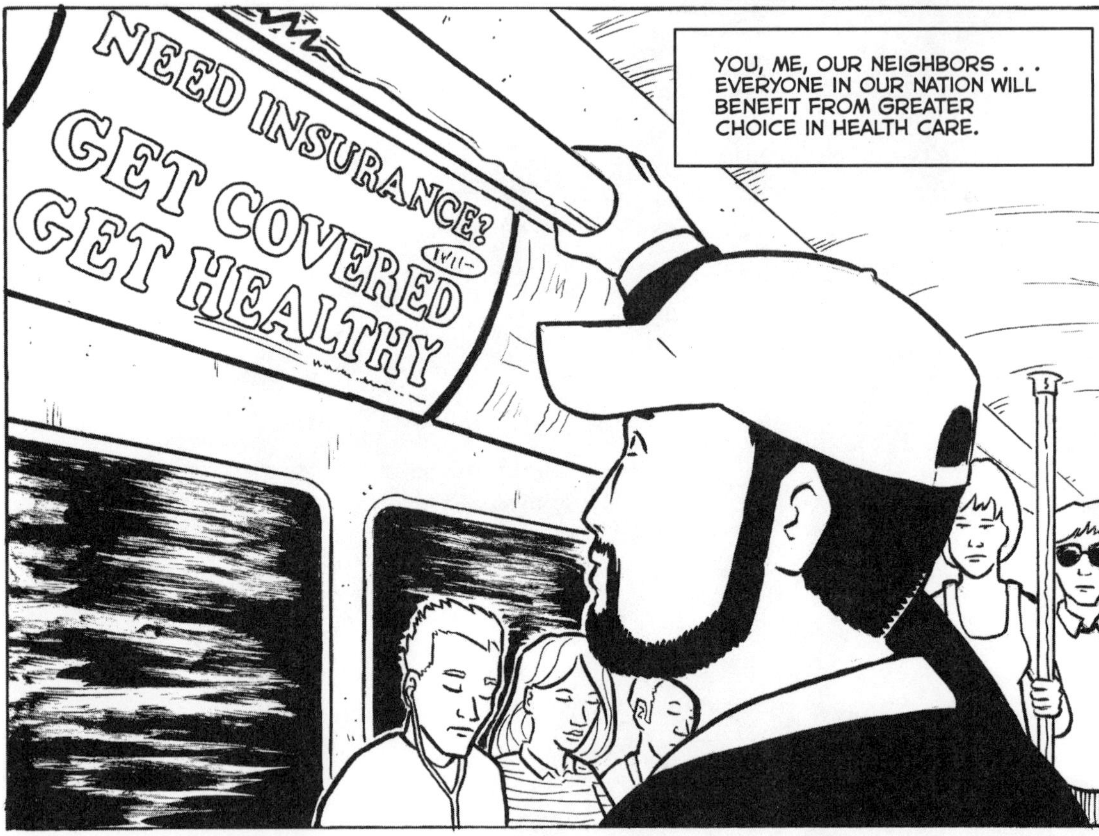

YOU, ME, OUR NEIGHBORS . . . EVERYONE IN OUR NATION WILL BENEFIT FROM GREATER CHOICE IN HEALTH CARE.

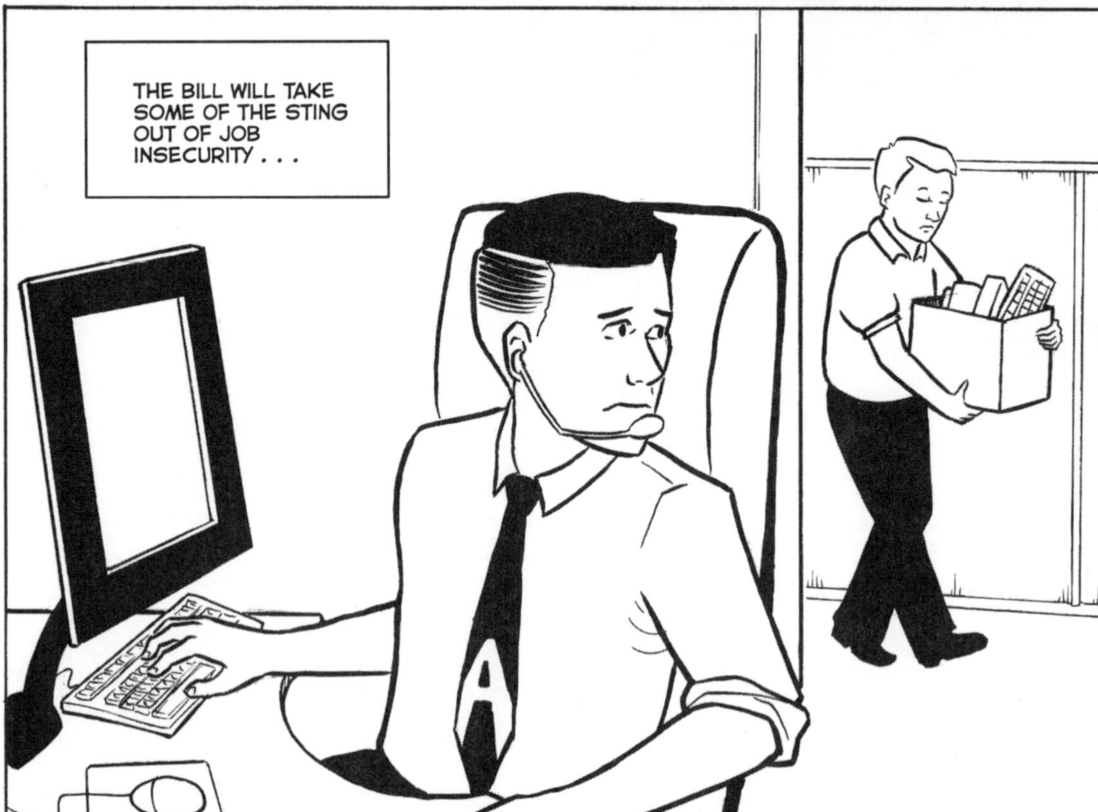

THE BILL WILL TAKE SOME OF THE STING OUT OF JOB INSECURITY . . .

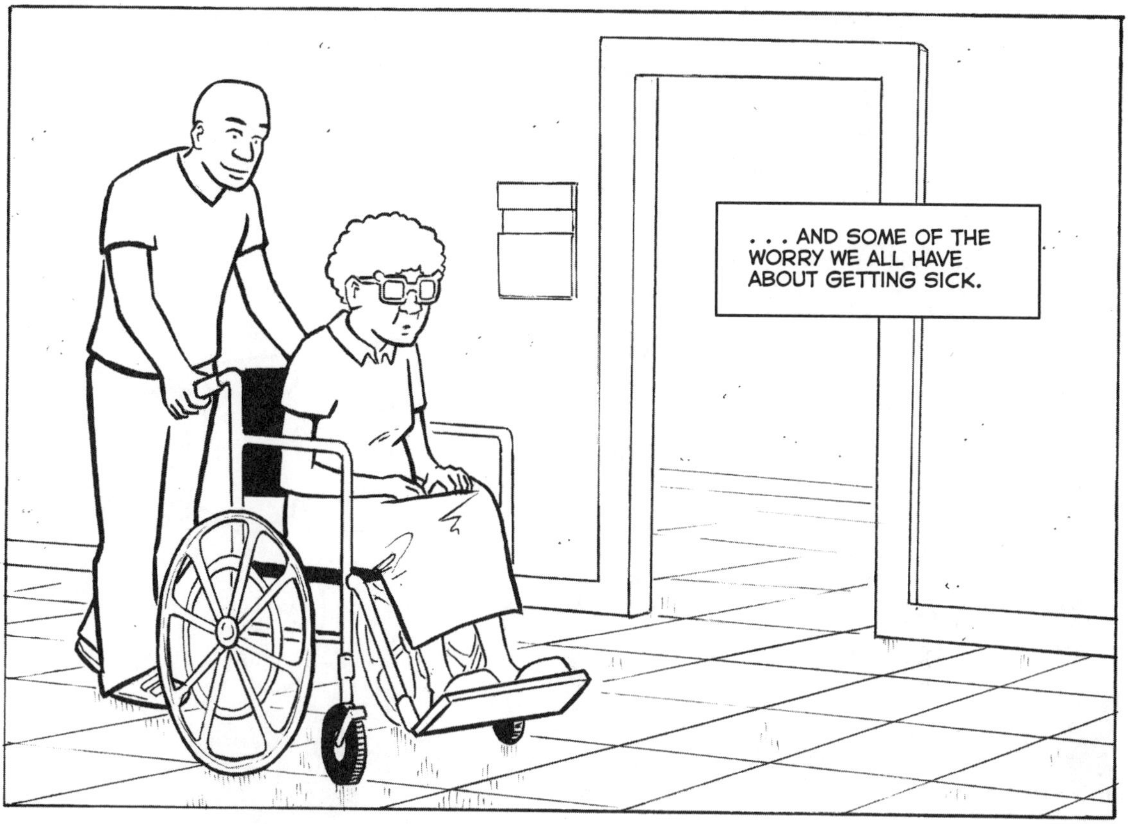

. . . AND SOME OF THE WORRY WE ALL HAVE ABOUT GETTING SICK.

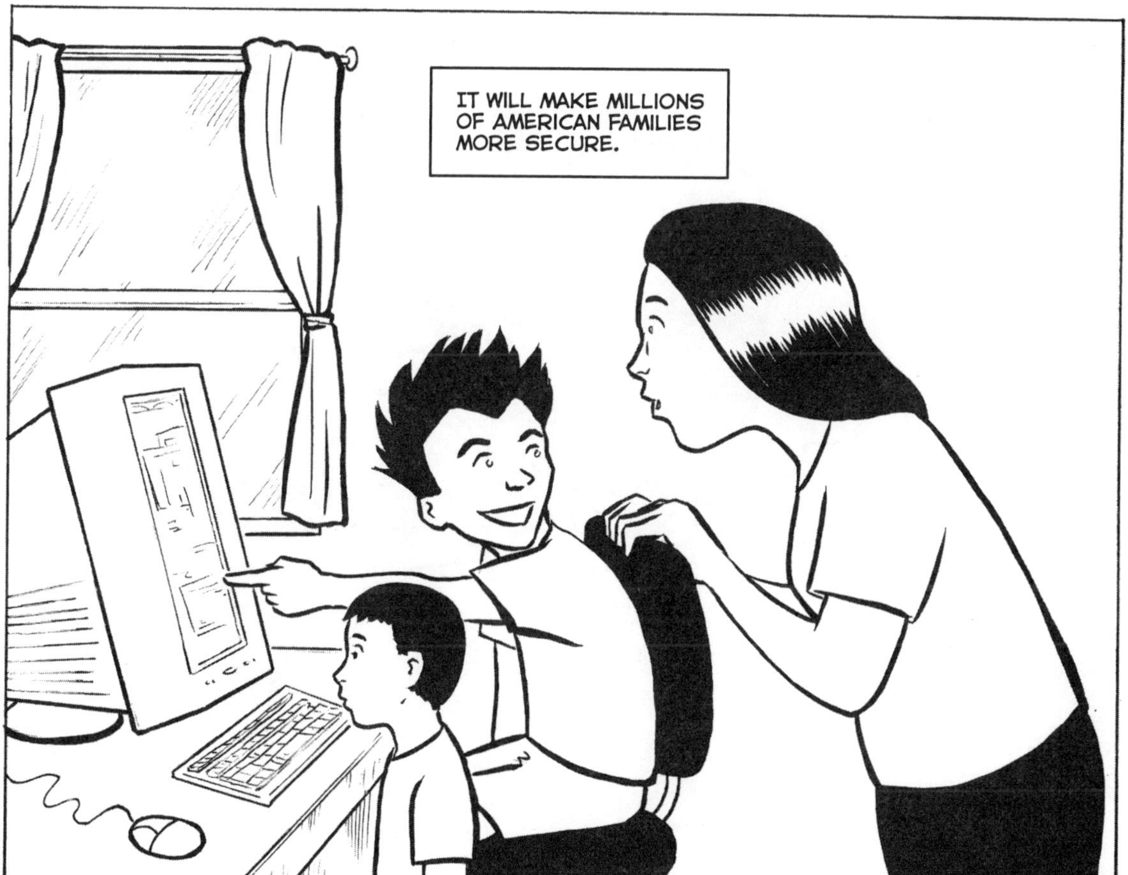

IT WILL MAKE MILLIONS OF AMERICAN FAMILIES MORE SECURE.

BETTER HEALTH CARE OPTIONS MEAN HEALTHIER PEOPLE.

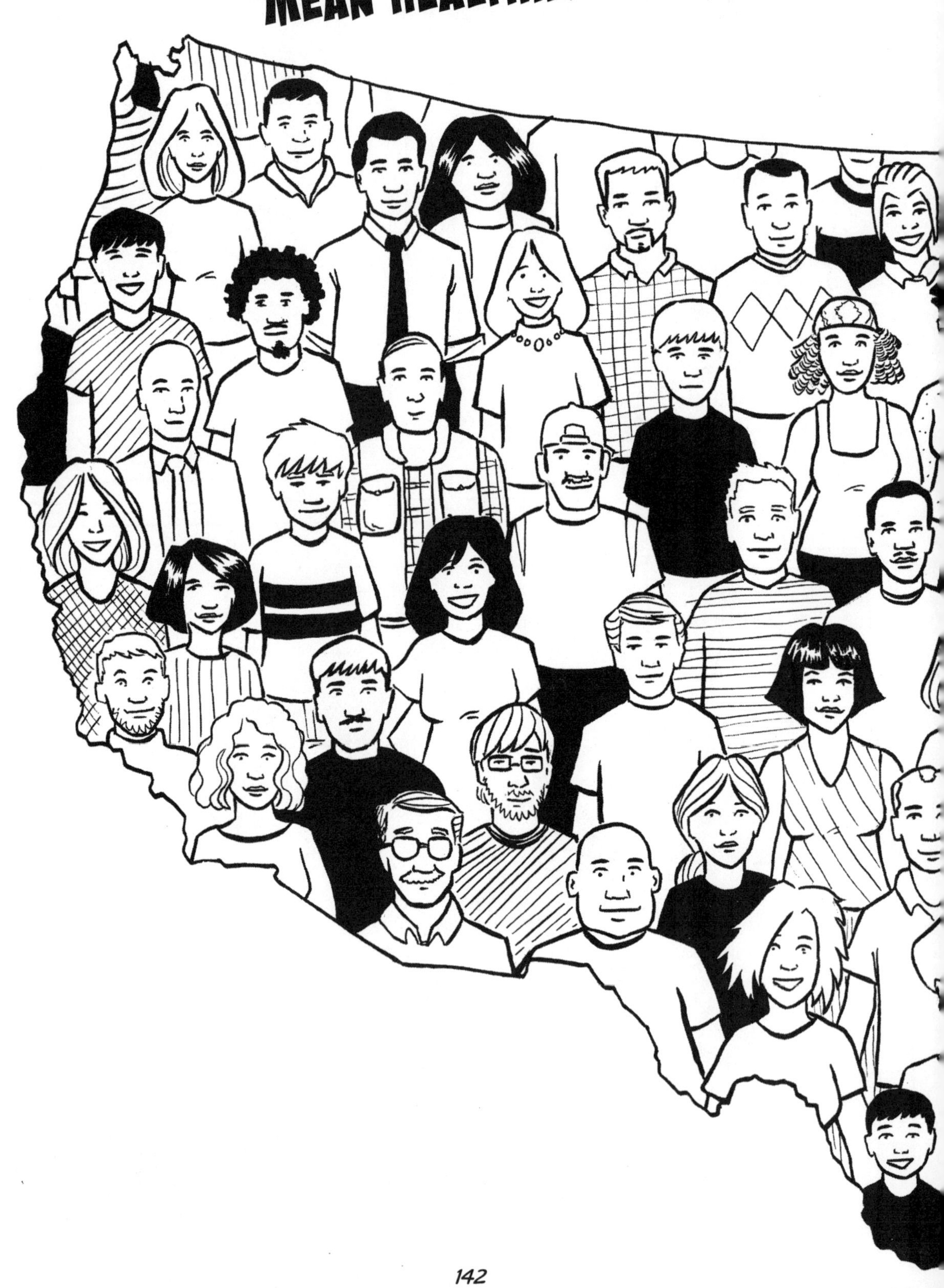

AND WHAT'S GOOD FOR US AS INDIVIDUALS IS GOOD FOR US AS A COUNTRY.

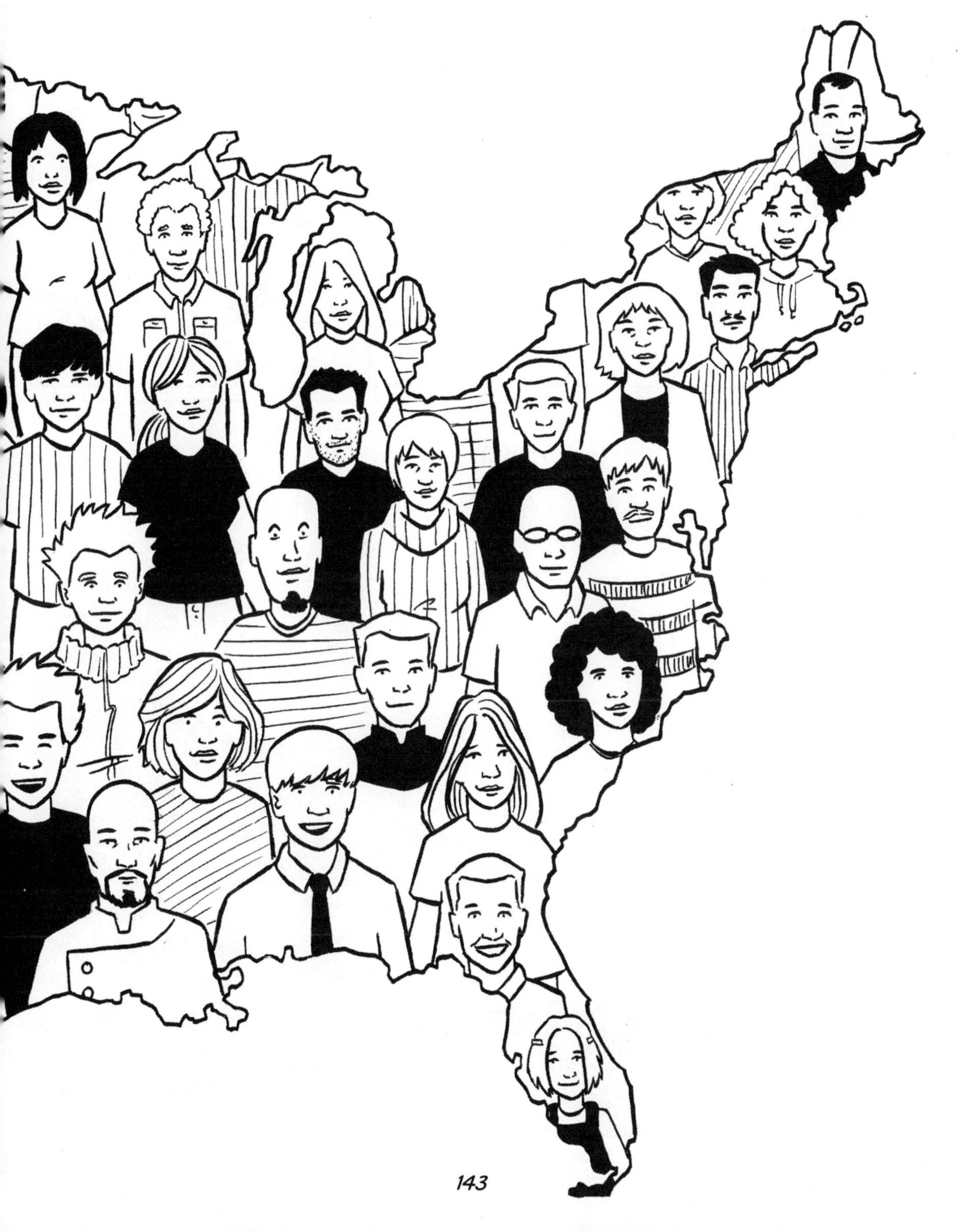

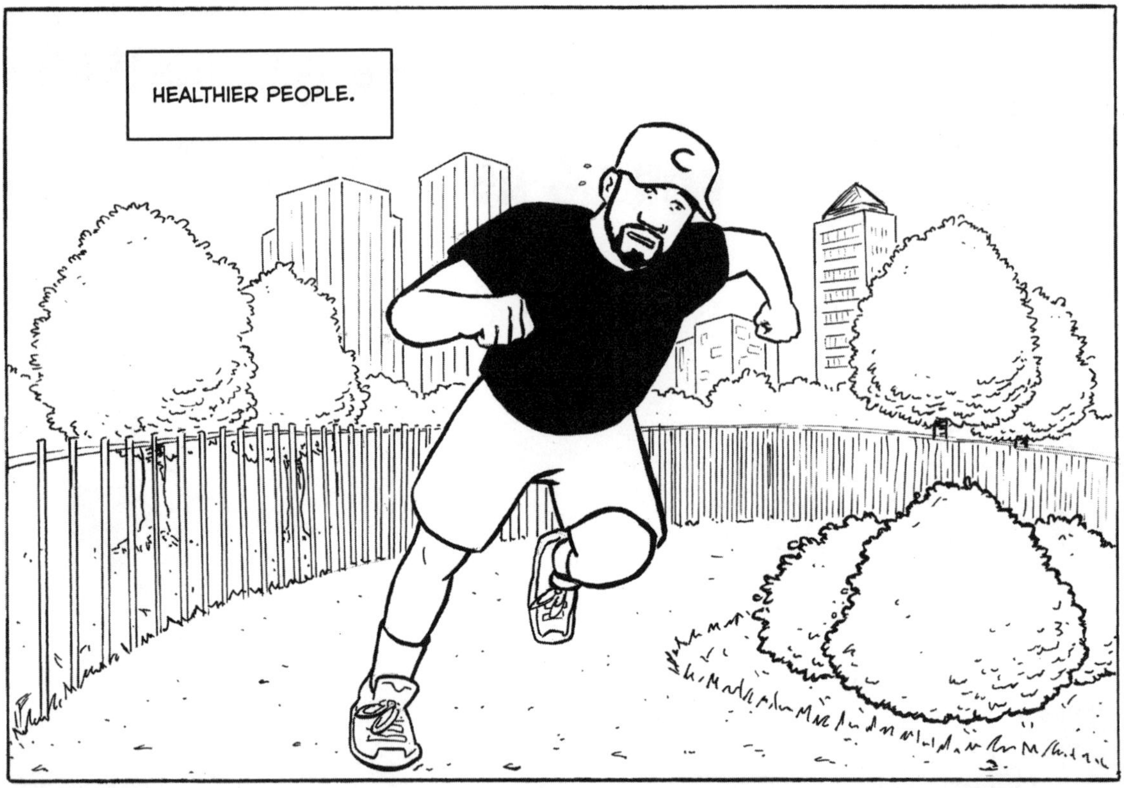

HEALTHIER PEOPLE.

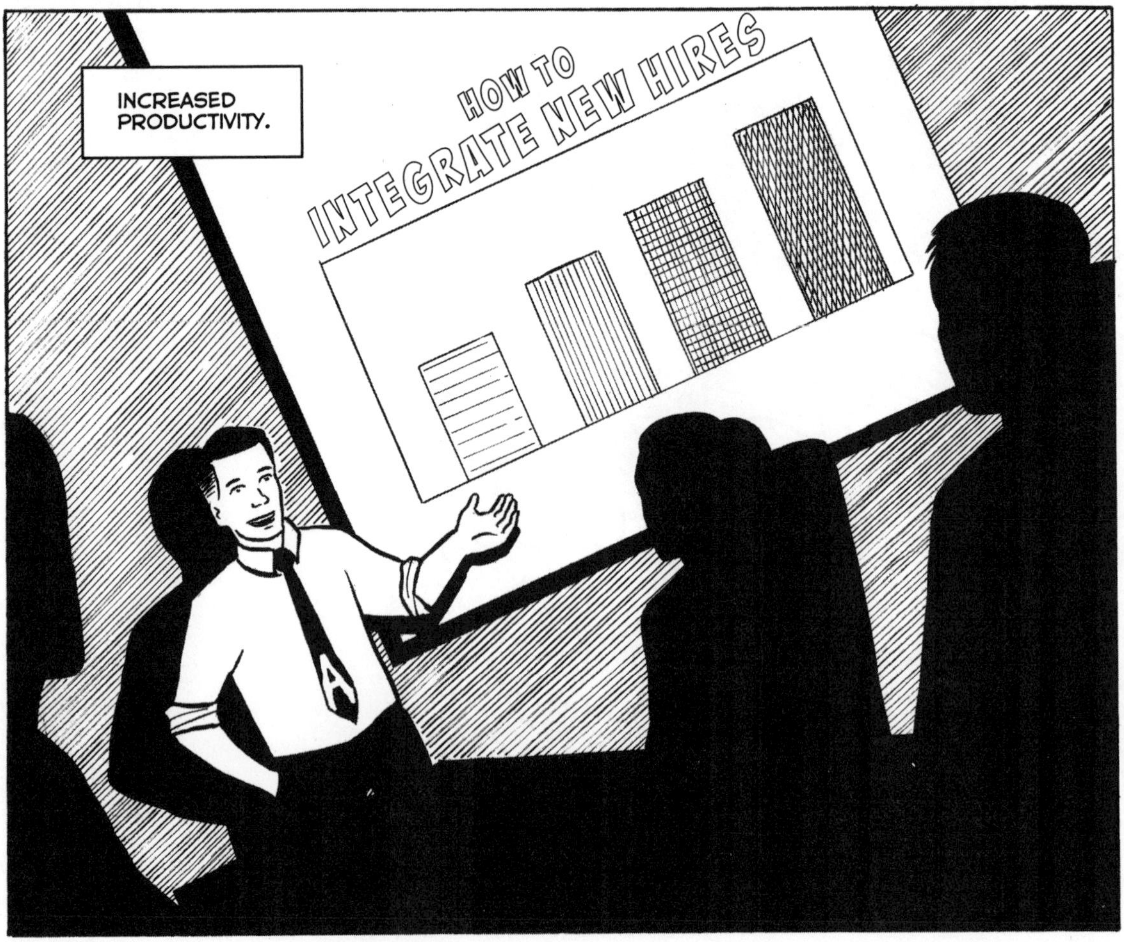

INCREASED PRODUCTIVITY.

HOW TO INTEGRATE NEW HIRES

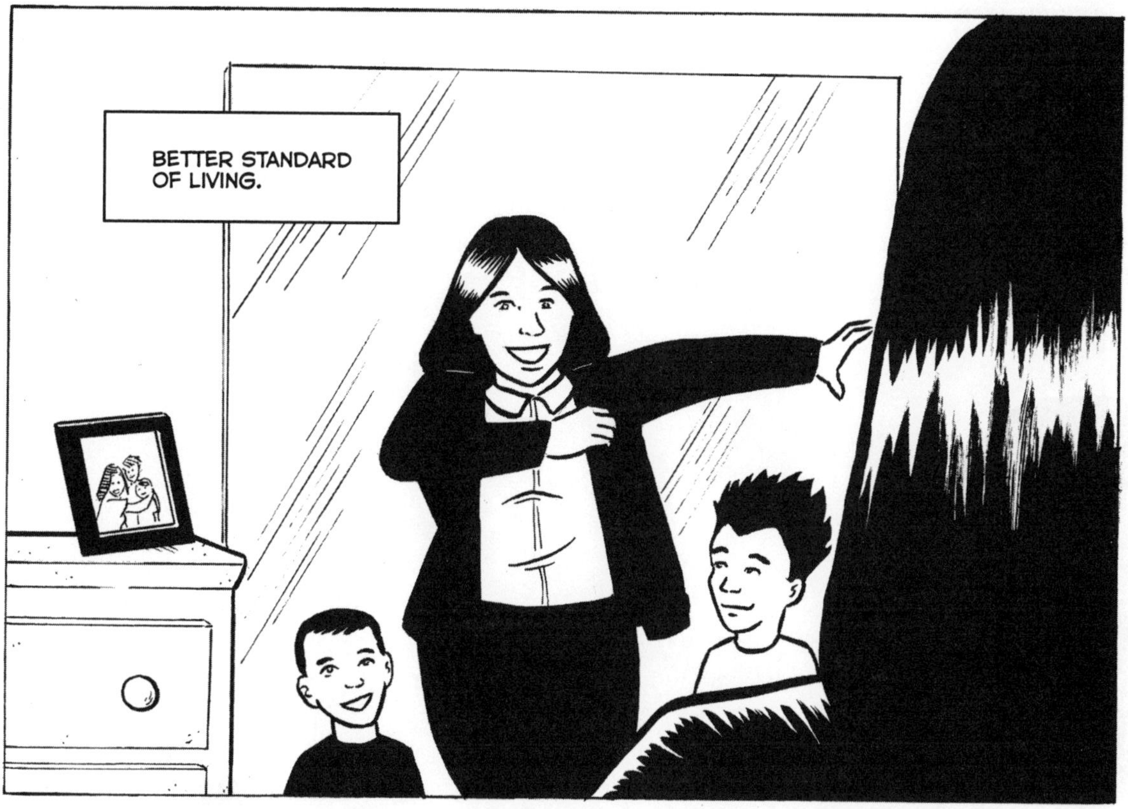

BETTER STANDARD OF LIVING.

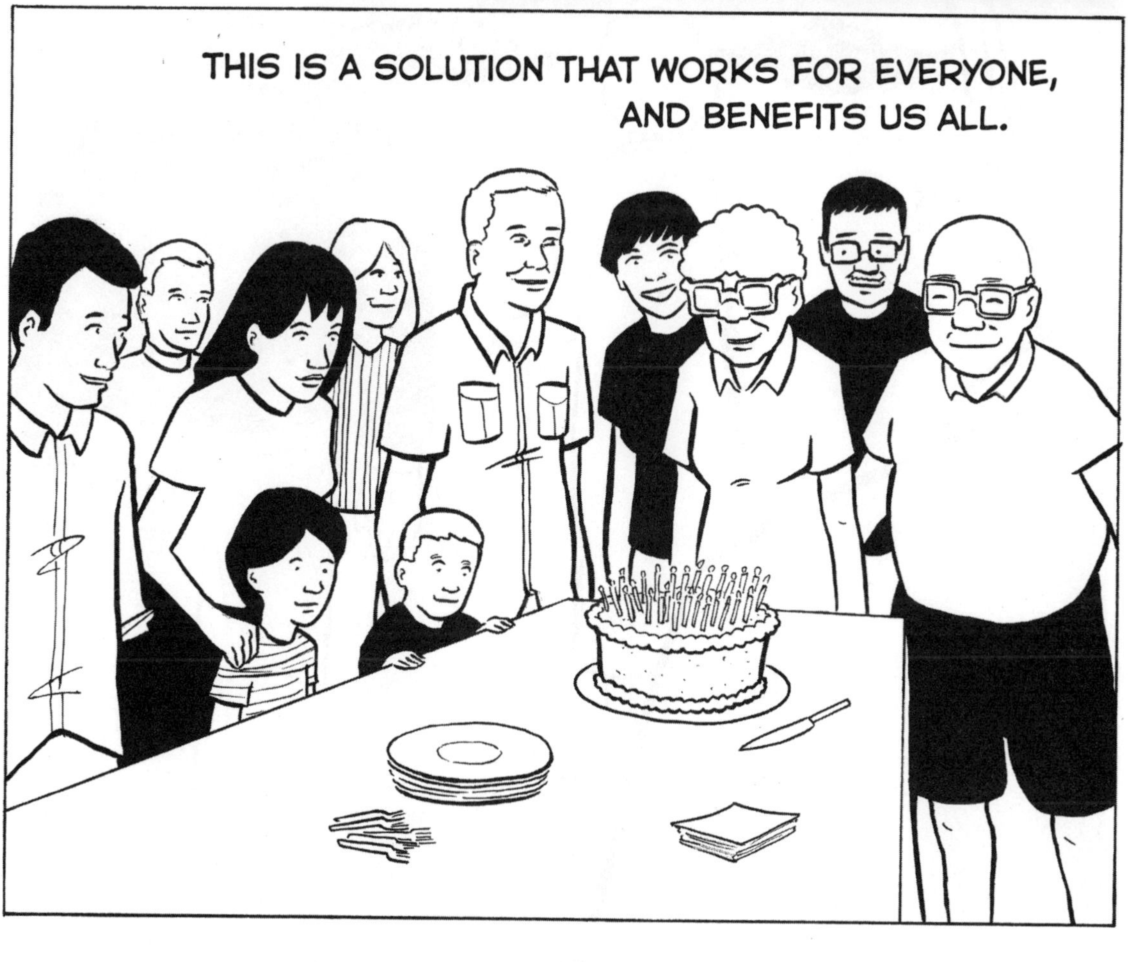

THIS IS A SOLUTION THAT WORKS FOR EVERYONE, AND BENEFITS US ALL.

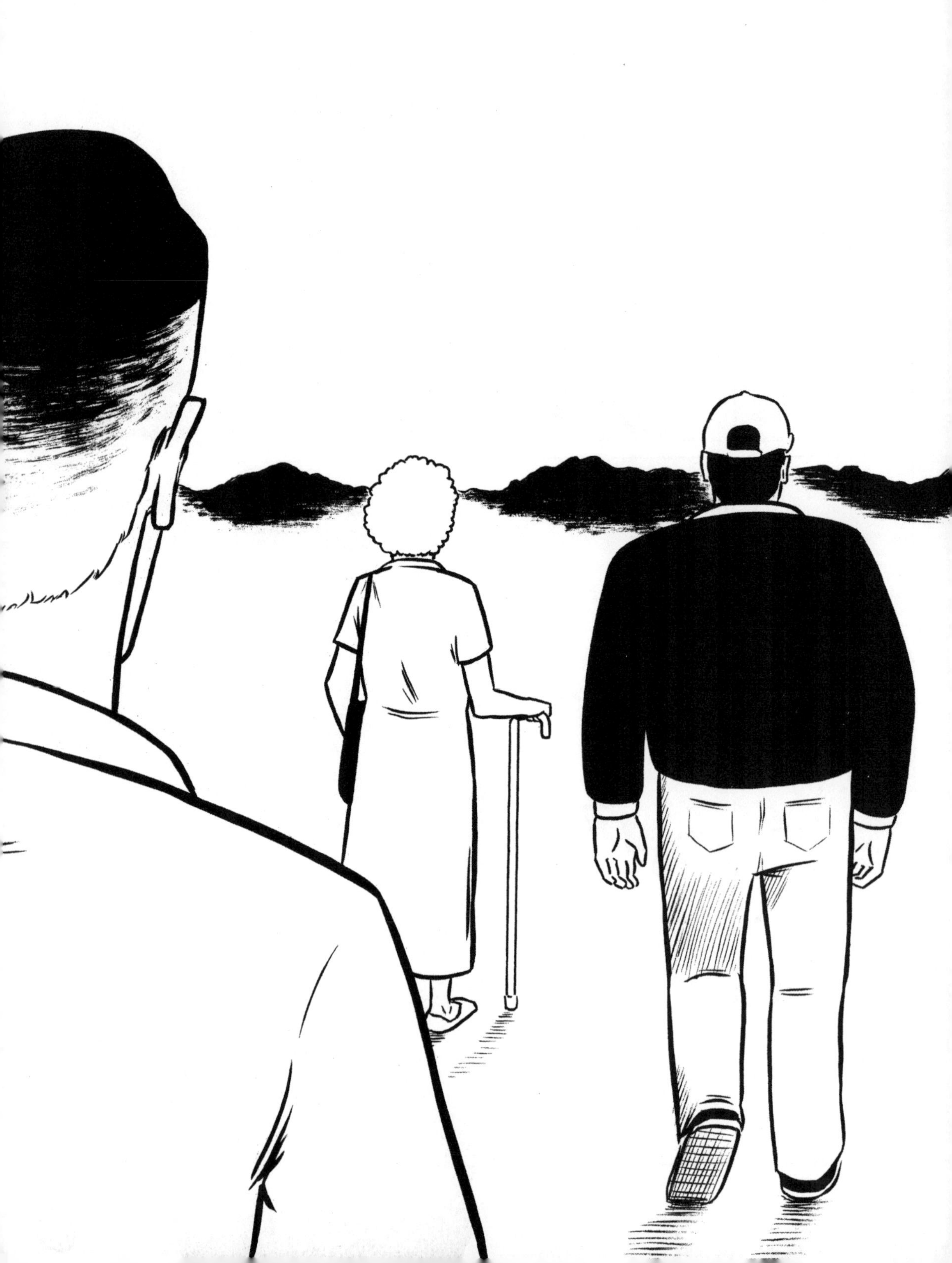

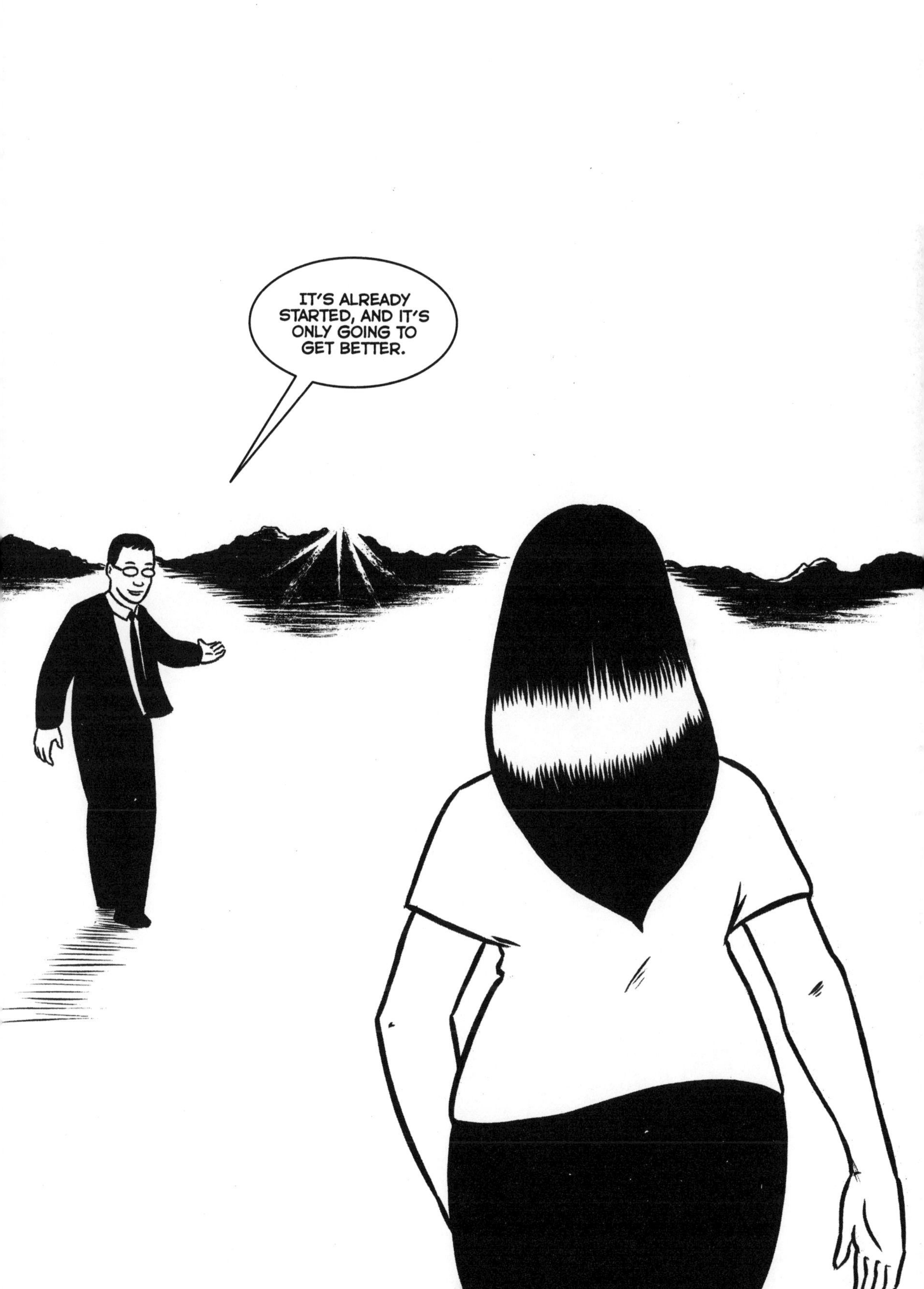
IT'S ALREADY STARTED, AND IT'S ONLY GOING TO GET BETTER.

RECOMMENDED FURTHER READING

A GOOD SOURCE OF ADDITIONAL INFORMATION, ANALYSIS, AND RESEARCH CONCERNING THE PATIENT PROTECTION AND AFFORDABILITY CARE ACT IS PROVIDED BY THE HENRY KAISER FAMILY FOUNDATION AND IS VIEWABLE HERE: HEALTHREFORM.KFF.ORG.

ANOTHER HELPFUL SOURCE IS THE COMMONWEALTH FUND'S SITE: WWW.COMMONWEALTHFUND.ORG/HEALTH-REFORM.ASPX.

ALSO RECOMMENDED IS WWW.HEALTHCARE.GOV, A FEDERAL GOVERNMENT WEBSITE MANAGED BY THE U.S. DEPARTMENT OF HEALTH AND HUMAN SERVICES.

FOR FURTHER DISCUSSION OF THE IMPACT OF THE MASSACHUSETTS HEALTH CARE INSURANCE REFORM LAW AND IMPLICATIONS FOR THE PPACA, SEE MY OWN "THE IMPACTS OF THE AFFORDABLE CARE ACT: HOW REASONABLE ARE THE PROJECTIONS?," NBER WORKING PAPER #17168, JUNE 2011.

ACKNOWLEDGMENTS

I AM EXTREMELY GRATEFUL TO THOMAS LEBIEN, WHO FIRST APPROACHED ME AND CONVINCED ME TO UNDERTAKE THIS BOOK. THOMAS MADE A COMPELLING CASE AND BACKED IT UP WITH WONDERFUL SUPPORT THROUGHOUT THE PROCESS.

I AM ALSO GRATEFUL TO MY COLLABORATORS ON THIS PROJECT. NATHAN SCHREIBER'S PICTURES MADE THESE ABSTRACT CONCEPTS UNDERSTANDABLE IN A WAY THAT WORDS ALONE COULD NOT. HARVEY NEWQUIST WAS A TERRIFIC COAUTHOR WHO MANAGED TO TAKE MY BROAD DESCRIPTIONS AND ECONOMIC PLATITUDES AND TRANSLATE THEM TO HIGHLY UNDERSTANDABLE TEXT. HOWARD ZIMMERMAN WAS A GREAT PROJECT MANAGER, WHO KEPT THE TRAINS MOVING ON TIME WHILE MAINTAINING THE QUALITY AND INTEGRITY OF THE PROCESS.

I AM ALSO GRATEFUL TO THE ENTIRE TEAM AT FARRAR, STRAUS AND GIROUX WHO HELPED PUSH THIS PROJECT TO COMPLETION.

I AM ALSO GRATEFUL TO MY MANY FRIENDS AND COLLABORATORS IN THE WORLD OF HEALTH CARE POLICY WHO ALLOWED ME THE HONOR OF WORKING ON THESE EXCITING POLICY ISSUES OVER THE PAST FIFTEEN YEARS. THE SUCCESSES OF U.S. HEALTH POLICY AT BOTH THE STATE AND FEDERAL LEVELS ARE DUE TO THE ENORMOUS DEDICATION OF THESE INDIVIDUALS TOWARDS IMPROVING THE FUNCTIONING OF OUR HEALTH CARE SYSTEM. CONGRATULATIONS TO ALL OF YOU ON YOUR HISTORIC EFFORTS.

A NOTE ABOUT THE AUTHOR

DR. JONATHAN GRUBER IS PROFESSOR OF ECONOMICS AT THE MASSACHUSETTS INSTITUTE OF TECHNOLOGY AND DIRECTOR OF THE HEALTH CARE PROGRAM AT THE NATIONAL BUREAU OF ECONOMIC RESEARCH. HE WAS A KEY ARCHITECT OF MASSACHUSETTS'S AMBITIOUS HEALTH CARE REFORM EFFORT AND CONSULTED EXTENSIVELY WITH THE OBAMA ADMINISTRATION AND CONGRESS DURING THE DEVELOPMENT OF THE AFFORDABLE CARE ACT. *THE WASHINGTON POST* CALLED HIM "POSSIBLY THE [DEMOCRATIC] PARTY'S MOST INFLUENTIAL HEALTH-CARE EXPERT."

A NOTE ABOUT THE ILLUSTRATOR

NATHAN SCHREIBER'S COMICS HAVE APPEARED IN *L'UOMO VOGUE*, *OVERFLOW*, AND *SMITH MAGAZINE* AND ON ACT-I-VATE.COM. HIS COMIC *POWER OUT* WON A XERIC AWARD AND HAS BEEN NOMINATED FOR AN EISNER AWARD AND MULTIPLE HARVEY AWARDS.